CONTENTS

PART ONE

Lupus: An Overview

PART TWO

Living with Lupus

PART THREE

Lupus and Your Emotions

PART FOUR

Lupus and Relationships

PART FIVE

Hoping . . . and Coping!

ACKNOWLEDGMENTS

Appreciative words of thanks must be accorded some very special people who provided invaluable assistance in the preparation of this book. Thanks to Betty Diamond, M.D., Robert Lahita, M.D., Lawrence Phillips, M.D., Yehuda Schoenfeld, M.D., and Harry Spiera, M.D., for their knowledgeable suggestions for the manuscript.

Thanks to the thousands of members of the Lupus Foundation of America, Lupus Alliance of America, and other independent local and international lupus organizations who provided such essential insight into the critical aspects of living with lupus. Special thanks to all of the important past and present members of these organizations who have played a significant role in the development of public awareness of lupus. Unfortunately, I can't thank all of them by name or we'd run out of pages before the book even began.

I would like to acknowledge some special friends and colleagues, past and present, who have impressed me with their dedication and achievements throughout my years of involvement with lupus organizations. They include Gail and Steve Alberti, Glenda Amon, Kathleen Arnsten, Jane Bailey, Steve Balch, M.D., Mike Belmont, M.D., Barbara Bourgeois, Jane Bozarth, Ann and Reeve Bright, Jill Buyon, M.D., Michelle Callender, M.D., Steven Carsons, M.D., Karel De Ceulaer, M.D., Jo Dewhurst, Betty Diamond, M.D., Ann Dominger, Enid Engelhard, Julius Erving, Jeri Falk, Joan Finzi, Cindy Flower, M.D., Sandy Frear, Richard Furie, M.D., Carol and Alan Goldklang, Paula Goldstein, Susan Golick, Evelyn Hess, M.D., Rudolf Hocks, Judi Jones, Elaine King, Honi Kurzeja, Ginger Ladd, Bob Lahita, M.D., Pat

Leisy, Robert Marcus, M.D., Kellie Martin, Brenda McCormack, George Nicholson, M.D., Richard Nussbaum, Jenny Palter, Duane Peters, Sefra Pitzele, JoAnn Quinn, Sandra Raymond, Noel Rose, M.D., Ph.D., Yehuda Schoenfeld, M.D., Peter Schur, M.D., Goldie Simon, Christine Smith, Marilyn Sousa, Harry Spiera, M.D., Fredda Steidle, Roger Sturdevant, Norman Talal, M.D., Cathy Thomas, George Tsokos, M.D., and Shelley Weir. (I beg forgiveness of anyone whose name was inadvertently omitted.)

Thanks to Renee Glick for word-processing assistance, and to Miriam Rich and Megan Newman at Avery, who made it a pleasure to correspond with my publisher.

Finally, thanks to Daniel Wallace, M.D., for his professional contributions of the highest caliber—his expertise, wisdom, and guidance are greatly valued.

FOREWORD

Questions, questions, questions. Newly diagnosed lupus patients have lots of them. They don't want to bother their rheumatologist. After all, they need to be respectful of his or her time, so they limit themselves to a few queries that are very important. But how can they cope with the disease? How does it affect their life? Can they have a family? How much sun can a lupus patient be reasonably exposed to? What about relationships, diet, exercise? Are they going to die? "What can I do to live as normal a life as possible?" is one of the most common concerns patients express to me. There is no one-sentence answer. In fact, the true responses would take any knowledgeable practitioner hours to articulate. If one searches the topic "lupus" on Amazon, there are at least two hundred books on the subject. Which one should patients buy or rely on? Dr. Robert Phillips has had a special interest in lupus for decades. His skills in assisting lupus patients to cope demonstrate a consummate professionalism and competence that borders on breathtaking.

Coping with Lupus fills an unmet need. In our busy, anxious, hurried existence, Dr. Phillips is reassuring, thorough, organized, and informative. He takes one through major concerns one by one. He leaves all but the bare-bones science to the lupus physician and concentrates on the mind-body connection and practical applications of how the disease influences our life. The head bone is definitely connected to the lupus bone. Studies have demonstrated that we have varying degrees of control over our blood pressure, Raynaud's phenomenon, and our activities that directly influence inflammation of the joints. Adhering to a physician's admonitions; adopting a specific diet or exercise regimen; keeping appointments with one's doctor; getting screened for blood pressure, cholesterol, blood sugar; learning about a disease; asking questions; having twenty-four-hour access to a caring physician; being screened for osteoporosis—all these, among other factors, have a tremendous influence on outcome in systemic lupus erythematosus, or SLE, that is almost as important as any specific lupus medication regimen. I have treated more than three thousand lupus patients in the last thirty years, and frequently recommend that they buy Bob Phillips's book. The prescient wisdom that *Coping with Lupus* imparts makes my job a lot easier.

Daniel J. Wallace, M.D., FACP, FACR
Clinical Professor of Medicine
Cedars-Sinai Medical Center
David Geffen School of Medicine at UCLA,
and author of *The Lupus Book*

FOREWORD TO THE
THIRD EDITION

Lupus is a disease of the immune system that affects primarily women in their childbearing years, though children, men, and the elderly can also be affected. Many women develop the disease in the prime of their lives. Systemic lupus erythematosus (SLE) has a wide array of clinical manifestations, ranging from symptoms that are mildly annoying to symptoms that are life-threatening. It is also unpredictable in its course—a patient with only minimal symptoms can become acutely and dangerously ill, whereas another patient with a severe case may improve spontaneously.

While no cure is available, treatment is usually quite successful, and most lupus cases can be controlled to a large extent. Progress in the understanding and treatment of SLE during the past twenty-five years has greatly improved not only the life expectancy but also the quality of life for our patients.

In spite of this, however, life for the lupus patient is a constant battle.

Even patients with no major organ involvement may have generalized achiness and fatigue as a constant companion. Moreover, SLE is often an "invisible" disease, in which the patient, though feeling quite ill, may appear robust and healthy, particularly to the untrained observer. Patients with SLE may have their symptoms and concerns underappreciated by those around them.

Treatments used for SLE are not only expensive, but are often associated with side effects that may add to the disease burden, in terms of both health and self-image. The latter is true in patients taking corticosteroids, with which swelling and weight gain become a terrible problem, particularly for young women.

The goals of treatment in a patient with lupus are to relieve symptoms, prevent major organ deterioration, and allow the patient to live as normal and active a life as possible. All the skills and techniques available to physicians are utilized to these ends. Thus both the illness and its treatment are a constant battle for the lupus patient to fight. It is akin to what Leon Trotsky called "permanent revolution." He taught that it was necessary to keep battling to achieve one's chosen goals.

All these concerns necessitate the development of coping skills on the part of the patient. The coping skills comprise a combination of the patient's own resources, family and social support, and intelligent and concerned medical and psychological care.

Dr. Robert H. Phillips has devoted his professional life as a psychologist to aiding patients with all types of problems, developing their strengths and ability to cope. Through his Center for Coping, he has aided many patients directly. His series of books on coping with various diseases has spread his message to countless others and has greatly increased the ability of those with a disease to have a satisfactory and fulfilling life.

In this book, Dr. Phillips presents patients and concerned family members with a superb overview of SLE, as well as how it is diagnosed and treated. He then identifies issues of lifestyle, emotional problems, and social interactions for the patient. His keen insights and upbeat messages represent a unique resource.

There is ongoing progress in the understanding and treatment of SLE. However, until a cure is found, the techniques and insights that Dr. Phillips shares will greatly improve the quality of life for all SLE sufferers.

Harry Spiera, M.D.
Clinical Professor of Medicine
Mount Sinai Medical Center, New York

FOREWORD TO THE FIRST AND SECOND EDITIONS

Systemic lupus erythematosus (SLE), more loosely known as lupus, is a chronic disease involving the body's immune system. Individuals who are afflicted with this illness can suffer myriad varying manifestations that can affect almost any part of the body. The manifestations can be quite minimal or extremely severe and even life-threatening, and they can appear and disappear with frustrating unpredictability, lasting anywhere from a few days to several months or more. Thus, those with this illness frequently can go for months or even years while physicians vainly try to make the diagnosis, and it is not uncommon, especially in the milder cases, for such patients to be labeled as neurotics or chronic complainers. Even after the diagnosis is made and the appropriate therapy is instituted, the patient has to live with the knowledge that the illness is not yet curable, and even though treatment has improved dramatically over the last decade, it is still far from ideal since the drugs used in many cases have significant untoward side effects. Obviously, all of this creates a life situation in which significant psychological stress is a constant companion of the patient, not only in terms of the disease per se, but also because in the face of all of the above, the individual must still interact with family, friends, employers, and strangers, as we all do. It doesn't take much of an imagination to understand that lupus patients have to cope not only with internal stresses, but also with the responses of the people around them, responses which at times can be as infuriating and frustrating as the disease itself.

Although a number of books have been written about lupus, both highly technical for physicians and in lay language for the general public, there has been a crying need for a comprehensive source book for patients and their families on how to cope with the psychological problems that such an illness produces. Bob Phillips is eminently qualified to have written such a book. He is a practicing psychologist who counsels many lupus patients because he has developed a special interest in the problems of this disease. He is also on the medical council of the Lupus Foundation of America and has served as a member of the National Board of Directors of the Lupus Foundation. He has written this book with understanding and compassion, and has included not only a comprehensive discussion of the kinds of reactions patients must deal with, but also many practical suggestions to help them do so. Having read the manuscript, I would like to say that I only wish all lupus patients could be so lucky as to have access to someone like Dr. Phillips, and that by writing this book, he has given them, in some sense at least, that access.

Ronald I. Carr, M.D., Ph.D.
Associate Professor of Medicine and
Associate Professor of Microbiology
Dalhousie University Faculty of Medicine
Halifax, Nova Scotia, Canada

PREFACE

The diagnosis of systemic lupus erythematosus can have a major impact on you and your family. No kidding! Certainly, there are many misconceptions, fears, concerns, and myths about lupus and its treatment. Undoubtedly you have many questions about your condition. Physicians and other professionals can answer some of them. Others may be answered by the relatively few books or articles on the subject. However, many questions cannot be answered. Why? Scientists just don't know the answers. This can be upsetting. Also upsetting is the feeling of isolation you may experience, the feeling that you're alone because no one understands. Knowing that you have a chronic illness can be depressing.

Fortunately, medical science has been making a lot of progress in controlling lupus. There is every chance that this will enable you to lead a longer, more normal and productive life. But what about the psychological effects of lupus? A major factor determining your potential to lead a normal, emotionally stable life is how well you cope with the strain of having a chronic illness such as lupus.

In living with lupus, you'll find yourself facing many important decisions. Initially, one of the most essential decisions you'll be making concerns how you can best become a partner in the treatment program that's going to help you, and how you can take control over the rest of your life, rather than letting life control you.

Heavy stuff? You bet it is! But that's why this book was written in the first place. Chock-full of information, suggestions, and strategies, this book will help you, your family, and your friends learn how to cope with lupus.

The first part of the book presents basic information about lupus: what it is, what the symptoms are, how to treat it, and so on. The other sections deal with different aspects of living with the disease, including coping with the practical and medical components of lupus, your emotions, and your relationships. The final section includes information about lupus research, as well as a coping review. We will explore each aspect in detail and will provide and examine many suggestions and strategies, as well as provide illustrative examples. In fact, a lot of the information you'll be reading can (and does!) apply to any chronic medical condition. In this book, however, the main focus is on your life with lupus.

As you learn to cope with lupus, it's important to realize that you're not alone; others are experiencing a lot of the same things that you're going through. This can be reassuring. But you should also remember that each person with lupus experiences symptoms differently. Similarly, the psychological consequences of having lupus vary from person to person. Your own life with lupus—the way it affects you and the way you experience it—will not be exactly the same as anyone else's. You are a unique person. Therefore, it will be up to *you* to use the suggestions and strategies presented in this book to help yourself cope as well as you possibly can. The goal of this book is to help you become an active person, rather than a passive patient. Keep this in mind as you read this book, and go through life: you are a person who happens to have lupus. The only time you should think about yourself as a lupus patient is when you're in your doctor's office, or in the hospital!

Researchers are working hard to find a cure for lupus. But until that time, you'll have to live with it. I hope this book will help both you and your family do just that, and do it comfortably. Remember: You can *always* improve the quality of your life.

Robert H. Phillips, Ph.D.
Center for Coping
Long Island, New York

PART ONE

Lupus: An Overview

1.

WHAT IS LUPUS?

Susan, a twenty-nine-year-old mother of one, had not been feeling well. She had been feeling very tired for a long time and was experiencing more and more pain in many of her joints. Seeing a number of different doctors had resulted in several different diagnoses, but no treatment was helping her to feel better. Finally, she went to yet another physician who gave her a complete physical, including all kinds of blood tests. After extensive analysis of the tests performed, he was now meeting with Susan in his consultation room to explain the findings. Susan nervously approached the chair by his desk and sat down. The doctor looked at her and wasted no time in telling her, "Susan, you have lupus." Susan's immediate reaction was very similar to the reaction of many individuals given the same diagnosis. Trembling, she looked at the doctor and exclaimed, "What's lupus?"

So, what is lupus? Lupus, the more commonly known name for *systemic lupus erythematosus* (SLE), falls into the category of diseases known as *autoimmune* diseases. To understand what this is, as well as what happens in lupus, it is important to be aware of how the immune system operates. This chapter explains what antibodies are, how they normally work and what goes wrong in lupus, and how this can affect the body. It also outlines the main types of lupus as well as the symptoms of the disorder, and answers some of the most difficult initial questions you may have following your diagnosis.

What Does Our Immune System Do?

The immune system is a very important part of our bodies. It is primarily made up of three categories of white blood cells—the B lymphocytes (the "B cells"), the T lymphocytes (the "T cells"), and the phagocytes. The B cells manufacture antibodies. The T cells normally work to help control the way the B cells do this job. The phagocytes assist in the action of the immune system by eliminating unwanted cells. Large, mature phagocytes, called *macrophages*, not only eliminate unwanted cells, but also signal the other white blood cells of the immune system when foreign invaders, called *antigens*, are present. The immune system is essential to protecting us from infection. It protects us from a variety of antigens including germs, viruses, bacteria, or fungi—anything the immune system believes is foreign to the body.

WHAT DO OUR ANTIBODIES DO?

Here's a very simplified way to start learning about the function of the immune system. (Remember: It's a lot more complex than this!) Imagine the immune system as a fort in a city. Inside the fort are thousands and thousands of soldiers who sit in readiness, waiting to go outside the fort and go to different areas in the city to fight evil and destroy the enemy. Normally, the immune system (the fort) produces antibodies (the soldiers) and cells (the tanks) that fight the antigens (the enemies), such as bacteria, viruses, and other germs throughout the body (the city). In lupus, there seems to be a malfunction in some of the cells of the immune system. For some reason that is not completely understood, there are soldiers inside the fort who try to destroy the city and perhaps the fort itself. This is what characterizes lupus. In lupus, normal, healthy tissue in the body is attacked by the increased amount of antibodies (the deranged soldiers). This attack leads to a kind of allergic reaction. You may be able to see evidence of inflammation in certain parts of the body where the attack is taking place. This is why lupus is also considered to be an inflammatory disease. The inflamed areas are usually reddish in color, tender to the touch, and often painful. Since individuals with lupus have such high amounts of antibodies that turn against their own bodies (auto), lupus is called an autoimmune disease.

WHERE DO OUR ANTIBODIES GO?

Normally, when we have foreign cells or substances in our bodies, the antibodies know where to go to control the invasion. The soldiers are very smart. They usually know exactly where to go and how to destroy the enemy. If an infection results despite the attempts of the antibodies to fight the germs, medications can be used to control it and to help the body return to a healthy state. This could be illustrated by saying that the soldiers have called in reinforcements—specialists to help deal with a specific problem that the soldiers can't handle themselves. However, in lupus, inflammations occur randomly, with no apparently predictable pattern of direction. It is not understood why these occasional inflammatory attacks occur. It is almost as if the soldiers have lost the ability to control their behavior. They run rampant, and they attack wherever it is convenient for them.

In lupus, tissue damage can occur in two major ways. First, the antibodies fighting selective tissue can damage it directly. For example, antibodies attacking red blood cells can destroy those cells, which would result in anemia. The second way damage occurs is from an inflammatory reaction resulting from the presence of *immune complexes*. What causes this? When an antibody in the blood mixes with the substances it is fighting, an immune complex is formed. Normally, the body eliminates this immune complex with the help of *complements*, a series of special proteins in the blood that help the antibodies to get rid of the immune complexes. However, in individuals with lupus, the immune complexes may not be eliminated normally, and they may be trapped in certain parts of the body. This causes an inflammatory reaction that is, among other things, primarily responsible for kidney disease in people with lupus, perhaps because the kidneys cannot filter out the substances. Damage from this type of inflammatory reaction can occur in other areas of the body as well. Once the immune complexes have been trapped, they trigger a sequence of events in which the body is actually trying to eliminate them, but can't. Unfortunately, in this process, the tissue in which the complexes are trapped also becomes damaged.

Inflammation resulting from the immune complexes can also occur in the connective tissues. Connective tissue, made up of a protein substance called *collagen* as well as fibers and supporting tissues, is the tissue that binds or connects the cells and tissues of the body together. There are connective tissues found in all parts or systems of the body. Therefore, any part of the body, or any connective tissue in the body, can be affected by lupus. Systemic lupus can affect virtually any organ in the body, including the heart, kidneys, brain, skin, joints, and lungs.

Who Gets Lupus?

Estimating the number of people in the United States who have lupus is a difficult—and controversial—activity. Some studies have suggested that approximately one and a half million people in the United States have lupus. Other estimates suggest that up to two million people, or even more, have lupus, and that up to five million people around the world have the disease! Regardless, the numbers suggest that more people have lupus than other well-known illnesses such as leukemia, multiple sclerosis, or muscular dystrophy (and there are *still* no telethons to raise money for lupus!). Estimates are that anywhere from 10,000 to 15,000 or more new cases of lupus are diagnosed each year.

The number of people being diagnosed with lupus seems to be increasing. Why is this so? Is it a true trend toward more people having lupus? Possibly. Is it because people are more health conscious and are seeing their doctors—who are better able to identify lupus—more often? Possibly. Improvement in diagnostic testing and increased public awareness of the disease also increases the numbers. Experts are still not sure how to explain this.

Lupus can occur in all races and ethnic groups, although statistics indicate a higher than average incidence in African Americans, Latinos, and Asians in the United States. More women than men are diagnosed with lupus. However, the percentages vary depending on what report you are reading or the expert that is citing the numbers! It is generally felt that up to 90 percent of all people with lupus are women.

Is age a factor in lupus? A very high percentage of individuals diagnosed with lupus are women in their childbearing years (the years between the start of menstruation and menopause). Their age at diagnosis usually ranges, therefore, from mid-teens to forties. Cases of lupus do occur earlier or later than these childbearing years, but not nearly as often. It is unusual for a child younger than five to have lupus. Scientists have been looking for answers as to why, both before and after childbearing years, the numbers of women and men who get lupus are more equal. Researchers hope that this may lead to a better understanding of what causes lupus.

What Causes Lupus?

Why does lupus occur? Why does inflammation occur in random areas of the body? Why does connective tissue become inflamed? Why, why, why? Although the causes of lupus are still unknown, researchers continue to try to come up with better answers to these questions.

At the present time, evidence suggests the existence of genetic, environmental, and hormonal components in the development of lupus. This supports the notion that there are a number of factors that come together in causing lupus. A tremendous amount of research continues to focus in this area. Much of the research that has been carried out is highly technical, dealing with scientific theories of the causes of lupus. Let's discuss the three main components currently believed to contribute to the onset of lupus.

GENETIC FACTORS

Could you have inherited lupus? Can your children inherit lupus from you? These are frightening questions. Evidence suggests that many different genes contribute to susceptibility to lupus; no one gene seems to be the culprit. The human genome project, in which scientists are learning more about the complete set of genes in a human being, has provided, and continues to provide, valuable information about the genetic role in the development of lupus.

Evidence suggests that some autoimmune diseases such as lupus do have a genetic basis, although this does not mean that lupus is an inherited disease. Rather, there may be a *genetic predisposition*, or a tendency, toward developing lupus that is inherited. For example, a history of lupus or other autoimmune diseases (such as rheumatoid arthritis, Grave's disease, Hashimoto's thyroiditis, or scleroderma, for example) in immediate blood relatives (parents and siblings) may increase the chances of lupus developing in a child. Once again, the percentages vary, depending on the study and the expert, but they are low. For example, estimates are that only approximately 5 percent of children of parents with lupus will develop the disease. So even if there is the possibility of a genetic predisposition to lupus, in most cases children still will not develop the disease. An interesting fact is that in identical twins in which one twin develops lupus, the other twin does not always develop the disease. In nonidentical twins and other siblings, the incidence of lupus is even lower. This clearly shows that genetics is not the whole story.

ENVIRONMENTAL FACTORS

Although it is believed that a hereditary factor may make certain individuals more likely to develop lupus, this genetic predisposition must still be triggered by environmental factors. Studies of identical twins in which one twin did not develop the disease support this. Scientists have considered, and continue to investigate, a number of environmental factors as potential triggers, including:

- Chemical agents (such as certain drugs, metals, and toxins)
- Sun exposure (UV rays can cause rashes and systemic lupus manifestations)
- Certain foods or supplements (for example, alfalfa sprouts contain an amino acid that can aggravate autoimmune problems)
- Infectious agents (such as viruses or bacteria that scientists suggest may disrupt normal immune system functioning)
- Stress (intense, prolonged stress or trauma has been frequently seen as a cause of lupus flares)

Additional research will focus on adding, or deleting, factors from this list.

HORMONAL FACTORS

The contribution of hormones to the onset of lupus has been intensely studied, primarily because of the disproportionate percentage of women who have lupus. In addition, the fact that lupus flares may be moderated by pregnancy or birth control pills also suggests hormonal involvement.

There are still far more questions about the cause of lupus than answers. Additional theories are introduced all the time. Hopefully, as you continue to live your life, research will provide more insight into the causes of lupus, which will ultimately help scientists find a cure.

Riding the Roller Coaster

When discussing lupus with her physician, Susan wanted to know if the disease would always cause the extreme pain she was feeling. She was told that her pain would probably come and go because lupus is a disease that is cyclical in nature. It's like a roller coaster, with its ups and downs. It rarely remains at the same level of intensity for long periods of time. On occasion, you may feel much better, but there are other times when disease symptoms may increase. When you're feeling good, there is no way of knowing how long it will be until another *flare* (an exacerbation, or worsening of symptoms) occurs. When you're in the middle of a flare and not feeling well, there is no way of knowing how long it will take until you are feeling better again.

FLARES AND REMISSION

So what exactly is a flare? At an international conference in 2010, a number of world-renowned experts gathered together to try to reach a consensus as to what constitutes a lupus flare. They finally agreed on the following definition: "A flare is a measurable increase in disease activity in one or more organ systems involving new or worse clinical signs and symptoms and/or laboratory measurements. It must be considered clinically significant by the assessor and usually there would be at least consideration of the change or an increase in treatment." Whew! What does all that mean?

In a flare, lupus is affecting your body more intensely. You may be experiencing more symptoms, more effects from the symptoms that you already have, or even new symptoms. (Each person experiences flares—and the symptoms of flares—differently.) Medication will be used to try to control the symptoms. When the flare begins to subside, the use of medications will gradually be tapered off. In a remission, the symptoms and signs showing that you have lupus subside, often to the point where they are no problem at all, even without medication or with minimal treatment. When you go into remission, you return to a virtually normal state of functioning, doing most or even all of the things that you used to be able to do. In addition, lab tests that are taken at that time will often be normal, although some, like the ANA (antinuclear antibody) test, may remain positive even during remission.

This flare/remission cycle may repeat itself a number of times during the course of your illness, and some individuals with lupus never go into complete remission. Their symptoms remain at a low level of intensity, controlled with medication, with occasional flares increasing the activity of the disease.

Symptoms of lupus may appear at any time. They may disappear for no apparent reason and reappear very soon in the future or after a long period of time has transpired; again, there is often no particular reason for their recurrence. Symptoms may even not reappear in the same form as when they last occurred. (Read more about lupus flares in Chapter 7.)

How Serious Is Lupus?

Any chronic disease can be serious. Does this mean that because lupus is a chronic disease, everyone with lupus has a serious case of it? No! The severity of lupus varies from being very mild (most common) to being life-threatening (relatively uncommon). How serious your case of lupus is depends partly on which systems of the body are affected by the disease. Certain organ involvement—kidney, brain, and heart, for instance—can have more serious implications than others, such as the skin.

It is important to remember that any illness, even a mild one, can become serious if it is not taken care of properly. Do you stay out until three o'clock in the morning three or four nights each week? Do you like to sit at the beach for hours at a time? Do you make sure that your reputation as a junk food junkie is firmly intact? Do you take your medication when you remember to take it, rather than when you *should* take it? Do you call your physician only when you receive a notice asking if you have moved to another town? If you use appropriate health procedures to take care of yourself properly, follow a well-structured treatment plan, take medication on schedule, and keep in close contact with your physician, you can increase the chances of lupus having a much milder impact on your quality of life. This is especially true if your doctor is carefully monitoring your disease and treats it more vigorously at early warning signs that underlying organ damage may be occurring.

The History of Lupus

Will knowing the history of lupus help you feel better? Probably not, but some people are curious about where things come from. Read on if you like. You will not be quizzed on names and dates!

Physicians had noticed symptoms of lupus for hundreds of years, even though the illness had not yet been named. Dermatologists were the first physicians involved with the illness, and they learned to recognize it simply by looking at the facial and scarring effects. The term *lupus*, however, has been applied to the illness only since the middle of the nineteenth century. Pierre Cazenave, a French dermatologist, believed that the rashes or scarred irritations on the skin looked as if the victim had been seriously bitten by a hungry wolf. In the nineteenth century, many illnesses were named according to what the symptoms looked like. So, in 1851, Cazenave named the illness *lupus*, meaning wolf. Since the skin inflammations were red, the name of the illness was expanded to *lupus erythematosus*, meaning "reddish wolf," to characterize lupus by its redness. This term was used to differentiate lupus from other illnesses that affected the skin but were infectious.

The red, bite-like patches and discoloration of the individual's skin, along with the resulting scars from the irritations, now are descriptive of, but not restricted to, the type of lupus called *discoid lupus* (also called *cutaneous lupus*). (See the following section for more about discoid lupus.)

In 1872, a dermatologist named Moritz Kaposi recognized that lupus could involve parts of the body other than the skin. In 1895, Dr. William Osler, a physician at Johns Hopkins Hospital, indicated that other organs of the body could be affected in many individuals with lupus, and skin problems were just one type of involvement. Upon realizing that other systems of the body were affected in lupus, he used the name *systemic lupus erythematosus* to differentiate it from discoid lupus, which primarily affects the skin.

Different Types of Lupus

As you have learned from this short history of lupus, there are two main types of lupus that we will be discussing in this book: discoid lupus and systemic lupus. (This doesn't take into consideration the other types of lupus, such as *drug-induced lupus*—which is not a focus of this book, since elimination of the drugs that induce lupus-like symptoms will often eliminate the symptoms—and *neonatal lupus*—which involves the occurrence of lupus symptoms in a newborn of a mother with lupus, and which, because it is rare, usually benign, and short-term, is not a focus of this book.) Symptoms of the two main types of lupus can follow the cyclical pattern of coming (flares) and going (remission). Even though this book deals primarily with the subject of coping with systemic lupus, it would not be complete without providing some basic information about discoid lupus as well.

DISCOID LUPUS

Discoid lupus primarily involves the skin. The word *discoid* is used to describe this type of lupus because the scaly, red patches, or lesions, on the skin are somewhat rounded in shape, almost like a disc. These lesions can be patchy, blotchy, or crusty. They may be present in the classic butterfly pattern, extending over the bridge of the nose to the upper parts of the cheeks below the eyes.

Discoid lupus usually affects the face and neck, and sometimes lesions appear on the upper part of the chest as well. Occasionally, there may be scaly, raised lesions on the skin of the arms, the trunk, or the legs. Lesions in discoid lupus usually occur on uncovered body parts. This does not mean, however, that you should dress yourself as a mummy; there are times when covered parts of the body get these lesions as well. The term *disseminated discoid lupus* describes those with lesions appearing in a generalized fashion over more of the body surface than just the face, neck, and upper chest. On infrequent occasions, the lesions can affect even the palms of the hands and the soles of the feet. It is also possible for lesions to appear on the scalp, despite the fact that these lesions may be hidden by thick hair. But when the scalp is involved, there may be a permanent loss of hair in the area, resulting in baldness (also called *alopecia areata* or *totalis*) in that area. Patchy lesions may also occur on the tongue, inside the mouth, or in the ears.

Other organs of the body are not affected by discoid lupus, and there are no internal symptoms. In addition, discoid lupus is considered to be a milder form of lupus—with no real threat to health. Does this mean that discoid lupus is a minor problem—something to be easily ignored? No. Discoid lupus can be painful, and in some cases, significant scarring can result.

In general, discoid lesions usually exist for fairly short periods of time, although they can remain for days, weeks, months, or even years. In extreme cases, lesions persisting for more than twenty years have been reported. It is very important that individuals with discoid lupus take care of lesions quickly and properly. With proper care, lesions may clear up in short periods of time. However, the longer the lesions persist, the greater the chance of permanent scarring and disfigurement. The two best ways to prevent serious disfigurement or unpleasant skin effects from discoid lupus are to use prescribed medications, such as corticosteroids or antimalarial drugs (your physician will guide you), and to protect yourself from the ultraviolet rays of the sun.

As with systemic lupus, the cause of discoid lupus remains unknown. Evaluation by a physician is necessary to determine if a skin condition indicates discoid lupus. Can this become systemic lupus? That is a big concern for most people who have been diagnosed with discoid lupus. But the consensus is that only a very small percentage of individuals with discoid lupus will go on to develop systemic lupus.

SYSTEMIC LUPUS

The main type of lupus we'll be discussing in this book is systemic lupus erythematosus. As we've already discussed, this type of lupus may attack any part of the body, including internal organs. The severity of this particular type of lupus depends on which part or organ of the body is affected. Like discoid lupus, systemic lupus may affect the skin. But unlike discoid lupus, internal symptoms may develop. Systemic lupus can be mild, but it can become more severe if some of the more important organs of the body, such as the kidneys, brain, heart, and lungs, are affected.

Frances, a thirty-seven-year-old woman, was frantic. She had been diagnosed six months previously with systemic lupus and had slowly begun to adjust to this chronic illness. Out of the blue, she received a telephone call from a childhood friend who, it seemed, also had lupus. Her friend, Mona, complained that she had a very severe case of lupus and had been bedridden for months at a time. Frances hysterically called her physician to find out if this was going to happen to her. She was advised that because each person is unique, each person experiences lupus differently. You can even experience symptoms differently at different times with lupus.

When Frances asked if she was going to die because of lupus, she was told that the mortality rate for lupus had decreased significantly because of advances in medical diagnosis and treatment. Frances was also warned not to read any books on lupus that were more than five to ten years old because so much had changed in the understanding of the disease since then. She was also warned that if she was planning to obtain information from the Internet, she should make sure that she consulted only reputable sites—and not believe everything she read unless she had discussed it with her doctor. (You can read more about obtaining information on lupus in Chapter 5 and in the Appendix.) She was reminded to remain in frequent touch with her physicians. But Frances was still frantic; she was still not reassured. When she asked what usually happens with people who have lupus, her physician told her that most people with systemic lupus experience difficulty with low-grade fevers, fatigue, and occasional rashes, along with joint pain or swelling. Many people with lupus rarely experience any symptoms other than these more common ones.

What Are the Symptoms of Lupus?

The symptoms of lupus can be divided into several categories.

- *General symptoms.* This category includes symptoms such as weakness, fatigue, low-grade fevers, generalized aching, and chills. These symptoms are most often evident when you're in a flare, although you may experience them fairly commonly throughout the course of your illness.
- *Skin.* Skin problems include rashes, patchy lesions, and red inflammations (discoid symptoms). Scarring on the skin of the scalp may be related to hair loss. Skin rashes from exposure to sunlight may occur. Bruising occurs commonly and more easily in people with lupus.
- *Chest.* Symptoms involving the chest include *pleurisy* or *pleuritis* (an inflammation of the membranes lining the inside of the chest around the lungs) and *pericarditis* (an inflammation of the sac surrounding the heart). These symptoms may cause inflammatory fluid to accumulate (pleural fluid or pericardial fluid), interfering with the nearby lung and heart function. With either of these manifestations, difficulty in breathing may occur and pain is common. Shortness of breath or a rapid heartbeat may also result. Inflammation in the rib area or in the abdominal muscles may cause chest pain as well.
- *Muscular system.* Symptoms involving the muscular system primarily include weakness and aching pain (also called *myalgias,* such as *fibromyalgia*).
- *Joints.* Joint pain is common in lupus: arthritis-like pain, swelling in the joints, redness, and stiffness. These symptoms may involve one or more joints, but the arthritis in lupus is rarely deforming.
- *Blood.* Lupus may also affect the blood. A low red blood cell count (*anemia*) is common in individuals with lupus and can be one cause of fatigue. White blood cell counts may also decrease (*leukopenia* or *lymphopenia*), leading to an increased susceptibility to infection. On the other hand, if there is an infection in the body, the white blood cell count may significantly increase. Platelets—those blood elements

responsible for helping the blood to clot—may decrease (*thrombocy-topenia*), causing increased black and blue marks or tiny pinpoint red spots called *petechiae*. Increased amounts of gamma globulin (the general name for the protein portion of the blood that contains antibodies) in the blood may also be seen with lupus, and blood tests may indicate a false positive test for syphilis. People with lupus may test positive for syphilis even though they do not have the disease.

- *Cardiac or circulatory involvement.* It is sometimes difficult to tell if you have cardiac involvement. You might notice increased swelling in your extremities, such as your feet, and feel shortness of breath. Or doctors may determine that you have an accumulation of fluid in the sac surrounding your heart. Cardiac involvement can be dangerous but does clear up when treatment is effective. The most common circulatory problem is Raynaud's phenomenon, in which spasms in the small blood vessels restrict the flow of blood to the extremities (most often affecting your fingers, toes, ears, or nose). This may result in pain and color change in the digits.

- *Digestive system involvement.* Stomach pain, cramps, nausea, vomiting, diarrhea, and constipation are occasional symptoms of lupus occurring in the digestive tract.

- *Kidney involvement.* Your kidneys may be less efficient in filtering waste out of the blood. Waste products remain in circulation, and *uremia* (an increase in waste products in the blood) may occur. In addition, there may be excessive amounts of protein lost in the urine, a condition called *proteinuria*. Since there is no pain associated with these changes, it is important to see your physician regularly so you can be tested for abnormal kidney function. Progressive swelling in the feet and legs may indicate edema, a sign of kidney involvement.

- *Nervous system involvement.* Various parts of the nervous system including the brain, spinal cord, and nerves may be involved. This may result in headaches or, in more severe cases, in symptoms such as seizures, temporary paralysis, psychotic behavior, or even strokes.

There are many symptoms of lupus. You may have only one, or you may have several. No one ever has all the symptoms. Some people have some of them, but most have only a few of them. You may have the same ones all the time, or they may change.

Experts have divided symptoms of lupus into two categories:

- *Non-organ-threatening disease.* People in this category experience symptoms such as achiness, fatigue, pain when taking a deep breath, fever, swollen glands, and signs of swollen joints or rashes, but their internal organs are not involved. Because these organs are not affected, a normal life expectancy is more likely. It is also unusual for their major organs to be affected if this has not happened after the first five years of lupus.
- *Organ-threatening disease.* People in this category, on the other hand, have lupus that does affect major organs, such as the heart, lungs, kidneys, or liver, or they have lupus and serious blood problems that suggest that their lupus may be organ-threatening. This category is more serious, and may become life-threatening, if treatment is not aggressive and effective.

So there's no way of knowing how your life with lupus will proceed and what symptoms you'll experience. There are a lot of questions, and far fewer answers. The only sure thing about lupus is that there is no sure thing about lupus!

Is Lupus Contagious?

One of Susan's primary concerns when she was first told that she had lupus was that she would be unable to stay with her husband and children because they might "catch" her disease. Many people who are newly diagnosed with lupus are concerned that it may be contagious. This is also a major concern of friends and relatives who do not know anything about the illness. Because lupus sounds frightening, some friends may be very concerned about being with you because of their fear of catching it from you! Worry not. People don't catch lupus! Since lupus is far from a rare disease, if it were contagious, such cases would certainly have been reported by now. And how

about physicians? Wouldn't they be at risk if lupus were contagious? Be
assured that physicians are no more likely to have lupus than anybody else.

Is Lupus Fatal?

Lupus is a chronic disease with no known cure at the present time, which
means that it can last as long as you are alive. Obviously, it is important to
remember that any illness, even a mild one, can become serious if it is not
taken care of properly. However, lupus is not generally considered to be a
progressive disease, and it is usually not fatal. (If you have read books and
articles stating that lupus is fatal, make sure you check the copyright dates
of the books or the publication dates of the articles. You'll probably find that
you're not reading current information.) Recent medical advances have been
able to provide better treatments, and happily, this has significantly reduced
the chances of lupus being fatal.

There are occasions, however, when lupus can be fatal. For the most part,
this occurs because of severe kidney disease, infections, severe central nervous system lupus, extreme cardiovascular complications, or blood clots.
Estimates of the mortality rate from lupus vary (most agree that they are
between 5 to 10 percent), but all the experts agree that mortality rates are
significantly lower than they were ten years ago. These statistics continue to
decrease with earlier diagnosis and more effective treatment.

Can You Predict the Future Course of the Illness?

Despite the fact that treatment for lupus has been more and more successful,
it is impossible to predict the future course of the disease. There is no pattern. Serious problems with lupus occur when the disease has a destructive
effect on important internal organs. So it is essential to diagnose and aggres-
sively treat lupus as quickly and efficiently as possible.

It still is not known what leads to a remission, how long any remission
will last, or whether you will ever be symptom free. What other reasons are

there for the difficulty in predicting the future course of your condition? Lupus is never a constant illness; it is always changing. Different systems and organs can be affected. Your age and attentiveness to your treatment program may also play a role in the severity of the disease.

Medical advances have been able to provide better management, so now many people can live long, reasonably normal lives. However, some cannot totally escape the pain that, despite treatment, may continue to range from mild to debilitating. In order to best live with lupus, it is essential to go beyond your medical treatment and do everything you can to deal with the pain, other symptoms, and emotional stress in your efforts to carry on your normal business and personal activities.

2.

HOW IS LUPUS DIAGNOSED?

After getting over the initial shock of being diagnosed with lupus, you may want to understand more about how your doctor finally concluded that you have the disease. It is often a very difficult and lengthy process, one that can take up to several years before the correct diagnosis is made. Several years! This doesn't mean that it takes that long for you to drag your symptom-laden body to the doctor! Because the initial symptoms of lupus may not be very noticeable or serious, you may not even be inclined to go to the doctor to have them checked out. As the symptoms worsen and you are more aware of your fatigue and joint pain, for example, you may then decide to go to the doctor. As you have the disease for longer periods of time, more symptoms of lupus may occur. (Remember, you may not be receiving any treatment yet.) This can make the eventual diagnosis easier because the package of symptoms will paint a suggestive picture for the diagnosing physician. But if your doctor doesn't come up with the right diagnosis, or if you run out of patience, you may end up going from doctor to doctor, trying different medications and treatments until you finally get the proper diagnosis or the correct treatment.

Lupus has frequently been called the great imitator. As you've already seen, there are an incredible number of symptoms you can have with lupus. Therefore, physicians who are trying to diagnose you may initially believe that another illness is to blame for your symptoms. Treatment may be started for the other illness. Only after seeing that the symptoms continue unabated may further investigation take place. In some cases, you may meet the criteria for lupus and for another autoimmune disorder (such as rheumatoid arthritis, scleroderma, or polymyositis). This confusion may lead to a diagnosis of mixed connective tissue disease in some cases, or crossover or overlap syndrome in others. So it may take some time to be able to narrow down the diagnosis to lupus.

What else makes it hard to diagnose lupus, especially in its early stages? Even though laboratory tests are only one component of the diagnostic process, results from these tests are not always correct. In a small percentage of cases, the findings are totally wrong! The tests may show no existence of lupus in someone who, using other criteria, has been diagnosed with lupus. This is called a *false negative test* (the test saying, "No, you don't have it," when you really do). On the other hand, some people who do not have lupus will show a weak, but nevertheless existing, positive lupus reaction to some of these blood tests. This is called a *false positive test* (the test saying, "You have it," when you really don't). Lab tests are only suggestive. A rheumatologist never makes a diagnosis of SLE on the basis of lab tests alone. Your doctor will be obtaining information about your whole medical history as part of the diagnostic process.

Researchers are still trying to come up with the perfect lab test for lupus. Maybe someday . . .

Setting Up Diagnostic Criteria

So what is necessary to reach a correct diagnosis of lupus? If lupus mimics other diseases, and laboratory tests for it are sometimes inaccurate, how do physicians ever determine if someone has lupus? After a lot of deliberation and analysis, the American College of Rheumatology (ACR) established fourteen criteria for lupus in 1971. Physicians generally agreed that it was likely that you had lupus if you had a positive response to four or more of the fourteen ACR criteria for lupus.

Our understanding of lupus is constantly changing. When the initial manuscript for the first edition of this book was written, physicians were still following the fourteen criteria. By the time the final revisions were being completed, the ACR had condensed the criteria to a revised list of eleven items. Much research has gone into the refinement of the list. It was revised and updated in 1982 and in 1997.

As important as these criteria are for the diagnosis of lupus, they are still considered a work in progress. Experts continue to work to establish criteria that differentiate lupus from any other condition so that the presence of the criteria will, with an increasingly high reliability, confirm the diagnosis of lupus.

Will these eleven items occur only in a person who has lupus? No. Anyone could have a positive response to an item, so satisfying any one particular criterion certainly does not mean you have lupus. That is why at least four of the criteria must occur. (Keep in mind, the criteria were really not established for clinical, diagnostic purposes; rather, they were primarily established for research purposes—for example, to include individuals with at least four criteria in a study of a new medication.) As you read through the criteria, see which ones apply to you.

The Eleven Criteria

It is necessary to meet *at least four* of the following eleven criteria to be diagnosed with lupus. The first four have to do with the skin, the next four have to do with systemic manifestations, and the final three are lab test results:

1. Facial redness or a rash on the face (often called the *malar* rash). This frequently appears in the form of the familiar butterfly configuration. The rash may be on both sides of the face or just on one side. It is usually flat.
2. A more extensive skin problem that may show as a rash, blotches, or raised scaly lesions. Scarring may result. These thick, raised patches are shaped somewhat like disks, and may occur on any part of the body. This is the main symptom of discoid lupus.
3. Photosensitivity—experiencing some kind of harmful physiological reaction to sunlight (more severe than just a sunburn!). Many people besides

those who have lupus are sensitive to sunlight, especially those with fair complexions. So, in order to meet this criterion, your reaction to sunlight (even with minimal exposure) should be more severe than just sunburn.

4. Ulcers (sores) in either the mouth or nose, or the throat. Although many people have had sores in their mouths from time to time, what is relevant in lupus is how often these sores recur.

5. Arthritis-type symptoms in two or more joints. Arthritic inflammation or pain must not be accompanied by any noticeable or marked deformity of these joints to meet this criterion. Arthritic problems in a joint show up as swelling or tenderness, or pain if the joint is moved. The joints that may be affected include the feet, ankles, fingers, knees, hips, elbows, shoulders, wrists, and jaw.

6. Either pericarditis or pleurisy. As we've discussed, pericarditis is an inflammation of the sac or lining surrounding the heart, and pleurisy involves inflammation of the membrane that lines the inside of the chest cavity surrounding the lungs.

7. One of two possible kidney problems, caused by inflammatory damage inside the kidney. One is the existence of excessive protein in the urine. This is called *proteinuria*. The other is the existence of blood cell "casts." These are fragments of cells normally found in the blood. If you have kidney disease, however, they may be found in the urine.

8. A neurological disorder, either convulsions (seizures) or psychotic behavior, without it possibly being caused by drugs or a metabolic problem.

9. One or more blood disorders. One blood problem that can occur with lupus is hemolytic anemia. *Anemia* is a common blood disorder. But if you have *hemolytic anemia* (in which the red cells are coated with antibodies that cause them to break down and break apart), this is one indication that you may have lupus. It is important to remember that red blood cells normally live, die, and are eliminated naturally. In hemolytic anemia, the blood cells are destroyed because of this antibody coating, and so they are eliminated too rapidly and prematurely.

A second potential problem with the blood may be a low white blood cell count resulting from destruction of your white blood cells. This condition is called *leukopenia*. White blood cells fight infection in the body. Since individuals with lupus frequently do have a low white blood cell count, this is an important criterion for diagnosis even if it occurs early in the disease.

A third blood disorder is *lymphopenia*, in which there is a decrease in the number of lymphocytes (a subset of white blood cells) in the blood. Lymphocytes are the main cells of the immune system.

Leukopenia or lymphopenia must be detected on two or more occasions for this to be a positive criterion in the diagnosis of lupus.

A fourth type of problem with the blood is called *thrombocytopenia*, in which there is a decrease in the number of platelets in the blood. This causes difficulty forming clots if you get a cut or a wound. As a result, bleeding may be more difficult to control. Thrombocytopenia must be detected in the absence of medications that can lower platelet counts.

10. A disorder in your immune system as shown by blood tests. One possibility might be the presence of the LE cell. The LE (for lupus erythematosus) cell contains two nuclei rather than the one nucleus usually found in cells. Two nuclei are present in the LE cell because people with lupus have antibodies in their blood that can "bind" with the nuclei of cells. When the antibodies bind with the nuclei, they increase the likelihood that a scavenger cell will ingest or consume this antibody-coated nucleus. So the cell with two nuclei is simply a cell that has its own nucleus along with a second nucleus that it has ingested because of the antibody coating the second nucleus.

    LE cells are found in about 60 percent of all people who have lupus, especially when the disease is in a flare phase. At the same time, LE cells are rarely found if you don't have lupus. So the presence of LE cells is an important indicator. In order for this criterion to be met, lab tests should show two or more LE cells on any particular occasion, or one LE cell should be microscopically observed on two or more occasions. However, in many centers, this test is not being used primarily because it is difficult to do accurately, it is very time consuming, and in over one-third of the cases, it would give a false result anyway.

    Another way of satisfying the tenth criterion is to obtain a false positive reaction to the test for syphilis. The reason that this item is included in the list is because of the frequency with which individuals who have lupus do show a false positive reaction to this test. It may suggest the presence of antiphospholipid antibodies, making it an important diagnostic test.

Other immune results that satisfy this criterion include the presence of other antiphospholipid antibodies, including anticardiolipin or lupus anticoagulant, anti-DNA, or a positive anti-Smith antibody result.

11. The production of antinuclear antibodies (ANA). If your immune system has been destructively overactive, which is common in lupus and other autoimmune diseases, you may have a positive result for the presence of antinuclear antibodies produced by your immune system. Your immune system normally produces antibodies. These are used to help fight infection. An ANA test that is positive suggests that your immune system is producing antibodies that fight your healthy tissue. Because many individuals with lupus do produce antinuclear antibodies, a positive result on the ANA test satisfies this criterion.

EVALUATING THE CRITERIA

So, how many criteria did you meet? Remember, any *one* of the above criteria may exist in anyone, with or without lupus. It is the *combination* of the criteria and the severity and duration of a symptom that may help determine whether or not you have lupus.

Although they are currently the best accepted guidelines, these criteria are not unchallenged. Some physicians feel that this list is not comprehensive enough, or that there are still some important factors that have been left out. Some items on the list are not considered to be as important as other items on the list. Some physicians question whether certain items should be included at all. More revisions of the list will undoubtedly be seen in the future.

Another criticism of the established criteria is the requirement that four of the eleven be met. What if you clearly have been suffering from the symptoms of lupus, but meet fewer than four criteria? Does this mean you don't have lupus? No. What if you meet four or more of the criteria? Does this definitely guarantee that you have lupus? No. Obviously, these are valid criticisms. Not all cases will be diagnosed correctly. But when used properly, the criteria at least increase the likelihood of an accurate diagnosis.

Remember: A proper diagnosis of systemic lupus is made after careful consideration of your medical history, a detailed physical examination, and an assessment of appropriate laboratory test results.

Summing It All Up

Lupus is a very difficult disease to diagnose. There is no one factor that can accurately diagnose the illness. But regardless, now that you have been diagnosed, it's important to learn about how lupus is treated. Read on to learn about the basics of lupus management.

3.

HOW IS LUPUS TREATED?

S o far, we have discussed what lupus is, who may get it, what some of the symptoms of lupus are, and what criteria may be used to diagnose the illness, as well as other details about the disease. Terrific, but the more important question now is "What can be done to treat it?" You probably have some important questions. What can your doctors do for you? What will doctors tell you to do? What are the treatments for lupus, and how will they affect you? How do you control your symptoms? How do you help yourself get back into the mainstream of life? Let's begin to answer some of the questions you may have about the treatment of lupus.

Treatment for lupus varies from person to person and depends on the symptoms being experienced. This chapter will discuss the goals for people with lupus when they undertake treatment, and the factors that most lupus treatment programs have in common.

Goals of Treatment

Because there is no known cure for lupus, treatment aims at a suppression of symptoms. You want to feel better, right? Well, that's the primary intent of treatment, along with protecting and strengthening your body.

Experts believe that people with lupus do best to follow a comprehensive treatment program and, at the same time, determine what they need to change about their lives. Most important, you must develop a greater under-standing of what is needed for true healing, not just for masking your physi-cal symptoms.

You want to reduce the impact of your symptoms. Adjusting your general lifestyle, changing your behavior and activities, and learning to cope with the many emotional reactions you may be experiencing can be very help-ful. However, this is not the ideal outcome. The ideal outcome is remission, where symptoms no longer exist. Although your active treatment of lupus with medication and lifestyle changes aims to suppress symptoms, hope-fully, these symptoms will completely disappear and you'll go into remission.

Developing an Individualized Treatment Program

You are a unique individual. And your experience with lupus is unique. No one else has the same set of symptoms or reactions to the disease. To be effective, your lupus treatment program must be designed specifically to meet your special needs. This means that you have to be involved in devel-oping your care plan. By being an active participant in your treatment plan-ning, you'll be able to tailor your program to fit your lifestyle.

Each physician usually has his or her own idea as to what types of treat-ments work best. If you went to five different physicians and described the same symptoms to each, each of the five physicians might well prescribe a different treatment program for you. There may be no one specific approach that is right. A lot of trial and error goes into developing the best treatment program for you, and you may feel like a human guinea pig. But remember, this is only because the goal is to find the package that works best for you. Because of the number of unknowns concerning lupus and how it affects you, it may take some time before your physicians find the best way to treat you. Because there is no absolute treatment, modifications may be necessary before your treatment program works best. Does that mean that there aren't any physicians who agree on how lupus should be treated? No. There is a lot of agreement. Most physicians do prescribe a similar treatment program for their patients, adjusting it appropriately for each individual.

In designing your treatment program, you and your physician will take into account numerous factors, including:

* The symptoms of lupus that you're experiencing, and their severity
* Your overall general health
* How active you are
* Your school or work schedule
* Your age
* Your family and social situation
* Other medical conditions you may have
* Your financial and insurance coverage considerations

You want to have confidence in the treatment program prescribed for you. Accordingly, it is very important for you to feel at ease with your physician. What if you heard that somebody else with lupus was receiving different treatment from a different physician, and you started to believe that the other treatment program might be better? You might start losing confidence in your treatment plan and then in your own physician. Not a great feeling, is it? Remember, there is no one answer! What works for somebody else may not necessarily work for you.

Rarely will your treatment program remain constant throughout the course of your illness. If your symptoms become more pronounced or severe (let's hope not), treatment programs may become more active and intensified. If you develop side effects or have other underlying conditions, your treatment may be much more complicated. If your symptoms become less intense (let's hope so), the treatment program may become less active and more relaxed.

What are your symptoms? Treatment will be aimed at the symptoms that are specifically affecting you. Frequently, carefully structured treatment programs can be successful in controlling symptoms to the point where you can really be yourself. However, there are times when the treatment program is not able to reduce all symptoms. Medications or other therapies may not successfully control a symptom of lupus in one particular part of the body or another, or complications may arise. But you'll work with your physician, and you'll cross that bridge if and when you come to it.

If you are in a flare, think about what may have caused it. If you are doing something that gets you sick every time you do it, then stop doing it! For example, consider sunbathing (or maybe you shouldn't consider it!). If every time you go out in the sun, within a day or even a few hours after exposure you get a rash and a fever, part of your treatment should therefore include restricting your exposure to sunlight and using an effective sunblock.

What Are the Components of Treatment Programs?

Professionals involved with the treatment of lupus recognize that the best, most effective treatment program incorporates five major components:

1. Adjustment of general lifestyle, involving changes in behavior and activity necessitated by lupus (see Part Two).
2. Coping with emotional reactions, because it is so important that stress and negative emotions be controlled, and for you to maintain a positive mental attitude, to avoid further problems with your health (see Part Three).
3. Proper medication, which plays such a major role in suppression of symptoms (see Chapter 10).
4. Attention to day-to-day living, such as including the most health-enhancing amounts of rest, exercise, and energy-conserving strategies in your daily life (see Part Two).
5. Attention to diet and nutritional needs (see Chapter 11).

Each of these components will be discussed in detail in subsequent sections of the book.

Your Role in Treatment

Regardless of the components in your treatment program, you play the most important role of all because you are the one who lives with lupus every day.

There are always things that you can do to help yourself. It doesn't matter how much medical knowledge you have. There are also things you can do that will make your condition worse, but obviously those are things to be avoided. To start helping yourself, identify those things that improve your symptoms and those things that make them worse.

As you follow your treatment regimen, do your best to adhere to it completely and accurately and be as active a participant as possible. Be alert to the progress you make, and keep an open mind. Feel free to learn about other options and discuss them with your physician if the treatment you're using either isn't working or seems to be working against you.

Physicians can provide much in the way of medical information, medication, and expertise. Family and friends can provide emotional support, caring, and guidance. But you are the only one who can make the many small decisions necessary to organize your lifestyle as much as possible. These decisions may be small, but they may be critical in determining how lupus affects you and your family. Obviously, you play a key role in influencing the way you feel. But that's not enough. No single factor is enough. A whole package approach is essential, where you help yourself in as many ways as possible, both medically and psychologically. The rest of this book will be discussing dozens of ways in which you can help yourself to improve your life with, or despite, lupus.

Final Treatment Notes

Becoming knowledgeable about lupus and its treatment is an important part of learning to feel comfortable living with the disease. There are numerous books available in bookstores and libraries that cover all aspects of living with lupus. Check out the For Further Reading section at the back of this book for the titles of many excellent publications on lupus and related topics. The Resource Organizations and Websites sections also list a number of Internet sites that offer loads of valuable information about your life with lupus. In addition, you'll find contact information for national lupus organizations such as the Lupus Foundation of America, Lupus Alliance of America, and major regional organizations such as the S.L.E. Lupus Foundation and Lupus LA, all of which are excellent resources. Also remember the importance of maintaining open lines of communication with your health care professionals. They are there to support you, and this includes answering any questions you may have about lupus and lupus treatment. Being informed and educated is the best way to start taking charge of your lupus.

Treatment will change as symptoms decrease in intensity or other symptoms occur. This requires that you work in partnership with your physician. Let the physician know of any changes in symptoms, whether they're better or worse, so that treatment is changed accordingly. Never change your treatment on your own.

As important as it is to know as much as you can, you cannot learn everything there is to know about lupus overnight! Learning is a *process*—it's not instantaneous. Take the time to become more and more knowledgeable, recognizing that you can continue to refine and enhance your self-care skills.

The speed with which your treatment brings about results varies. Don't expect immediate success. However, with patience and proper adherence to a treatment program, you can reap the rewards of your efforts.

PART TWO

Living with Lupus

4.

LIVING WITH LUPUS: AN INTRODUCTION

So now you're living with lupus. What are you going to do about it? The goal is to live successfully with it, right? The goal is to be a person who happens to have lupus, rather than a lupus patient, right? Living with lupus is what this chapter (like this book!) is all about. How do you get started? Remember that learning how to live with lupus is like peeling an onion. You peel the onion one layer at a time. You learn how to live with lupus one step at a time.

It's hard enough to live with lupus. It's even harder if you fear that lupus will take (or already is taking) control of your life. The degree to which lupus symptoms affect your *body* may depend on the disease and its treatment. But the degree to which you let it control your *life* is still up to you. Your goal, always, is to be in control of as many aspects of your life as you can.

Lupus can affect many things, such as personal relationships, vocational capabilities, financial matters, mood, self-esteem, as well as physical and emotional health. But there's a difference between *affect* and *control*. That difference is you! The more control you have over your life, the healthier you will be, *regardless* of the ways that lupus may be affecting you.

What things can help you be more in control? There are plenty. In fact, this whole book is about feeling more in control of your life with lupus. Here are just three ideas to illustrate the point, and to whet your appetite:

- *Work on your attitude.* Even though a positive mental attitude may seem like an "intangible," it often distinguishes between those who cope successfully with lupus and those who don't. And whether your attitude is intangible or not, there's a lot you can do about this (see Chapter 22).
- *Develop new interests.* Even if lupus results in some changes in your life, and possibly interferes with your being able to continue some of the things you used to enjoy, there are always new things you can do. By focusing on that, you will feel more control of your life (see Chapter 13).
- *Join a support group.* The strategies and support included in such regular meetings can be invaluable (see Chapter 33).

This is just the beginning. There's so much that you can do. Lupus does not have to be the end of your life. It really is a new beginning. Don't let lupus be who you are. Let lupus just be what you have. You may feel that you're different because of lupus. The better way of looking at it is that lupus is something different about your life, but the person you were is the person you are. You still have the same likes and dislikes. You still have the same preferences. Lupus is an addition, even if you look at it as an unwelcome one. It is up to you how you accept that it is now a part of your life.

Take responsibility for your life with lupus: You want to be the director of your physical and emotional health, as well as your social, vocational, and family life. Remember: Happiness does not just come from feeling well; it comes from dealing well!

Moving Forward

Let's start this section with your initial reactions, how you may have felt at the time you were diagnosed. Then we'll talk about the steps you can take to move forward with your life. (You'll use many of the steps time and time again during your life with lupus, so you'll want to refer to them frequently.) After that, we'll deal with some of the most important issues people with lupus face, including physical symptoms, treatments, and day-to-day matters. Not only will you learn important information, but you'll learn proven, effective strategies to help you feel better, be healthier, and cope more effectively. Onward . . .

5.

YOUR DIAGNOSIS

When you first found out that you had lupus, how did you feel? How did you react when your doctor finally told you the news? It's only natural to feel overwhelmed after learning that you have a condition such as lupus. After all, there's no easy way to accept the fact that your life is going to change. Initially, your mind may be filled with questions about what lupus is and what the possible complications may be. So how can you possibly begin to cope? Calm down, take a deep breath, and be comforted with the knowledge that there are many things you can do.

Initial Reactions

When first diagnosed, you may not be able to react at all, since it may not seem "real" to you. But some people go through a hard time from the very beginning. It can be shocking to be told that you have lupus, especially if you'd never even heard of it beforehand.

Emotional reactions to lupus are not always rational. As a matter of fact, in many cases, they are completely irrational. And as the full impact of the diagnosis sets in, you may experience a whole variety of feelings, ranging from sadness and anxiety to anger and frustration. You may feel upset because you'll have to make some lifestyle changes. You may be fearful that you'll never adjust to living with lupus. No one—not even you—can predict how you'll react to the diagnosis, because no two people react in exactly the same way.

Let's look in greater detail at some of the more common reactions to the diagnosis. Later on in the chapter, we'll look at how you can begin to cope with these emotions.

YOU MAY BE IN SHOCK!

Being diagnosed with lupus may be shocking. And as the intensity of the shock wears off, it is quickly replaced by feelings of disbelief. It's hard to believe that you've got a *disease*! This disbelief, though, is actually a calmer sensation than the initial shock and subsequent emotions. It gives you a chance to adjust to what you have heard—to get used to it in your own way, at your own pace.

Give yourself time to get used to the diagnosis. Get a second medical opinion, if that would make you feel more secure (more about second opinions in Chapter 32). Don't feel that you have to absorb it or, more important, accept it all at once. This takes time.

YOU MAY BE IN DENIAL!

Why do some people deny that they have lupus, even when they've just been diagnosed? It's probably because the reality of the situation is simply too painful to acknowledge. Regardless of the symptoms you've been experiencing, hearing that you have lupus may provoke denial. You may protest, "Oh, come on. It can't be true," or "I'm sure the problem will go away by itself," or even "#!&^*X#, leave me alone!" It's really not at all unusual to deny that a problem exists. You may not want to deal with the potential consequences of the situation . . . all the ways in which it may change your life.

Did you ever ask yourself, "Why can't I go back to the way things used to be?" Do you ever wish you could wake up one morning and find out that this was all just a bad dream? This is very common, but also very counterproductive. The more you keep hoping the situation will go away, the slower your adjustment will be. Why? Because you're not really admitting to yourself that you've changed—perhaps permanently. Rather, you're trying to push it out of your mind, hoping that things will return to the way they were. Try to recognize that your condition does exist now, that it affects you, and that it will remain with you. Then aim your efforts in the *right* direction. Try to plan your activities and structure all of your thinking toward handling your situation as effectively as you can.

If you're reading this book, chances are that you're probably not totally denying your condition. But if you are denying it, somewhere along the line you're going to have to start facing reality. Speak to professionals who know about lupus, and have them explain it in further detail. Let them tell you about the treatments available for your condition. Read about lupus. Or talk to others with lupus and listen to what they went through when first diagnosed. You will find that many of their experiences parallel your own. You'll also find that many of them have learned to adjust—just as you'll eventually adjust!

As you'll read in more detail shortly, there are times when denial can be positive. How? It can be helpful by keeping you from dwelling on problems that worry won't help. In other words, if there's nothing you can do to improve a situation, why keep thinking about it? Remember that although denial does distort reality, there may be times when distortion is necessary. So denial can be helpful early on, following diagnosis, as you get used to dealing with that diagnosis. It may enable you to go about your normal routine while you're getting used to these unpleasant circumstances. But the appropriateness of denial can turn to inappropriateness if it keeps you from doing what you have to do in order to help yourself.

YOU MAY FEEL CALM!

Frequently, as with any traumatic event, you may feel numb at first. You may sit quietly in the doctor's office, listening to everything that is being said. But you may not really be absorbing it. You may hear your doctor talking, but the words are not penetrating. You might even actively and calmly participate in the discussion without any emotional reaction. That may come later!

YOU MAY FEEL ANXIOUS!

Following the diagnosis of lupus, a commonly experienced reaction is anxiety. Even terror, or sheer panic! You may think, "Oh, no, I have lupus!" "What is it?" "Where does it come from?" "What's going to happen to me?" Or you may ask, "How will the disease affect me?" "Will I ever get better?" "Who will take care of me?" "Am I going to be confined to a wheelchair?" "Am I going to die?" These are all difficult questions that may pop up when you're diagnosed. Family members and loved ones may ask them (and panic) as well. You may believe your life will never be the same again, because it will now include lupus.

Let's talk about this reaction. Nobody enjoys pain or physical restrictions. It's normal to be upset and afraid. You probably don't understand the diagnosis. (Many people diagnosed with lupus didn't even know about the illness beforehand.) After all, lupus even sounds frightening! You may suddenly be hit with the fact that you are mortal and vulnerable. You'll realize you may have this problem for the rest of your life. Physically, it's not uncommon to feel faint or dizzy, or to experience other stress reactions at the time of diagnosis. Because of the tremendous fears that can immediately follow diagnosis—fear of loss of health or loss of independence—it's not surprising that this time is one of turmoil. The path to recovery from this turmoil is rarely smooth. A whole other group of emotions, such as rage, anger, and depression, comes into play as well.

Family members and loved ones may have the same fears and ask the same questions. They, too, may feel anxious. They may feel helpless because they don't know what they can do for you. This can certainly make things worse—for them *and* for you. (There is more about fears and anxieties in Chapter 24.)

YOU MAY BE RELIEVED!

You may be surprised to hear that some people actually are *relieved* when they are diagnosed with lupus. Why? Well, perhaps they knew they had a problem, but didn't know what it was. Or maybe they'd been experiencing a lot of pain and nothing seemed to help—making them question their sanity. Or maybe they had tried to get a diagnosis for a long time. Amazingly, research has shown that it can take years to diagnose lupus in some people. That's a very long time to wonder what's wrong, especially considering how sick you may be feeling.

If you were experiencing different symptoms and nothing seemed to help, then the diagnosis of lupus may give you hope—hope that treatment will improve the way you're feeling. Maybe you were afraid to go to the doctor, for fear that you would be diagnosed with a fatal illness. Then you're probably relieved to find out that your condition can be managed and that you're not going to die. Perhaps you thought that your symptoms were purely psychological. Or maybe your family members didn't believe that you were experiencing physical symptoms. Well, then, isn't it good to learn that there's a reason why you've been feeling this way—that it isn't "all in your head"?

YOU MAY BE ANGRY!

You may utter the inevitable words, "Why me?" You wonder what you did to deserve this. Your anger may be directed toward the doctor, family members, your spiritual leader, or anyone else that you can "blame." This doesn't have to make sense. It's not as though they *did this* to you. But the reality is that you're just angry, angry that this is happening to you and affecting your life. (You can read more about anger in Chapter 25.)

YOU MAY BE DEPRESSED!

As, more and more, reality sets in and you realize you can't deny what you have, and you can't do anything to make it go away, you may get more depressed. You may withdraw from normal relationships and normal activities. You may not feel like doing anything. You may sleep too much, more than what is necessary to rest your body. You may lean on inappropriate coping strategies such as drinking or taking pills (more about depression in Chapter 23).

Other Reactions

There are other reactions that some people experience following the diagnosis of lupus. Let's discuss a few of these.

DAMAGED SELF-ESTEEM

One of the most important characteristics that each person has is self-esteem. The way you feel about yourself is very important and helps you get through each day. Unfortunately, a diagnosis of lupus may have a damaging effect on self-esteem.

Have you liked yourself less since your diagnosis? Previous feelings of confidence can be quickly shattered, and this can have a very unpleasant effect. You may not feel or behave like yourself. You may feel embarrassed that you're not able to do the things you used to be able to do. You may now have difficulty with things you always used to take for granted. You'll want to deal with this right away in order to return to effective, efficient functioning.

One problem that can affect your self-esteem is the feeling that you're no longer independent and that you've lost a certain amount of control over your life. For example, you may feel there is little you can do about the pain. The degree to which this feeling exists varies from person to person. Medical visits, medication, treatments—all these things, and more, make you more dependent on the medical system. And this may continue for the rest of your life. If you allow it, your self-esteem may suffer because you feel more dependent on others in the health care system or in the hospital, where others control virtually every aspect of your life.

What can you do about this? Instead of being upset by the things you can't do or the ways in which you are dependent on others, focus on the things that you still *can* do! Try to maintain as normal a routine as you can. As we discussed earlier, take control over as much of your life as possible. Get involved in support groups. Speak to others to find out how they handle these very important issues. If necessary, speak to professionals for additional tips.

CHANGING BODY IMAGE

Changes in body image may occur because of lupus. In fact, just knowing you have lupus can change the way you feel about your body. This, too, can have a very profound effect on your self-esteem.

What can you do to improve your body image? Remind yourself that you can control how you feel about any changes that have affected your body. If you choose to do additional things to enhance your appearance, you may want to contact professionals about what you can do. For instance, you might wear a different style of clothing to refocus the attention of others, or follow dietary programs designed to stabilize weight. The most significant step you can take may be to work on your attitude. Remind yourself of who you are, and who you've always been. Feel good about the things that are truly important, and minimize the rest.

SELF-BLAME

Do you feel as though you "set yourself up" for lupus? Do you worry that you're being punished for something you did—that this disease is the result of some wrongdoing? What's the point of thinking this way? Does it really help you? It isn't true, so why let these thoughts overwhelm you?

There's no question that there is a connection between mind and body. The way you feel can certainly contribute to the way your health thrives or suffers. But rather than spending valuable energy blaming yourself for ways in which you may have let yourself down, doesn't it make more sense to focus on ways in which you can build up your body, correct any problems that you can, and move on? One of the best ways you can do this is to improve the way you deal with your emotions. Therefore, you'll want to recognize and let go of any self-blame. Not only do you want to be compassionate toward others, but you also want to be compassionate toward yourself! Try to focus on what you can do to improve yourself, both physically and emotionally.

NEGATIVE THOUGHTS

It is as important to push away negative thoughts as it is to eliminate self-blame. The less room there is in your mental attitude for negativity, the more room there will be for positive feelings. This will provide you with an important foundation in your efforts to cope better.

Everyone has negative thoughts—thoughts that lead to the growth and intensity of negative emotions. However, there is no law that says you have to let these thoughts continue! Don't allow them to remain in your head and overwhelm you! Keep challenging these thoughts. Work to turn them around and make them more rational, realistic, and positive. In this way, you'll continue to focus on the positive feelings that are such an essential part of successfully living with lupus.

It is a waste of valuable energy to be angry, guilt-ridden, self-blaming, or self-critical. It's now time to harness the energy that goes into these negative emotions and to turn it into positive energy that can strengthen you.

DEATH WISH

Did you ever wish you could die after being told you have lupus? Some people do. Emotionally, they exclaim that they'd rather die than have to go through this. If you've ever felt this way, don't feel guilty about such thoughts. You're not alone. Although you may feel like giving up from time to time, these feelings can go away, and even more quickly if you work on them. If, however, these thoughts really reflect suicidal wishes, please reach out immediately for professional help. Don't feel that these more intense thoughts will just go away over time, or if you work hard enough on them. Sure they might. But if they don't, others can help. This does not suggest that you're a failure. In fact, you're a success if you recognize a problem that may benefit from professional help, and reach out to get it. Caring counselors are trained to help you straighten out your thoughts and feel more positive about being . . . and staying . . . alive.

How Can You Begin to Adjust?

You may have many questions immediately following your diagnosis. However, the most important question is one that only you can answer: "Will I give up living because of lupus, or will I continue to live despite lupus?" The following steps should start you on the road to living successfully with lupus.

TAKE CHARGE

You must take the reins and begin to help yourself. Sure, you can receive love and support from your family and friends, and you can obtain guidance and expertise from professionals. But that's never enough. *You* are the one who is going to have to come to grips with lupus. At first, adjusting may be a difficult struggle that requires tremendous effort. You may go through a lot of emotional turmoil. But there is no other way to deal with your illness successfully. You must face it.

When you are learning to cope with lupus, it's important to have a sense of empowerment—to be in control of as many factors in your life as possible. Yes, we've discussed this before. But it's important enough to bear repeating. Because of the important role you play in managing your lupus, you have the power to regain control of your health and live your life to the fullest.

INFORMATION, PLEASE!

Many of your initial reactions were probably the result of not knowing enough about lupus. So you'll want to learn as much as possible. It's very easy to let your imagination run wild. Initially, you'll probably keep thinking about all the things that can possibly go wrong. You'll worry about every symptom. You may also become frightened about developing lupus-related complications. So learn the facts about your condition. This is a great way to alleviate some of the anxiety caused by the diagnosis.

Your physician will be helpful in providing information or will at least suggest ways of getting it. Read a lot, but make sure the information is not outdated. Not only can older books and magazines be misleading, but also they can be downright dangerous and depressing. Many times people have been devastated because they read old information that gives very little hope for a happy life with lupus.

After reading general, consumer-oriented information, you might want to move on to more technical material. Ask questions about anything you don't understand. And certainly ask questions about anything that frightens you! After all, medical writing merely states medical facts and statistics—it's not necessarily written to comfort people with lupus. Don't forget this, or you may become unnecessarily alarmed!

It probably wasn't a lifelong goal of yours to become an expert on lupus, but think about how much this information may help you. Doctors will respect your questions more. And you'll understand exactly what's going on in your body. These are just two of the many advantages that can come from reading about your condition.

Should you believe everything you read? Of course not! There's no shortage of miracle "cures" and alternative treatments for lupus. If a claim seems too good to be true, check it out to be sure the source is indeed reputable. New procedures and treatments must undergo rigorous scientific study to be proven effective. If you can't find credible scientific evidence to back up a claim, then you would be wise to stick with your current program.

As we've previously discussed, lupus organizations and other comparable health organizations are committed to providing current information about lupus and promoting public awareness of the illness. Many of these institutions also sponsor forums, recruit guest speakers, and organize clubs and self-help classes. Take advantage of these valuable resources.

INFORMATION ONLINE, THANK YOU

How far we've come! Estimates are that more than 80 percent of all people have tried to get health-related information online. There is a huge amount of information about lupus available on the Internet. Virtually anything you might possibly want to learn about your life with lupus (yes, even about coping!) can be obtained online. For example, all you'd have to do is search for the word *lupus* using Yahoo! or Google or another search engine, and you will immediately be overwhelmed with thousands if not millions of links to other sites containing information. (Try it; it's amazing!) But with so much information being so readily accessible, problems may arise if you're not careful. Are you suggestible? If you are, if you believe everything you read, you need to carefully consider the validity of everything that comes up on your screen.

Lorraine was scared. She didn't know much about lupus and had just been diagnosed. So she went online. Because she was such a nervous person she did a search for *lupus and anxiety*, and found many links. She clicked on one, started reading it, and read, "Anxiety has also been proven to cause lupus . . ." "Oh, no," she immediately thought, "what did I do to myself?"

No, Lorraine did not *cause* her lupus by being nervous. But what she *did* do to herself is cause more anxiety . . . needlessly! Consider carefully anything you read online. Don't accept it as gospel. Get the facts, and don't jump to conclusions based on anything you read, especially if you're not sure about the qualifications of the authors. This does not mean you should immediately reject or disregard this information. Just be intelligent about believing what you read. Of course, this is true whether the information is available online, or in a book, an article, or anything else! Anything you read that differs from what you know or have already learned should, of course, be discussed with your doctor. Be selective, know how to search out the information you want, and use appropriate discretion in deciding what information you will ultimately use.

So now that you've agreed to be careful (you do promise, right?), what are the two main advantages of obtaining information online? You will usually get current, detailed, up-to-date information. And, you can become more knowledgeable from the comfort of your home (even your bed, if you use a laptop!). People often learn things online that they don't read about anywhere else. For example, you may find out about new (and approved) treatments or clinical trials that would be beneficial to you.

The Resource Organizations and Websites sections at the back of the book list a number of Internet sites that may be of interest. (And if a listed website is no longer available, forgive me: the Internet changes every day.)

KEEP RECORDS

The longer you live with lupus, the more information you will have about your treatments, medications, symptoms, and doctors. It makes sense to keep all of that information in one place by detailing your entire medical history in a word processing document on your computer. Not only can this keep all of your essential information in one place, but it can help you with all of your medical appointments, and it can be especially helpful if you have to go to new doctors. Setting up files of your medical history also makes it easy to add new information, as necessary. So what details might you want to include? Keep a written record of your symptoms, treatments, medications, side effects, doctor visits, hospitalizations, and anything else that you think is pertinent. Don't feel as though you have to write your entire medical history in one sitting. Start by writing as much as you can, and then add as needed (and as remembered!). There's no time like the present to start putting all of your information in one place.

Some people set up additional spreadsheets containing more detailed information about their medications, including facts such as the date the medication was prescribed, the name of the medication, the dosage, the prescribing physician, anticipated and actual benefits of the medication, and side effects experienced. There are even flash drives (those small devices that plug into the USB port of your computer) that are specifically designed to hold all of your medical information. Examples of available flash drives prepared for this purpose include ER Card (ercardmember.com), MedicTag (medictag.com), and e*MedTag (americanmedical-id.com).

SHARE WITH OTHERS

Whom do you tell about your lupus? What do you tell them? Obviously, you want support. You may feel alone and different enough as it is. When you think about those you know, you can be reasonably sure that there are certain people who will be supportive. But you may also fear the kinds of reactions you might get when you share your news with other people. For example, you may be afraid to say something to your boss, or to someone you just started dating. But developing your support "network" is very important in living with lupus. In fact, much more information about this topic is found in Part Four of the book.

DEVELOP A POSITIVE RELATIONSHIP WITH YOUR DOCTOR

Obviously, you must work with health care professionals you can trust and who have had experience working with people with lupus. You have the right—in fact, the obligation—to learn as much as possible about the different treatments for lupus. And you can start by asking questions of your physician. If your doctor (or another member of your treatment team) does not seem receptive to your questions, try to make him or her aware of how important these concerns are to you. If no progress is made, then you may have to reconsider this relationship.

Because a chronic illness is ongoing, the patient–physician relationship will be ongoing as well. You will have much more contact with your physician, because of your lupus. Some say this relationship is like a marriage, but unfortunately, you're not entitled to 50 percent of your doctor's assets if you separate! (You can find more about dealing with your physician in Chapter 32.)

HELP YOUR FAMILY ADJUST

It is understandably difficult to adjust to the diagnosis of lupus and to cope with the many different emotions you are experiencing. This adjustment becomes that much harder when the people close to you also have difficulty with their emotions—especially if their emotions are different from yours!

Of course, it's easy to understand why family members might have trouble dealing with the diagnosis. They, too, will go through periods of denial—times at which they'll say, "No, everything will be fine," or "I'm sure the problem will clear up by itself." Unfortunately, this won't make things easier for you. For example, if you're trying to come to grips with lupus, but family members are not acknowledging its existence, this may affect your ability to cope successfully. We'll discuss denial a little bit more in the next chapter.

Ann Marie, a thirty-four-year-old nurse, had only recently been diagnosed as having lupus. After a few very depressing weeks, however, she began to learn how to cope. She was finally able to handle thoughts of lifestyle changes, concerns about reduced mobility, and some of the other unpleasant realities associated with lupus. Sound great? Not really. You see, Ann Marie's husband of fourteen years couldn't admit she had a problem, her children were afraid that she was going to die, and even her sixty-eight-year-old mother was considering selling her ranch in Texas to move closer. Although Ann Marie was learning how to cope with lupus, she could not cope with her family. They couldn't handle it and were making things very difficult for her.

It's a great idea for family members to seek out people to speak to—just as it may benefit *you* to seek help. Spouses, children, and others can find out more about lupus and learn how others cope with treatment. They can even join support groups or seek counseling. So encourage your family and any willing friends to learn as much as they can and to seek whatever help they need. Their adjustment will help your adjustment.

DEAL WITH YOUR EMOTIONAL REACTIONS

The emotions stemming from the diagnosis of lupus can be unpleasant. You may experience regret, sorrow, nostalgia, and anger, remembering the way life used to be. Many fears may come to mind, some of which can be overwhelming. Fears of incapacitation, of being handicapped, or of losing out on life are all very common. Begin facing them. They can and must be faced in order to move your adjustment along more smoothly. (Part Three contains a lot of information and strategies to help you deal with your emotions.)

A Diagnostic Departure

Start thinking positively about your life with lupus. Learn as much as you can about your condition. Use whatever support systems are necessary. Use all of the stress management and emotional control techniques you can learn. (Many good ones can be found in this book!) Start saying to yourself, "Lupus may be a part of my life, but I'm still alive, and I'm going to do whatever I can to help myself adjust."

After some time, learning more, and hopefully working on your thinking, you'll get to a point where you are starting to accept what you have. You may not like it. You may *never* like it. But the goal is to accept the fact that lupus is now part of your life. You're going to move forward with your life doing the best you can. You want to help yourself and others, and enjoy your life (and it can be pretty darn good!).

Once you have become more familiar with your condition and understand how it affects you, what can you do to deal with it? For one thing, you can find out what specific changes may have to be made in your lifestyle. There is no way of knowing how many changes you'll have to make to create the best possible life for yourself. But tell yourself that you will make them, and that you will learn to live with them! You're going to lead as complete a life as you can. The more quickly you can adapt your lifestyle to fit your needs, the more rapidly you'll be able to enjoy your life. This may be hard at first and will certainly take time. But you're not helpless, and you can take steps to make the most of your life *despite* lupus!

6.

COPING WITH LIFESTYLE CHANGES

So, you have to make changes in some aspects of your lifestyle because of lupus? Yes, that is all part of the package. But changes may occur in anyone's life for a number of reasons. If you began a new job, you might have to wake up earlier, commute in a new direction using a new form of transportation, or adjust to a different salary. And if your new job required you to move, you would have to learn your way around a new neighborhood.

In your case, it's lupus that has now changed your life. Although you may think it will be impossible to ever again lead a normal life, this is unlikely to be true. However, you must make certain changes that will let you lead a comfortable life despite lupus. Remember that you want to feel better, enjoy life, and do what you can. These goals are both reasonable and achievable.

To different degrees, lupus can affect work, family life, sexual activity, social activity, finances, and other aspects of day-to-day living. Make up your mind to accept and work through any necessary changes. But also be aware that there are always things you can do to improve the way you live.

Your lifestyle will, to a large degree, be of your own choosing. You'll automatically take many different factors into consideration when determining what your lifestyle is and what you want it to be. You can decide how full you want your days to be. You may also decide to put things off until you "feel better." But why wait? Why not try to see what you can do right now to improve the quality of your life, even while you're learning to live with lupus?

What Changes May Take Place?

Lupus can result in a change of lifestyle because of a number of different factors, including the following:

- Physical pain or other symptoms may affect your ability to work, go to school, play, or enjoy personal relationships.
- Physical pain or other symptoms may result in frustration, sadness, depression, anger, and even a strong sense of loss. You may miss the things you are not able to do. You may get angry with your body because you want to do everything the way other people do and you can't.
- You may have difficulty functioning both at home and at the office.
- Activities, travel, or everyday events may have to be changed, reduced, or eliminated due to pain or limited energy.
- Regular physical activity and exercise may be difficult.
- Your economic status may be affected if large out-of-pocket or non-insurance-reimbursable expenses are incurred for drugs and treatment.
- Feelings of instability—never knowing when you are going to feel sick, exhausted, or in pain—can interfere with daily activities, or such luxuries as vacations or trips.
- Your pain and other physical complaints may scare away your friends.

Making Changes

As we've already discussed, one very important part of coping with lupus is learning to take control over as much of your life as possible. This means taking an active part in treatment decisions and determining how all aspects of treatment can fit as comfortably as possible into your lifestyle. Keep in mind that there's a difference between taking control of your life and looking for a miracle, such as your lupus going away forever. Yes, this miracle would be wonderful, but hoping . . . and waiting . . . for it will not help you improve your life. In fact, it might slow down your adjustment. Ignoring your symptoms (a type of denial) can also slow down your adjustment and limit your ability to cope. So instead of looking for miracles, focus on doing the best you can to help yourself.

A diagnosis of lupus may seem totally negative. However, this diagnosis can be viewed as positive if it serves as motivation for constructive change or self-improvement. You see, people change and grow not only when things are going well, but also during times of adversity. By looking at your life from a different perspective, you may be able to start weeding out those things that have not been good for you and begin introducing better things. This will improve not only your own physical and emotional health, but also the well-being of those around you.

At this point, you want to alter your lifestyle to make things as easy as possible. It's important to make the right changes that will allow you to continue doing much of what you want to do without putting too much pressure on your body. In fact, as you modify your life to reduce or avoid discomfort and conserve energy, you should gradually begin to feel better. For example, try spreading out your most taxing activities. Pace yourself. If necessary, be sure to include rest periods during the course of the day so that you can "recharge your batteries." These changes should help you do many of the things you want to do while taking care of your physical needs. The following are some other suggestions that may prove helpful.

SET PRIORITIES

Look at yourself not as a person with unlimited strength, but as one of limited energy. Focus on the most important things you want to do in your life, and try to spend less time on those things that don't have as much significance.

Each day, prioritize your activities so that you can spend your energy on those tasks that are most important. Make up a list of the things that need doing, and then group them into "musts," "maybes," and "possibilities." On some days, you'll be able to do many of the tasks on the list; on other days, you may be able to do very few. During those times when your energy is limited, you'll be glad that you were smart enough to accomplish the most important tasks first.

Just as you must complete certain tasks each day, you should also make it a point to do something you enjoy. Spend more time with those people and on those activities that are more supportive of your physical and emotional well-being. This includes your family and others who truly care about you as a person. If it is hard to talk to your family, talk with a teacher, a clergy person, or a friend whom you can trust. Spend less time—or, possibly, no time!—with those people and activities that drain your strength and give you less pleasure. This will improve the overall quality of your life, better equipping you to deal with the stress of lupus.

Despite all the changes you may be making to better cope with your lupus, you want to maintain as much normalcy in your life as you can. Continue doing as many of the things that you enjoy as you can. Hobbies can help—after all, you need something to take your mind off this disease! Find an outlet for your emotions—music, writing, photography, movies, reading, the Internet, and so on.

As you work on adapting your lifestyle, also try to gradually modify your standards, requirements, and obligations. Don't feel that you have to live up to all of your previous standards—especially if lupus or its treatment has diminished your strength. There is no law that says you must keep your standards at the same level throughout your entire life. Be flexible and realistic, and change as necessary to make yourself more comfortable.

Life with lupus has its ups and downs. Changes may be necessary because of your emotional needs, treatment, pain, other symptoms, and a number of additional factors. The most efficient way to adjust is to anticipate as many of the ups and downs as possible, and ride them out as smoothly as you can.

SET GOALS

Life without goals is meaningless. Set short-term, intermediate, and long-term goals for yourself. For instance, you might choose the next book you'd like to read, find a new hobby or interest you'd like to pursue, or plan your next vacation. (Yes, you *can* plan a vacation. Learn more about traveling with lupus in Chapter 15.) Then keep moving toward these goals. This will help to put your life into a better perspective.

LIVE LIFE ONE DAY AT A TIME

Live each day one at a time. Although this may seem incompatible with having goals, it's not. You can continue to live one day at a time even though you have goals in the back of your mind, goals that you've set up to give your life structure and focus. Enjoy life as much as you can. Try to add pleasure to some of the ordinary, mundane things to which you previously gave little thought. If you go for a ride in your car, for example, instead of focusing on your destination, enjoy the process of getting there. Look at the scenery around you. Admire the beautiful things that life has to offer. At the same time, don't neglect planning for the future. All of this is important in developing a positive mental attitude.

Getting Used to Changes

What are some of the factors that will determine how well you'll adapt to changes in your lifestyle? There are many. For example, what were you doing before you were diagnosed with lupus? How satisfied were you with your work and leisure activities? How much education did you have? How supportive were the people close to you—both family and friends? How has your condition affected you, both physically and emotionally? These and other questions play a role in determining how you'll adjust to lupus, its treatment, and any changes it necessitates. But that doesn't mean your hands are tied. You can improve the way you deal with virtually every aspect of your life with lupus.

The changes you'll make in your lifestyle because of lupus require determination and self-discipline. At this point, your head may be spinning. You may fear changes that may have to take place in your activity schedule, job, or social relationships. You may also be apprehensive about dealing with physical discomfort, body changes, and medication. You may even worry that you won't be able to perform your normal chores and responsibilities. These concerns are in no way unusual. Most people with lupus do feel this way. But the fact that you can do much to improve your life should help you reduce your fears and approach change in a more positive way.

As you modify your lifestyle, be aware that the changes you make can affect your self-esteem. Your self-esteem is, at least to some degree, a reflection of the role you play in life: the ways you deal with the people around you, the activities in which you're involved, and the routine that you normally follow. When any of these things change, your self-esteem can change as well. By keeping this in mind, you may be more likely to make changes that will help you preserve—or improve!—your self-esteem.

HOW ABOUT DENIAL?

What happens if you decide not to make necessary lifestyle changes? This may indicate that you're trying to deny your situation. Why might you deny? You may be:

- Trying to avoid the reality of the situation. Whatever the facts are, you are not acknowledging them.
- Avoiding even acknowledging that a situation exists.
- Trying to minimize any possible consequences of your situation.

Denial is a very common coping strategy among people who are living with a medical problem. Sometimes it can even be positive. Why? It may give you the opportunity to work on improving your situation, or dealing with it better, without being overwhelmed by it. Denial is positive when it helps you to not think about something . . . when thinking about it wouldn't do you any good anyway! It also gives you an opportunity to get used to certain new realities at a pace that you can handle, rather than being overwhelmed all at once. But it's important to be aware of denial's negative side, too. What if denial keeps you from doing what you need to do? For example, what if you don't get enough rest, or you don't pace yourself, or you don't take all of your medication? These are examples of destructive denial, and this can hurt you. So continue to stay on top of this.

What Can You Do?

If you recognize that you are denying, try to address this from a more realistic, positive, comfortable perspective. Try to focus on the facts. Then ask yourself what exactly you are afraid of. Think about what the potential downside would be for continuing your denial, as well as how much better off you'll be when you finally accept your reality—and work to move forward.

If you know that this is a problem for you, get some support so that you don't feel alone in dealing with all of this. Consider joining a support group, or reach out to a mental health professional. Not only will this help you through the rough spots, but by doing this you've already signaled that you're working to move past denial.

What do you do if you're trying to help a loved one who you know is in denial? This, in some ways, is even harder. You may be seeing what's going on, but your loved one continues to block everything out. They may be resistant to any efforts you make to try to get through to them, and get angry at you for trying. Getting past denial may be gradual. Start by trying to talk to them. Even opening the door a little is a good first step. Let them know that you're there to support him or her in any way you can, but don't be pushy.

Ingredients for Successful Coping with Changes in Lifestyle

You'll be in the best shape to adapt successfully to changes in lifestyle if you:

- Become aware of how your body feels. How is it reacting to the things you are doing? Act accordingly.
- Understand what makes you tense, knowing what you can and cannot do to change or avoid the symptoms and problems associated with lupus.
- Pay attention to yourself, your goals, and your needs.
- Elicit the help of the people around you. Use relationships as a buffer. Join together with others to tackle the cause of your stress.
- Use laughter and humor to reduce stress.

- Build on the talents and activities you can still enjoy (and there'll be plenty of them).
- Concentrate on strengths and accomplishments rather than dwelling on negative thoughts and disappointments.
- Follow a healthy diet.
- Get enough sleep. Allow time for rest and quiet and don't try to solve problems at night or when you're overtired.
- Exercise to reduce the effects of stress by bringing blood to the muscles and the brain and stimulating production of the chemicals that give you a sense of well-being.
- Have fun in life. Spend time on hobbies that you enjoy.
- Realize that you need to do things for yourself and actively think of yourself separately from the symptoms of this disease.
- Think of yourself as a formidable person and not some tired, miserable, suffering person.
- Learn all you can about lupus and seek out appropriate professional help. It is important to recognize when to ask for help—medical, psychological, spiritual—whatever it takes.
- Work on enhancing your relationship with your partner—adapting to the symptoms and being able to experiment to find the best ways to enjoy intimacy.
- Relax to reduce your experience of pain.
- Have your mind, body, and spirit in the best shape possible, so you can conquer anything that comes along.

Guidelines for Change

There are a number of things you can do to make any changes necessitated by your condition easier and less stressful. The following are some general guidelines for living with lupus:

- Make your house user-friendly. Every bit of energy you conserve by making things easier for yourself around the house—including the use of appliances, structural changes, clothing modifications, and more—can be funneled into areas that will better enhance your overall lifestyle.
- If you anticipate that your mobility will be limited, even temporarily, obtain a temporary handicapped parking permit from your town. In most cases, you'll need a letter from your doctor saying that this is necessary. It may take time to get this permit, so act now so it will be available if you need it.
- Make resting more comfortable by using support and positioning aids, made of foam, elastic, or some other material. Some people use magnetic field therapy to promote a sense of well-being. Mattress pads, pillows, wraps, and other forms of these products provide cushioning, comfort, and support. They're light enough to be moved around the house as necessary or to take with you when you travel.
- Consider getting a cordless phone if you're going to be alone for any period of time. This will enable you to always have a phone close to you. Or make sure you have your cell phone next to you. If you're more concerned about a problem occurring when you're alone, consider getting one of those medic alert signals or pendants that can be activated in an emergency.
- Be aware of how your body feels—how it reacts to different activities. Then act accordingly, resting as necessary.
- Build on the talents and activities you can still enjoy—and there are sure to be plenty of them! Try to focus on the things that you still have, rather than what you have lost. This guideline can be applied to relationships, activities, abilities, and interests.
- Give yourself permission to indulge in the things you enjoy. There are probably enough negative things in your life right now! Allow yourself to enjoy the positive things without guilt.
- Simplify your life. Work to reduce the pressures that you place on yourself by focusing on the tasks that must be done and temporarily shelving those that are less urgent.
- Be more protective of yourself. Establish and follow routines that will supply you with the proper amounts of sleep, exercise, and nutrition. Take the precautions necessary to guard against accidents and infections. Improve your ability to communicate. Communication problems are the

main reason relationships dissolve. By learning how to best discuss important issues, not only will you decrease the chance that your existing relationships will fail, but you'll also increase the likelihood of establishing new, more enjoyable ones.

- Maintain control over your life, and do as much as you can—without exhausting yourself, of course. Research has suggested that people who continue as many of their normal routines and activities as possible feel better and live with their disease more comfortably.

Set Up a Coping Action Plan

There are always things you can do to improve your life with lupus. Your goal is to achieve more of the positives, and minimize the negatives. Here are certain things to remember as you plan and implement the coping strategies that you learn:

- Identify the things that you want to work on changing. Make sure that these are changes that you want to make rather than changes that you're being told to make. (Obviously, if your doctor is telling you certain things need to be changed, they become a priority.) You'll also want to improve your thinking as part of making these changes.
- Focus on the ways your changes are going to help you. The best motivation is being able to identify the realistic end results that you want—and shoot for them.
- Make sure your goals are realistic and attainable. Avoid the tendency to dream of turning your life around overnight, or in ways that may be physically or practically unreasonable.
- Break your changes down into small steps. Not only does this increase the likelihood of success, but it also increases the motivation you will feel as you achieve each step. Always remember: What's the best way to eat an elephant? One bite at a time!
- Anticipate ups and downs, and successes and misses. Anticipating them increases your motivation to conquer them, to get past the downs and back

to the ups. Not anticipating them opens the door to frustration, despair, depression, and a reduction of effort.

- Put everything in perspective. Look at your life as a whole. Keep focused on the positive reasons you have for getting up in the morning. Always look for ways to make your life better. If you have difficulty with this, you may want to talk with somebody who can help you to be more positive. Remember: A positive mental attitude is one of the best attributes to have for successful coping with lupus.

- Enjoy the changes you're making, and the process of making changes. Enjoy the ride, not just getting to your final destination. Periodically, when you look back, your goal is to happily compare where you are to where you were. This will justify—and motivate—your effort.

As We Move On

Yes, you may have to make some changes in your lifestyle. But why assume that all of them will be negative? Isn't it possible that some of them will be for the better? Maybe you've been such a hard worker that you've never spent enough time with your family. If you have to cut back on your work schedule because of lupus, perhaps you'll truly enjoy the increased time you'll be able to spend with your partner or children. It's possible that some of the medication you'll use to control lupus will also help control other pesty problems that have been troubling you for a while (whether related to lupus or not). Certainly, learning to take better care of yourself will pay off in the long run. So don't convince yourself that your life is ruined because you have lupus. Always look at the positive in any situation.

In the remaining chapters of this section, we'll look at ways to better cope with pain, fatigue, and other effects of lupus and its treatment. We'll also look at diet, exercise, and medication—in other words, at many of your lifestyle concerns. So read on, and remember: You are the most important ingredient in the recipe for successful adjustment to lupus. So do everything you can to help yourself. All of your efforts are sure to reap invaluable benefits in the form of greater health and happier day-to-day living.

7.

PHYSICAL SYMPTOMS
AND CHANGES

Caution: Reading this chapter may be hazardous to your health. Your emotional health, that is. Hazardous? Yes, if you start feeling that you're going to experience all the symptoms discussed in the chapter. Please, please, please remember: No one ever gets all the symptoms of lupus, and most people get only a few. Read this chapter and learn about any symptoms you do have. Don't be frightened when you read about the ones that you don't have, because you may never get them.

Any chronic illness can affect you in a number of ways, including physically, psychologically, socially, and economically. It is important that you know about the many different symptoms you may experience as part of living with lupus. Then you will not be surprised if you experience them. Of course, you should also know about ways to control them, either medically or with lifestyle changes, or both. Might there be physical symptoms that you *can't* improve? Unfortunately, yes. And in that case, you'll have to learn to simply accept them. This may seem like a tall order, but what choice do you have? Try to concentrate on the things you *can* control. Deal with the symptoms as they come, if and when they come. Don't anticipate the worst, because that won't help you. Instead, focus on what you *can* do, because it's far better to put your energy into more positive efforts.

So let's discuss some of the most common symptoms of lupus (other than fatigue and pain, which, because they are so common—and debilitating— will be discussed in chapters devoted specifically to them) and how to deal with them. When there are things you can do, we'll give you suggestions. If no treatments or management techniques are available at the present time, you'll at least learn more about the symptoms and know that you're not alone in experiencing them.

Joint Problems

Joint involvement is considered to be one of the most prevalent symptoms of lupus. Anywhere from 80 to 90 percent of all people with lupus will experience joint pain or arthritis-like symptoms at some point during the course of their illness. In fact, one of the first and most common complaints that bring people to physicians, and which may ultimately result in a diagnosis of lupus, is persistently aching joints (especially the wrists, fingers, or knees). More than half of all people with lupus will probably experience muscle aches as well. Which joints can be affected? The pain can occur in the hands, arms, legs, or feet, as well as in the shoulders, hips, lower jaw, and knees. Joint aches and pains are so common that, as you've already read, this is one of the criteria used by physicians in diagnosing lupus.

WHAT HAPPENS?

The joint pain you experience is due to inflammation. This inflammation occurs in the lining of the joints and may cause swelling. Because you never know where the inflammation is going to occur, you can rarely predict which joints are going to end up aching. You may be a good guesser, though, based on your previous experiences!

Individual attacks of joint pain may last from several hours to several days or weeks. During this period of time, you can become so sensitive to the way you feel that you may easily begin to predict when the joint pain will be more or less intense.

When does it hurt most? You may notice more intense joint pain or stiffness in the morning when you awaken, or in the evening prior to going to bed. For some people, the symptom tends to be less noticeable during the day, and you may notice improvement in your ability to move your joints comfortably.

Along with the discomfort that is felt, your joints may feel exceptionally tender. It may be painful to even touch the affected joints. Fluid may accumulate, and does so most often in the knees. Redness and warmth of the joints affected with arthritis-like symptoms also occur, but not as often as the tenderness. Often there is a lot of pain even if the joints are not red or swollen. Fortunately, joint involvement in lupus rarely results in a deformity of the joint.

Joint aches and pains are uncomfortable. They can make it harder for you to cope, and changes in lifestyle may be necessary. Walking may be more difficult, and certain physical activities may have to be curtailed when joint symptoms are intense. A positive note: Joint symptoms can decrease in intensity as your body responds to treatment for lupus.

WHAT CAN YOU DO?

If you're experiencing joint problems from lupus, there are usually two goals to try to achieve. You want to try to control any pain as much as you can, and you want to maintain as much efficient joint function as possible.

The use of drugs has been helpful in reducing the effects of joint aches and pains. Anti-inflammatory drugs, such as aspirin, other aspirin derivatives, and nonsteroidal anti-inflammatories (NSAIDs), are usually used at first, since arthritis alone is often not sufficient to justify the use of more powerful drugs such as corticosteroids. If you need steroids for treatment of other symptoms of lupus, the use of these drugs will also improve problems with joints (see Chapter 10 for more information about medication). Surgery is usually not necessary.

A warm (not hot) bath or shower may be helpful. Gentle exercises may help to loosen you up. (See Chapter 12 for more information about exercise.) If you experience any stiffness during the day, move your joints gently and consistently to work it out as comfortably as you can.

In a small number of more extreme cases, where joints have lost a good deal of strength or mobility, some people with lupus may use supportive devices such as canes, splints, braces, crutches, or even walkers. In some cases, they may be helpful for joints such as the hands, ankles, feet, hips, or knees. They preserve and protect them (sounds like the United States

Constitution!), and allow for as much functional mobility as possible. These devices may also help by spreading out the weight that would be placed on any weight-bearing joints. Discuss their use with your physician to see if there's any benefit to you.

AVASCULAR NECROSIS

A discussion of joint problems would not be complete without referring to *avascular necrosis* (also called *aseptic* or *ischemic necrosis*). It is one of the potentially serious consequences of the combination of inflammation, reduced blood supply, and lupus-related joint involvement. This is also called bone tissue death and results when blood supply to the bone diminishes. This can lead to more fragility and brittleness in the bone. It is often uncertain whether avascular necrosis results from the use of corticosteroids (which may produce blood supply–reducing fat clots) or from lupus activity itself (such as clots caused by lupus anticoagulants circulating in the blood). In extreme cases, the treatment requires surgical replacement of the affected joint. Although avascular necrosis occurs relatively infrequently (it is estimated that up to approximately 10 percent of people with lupus develop avascular necrosis symptoms), it can be serious because it usually involves the weight-bearing joints. The most common location of avascular necrosis is the hip bone, although other bones, such as the shoulders, knees, or ankles, can be affected as well, since these are the joints that tend to be more affected by loss of blood supply.

Rashes

Rashes are one of the more common symptoms of lupus. They are the major symptom of discoid lupus, but they also are very common in systemic lupus. The classic butterfly (malar) rash (redness across the bridge of the nose that spreads out onto each cheek below the eyes) has long been one of the most noticeable signs of lupus.

Lupus rashes may appear virtually anywhere on the body. In fact, arm and leg rashes are almost as common as malar facial rashes. Rashes are usually reddish in color and may or may not be raised and scaly. More than two-thirds of all individuals with lupus will eventually have some type of skin rash.

There's no way of knowing how long any rash will last, how dark the reddish color will be, or even what it will actually look like. Rashes or redness are usually more noticeable during flares and may be less so or may go away altogether during remission. But the rash is not a barometer measuring the intensity of your flare. ("The worse the flare, the more the rash" is not true!)

Rashes may itch! That can be even more unpleasant than the unsightliness that you dread. Not all rashes are itchy, though. Your itchiness may be caused by something other than a rash. Sometimes dry skin is the culprit. Your skin may be dry because of lupus, because of medication that you are taking, or even because of age. The cause of the itchiness determines how it should be treated. If you think medication may be causing the itchiness, check with your physician to see if changes in the dosage can help. Otherwise, applying lubricants or ointments to the skin may be helpful.

Rashes can be upsetting because you may feel that they distort your appearance. You may feel that they attract attention to you, and certainly not the kind that you want. You may be apprehensive that people will shun you, fearing that your lupus and its rash are contagious (which they definitely are not). You can tell them about lupus, but they may still be uncomfortable. Therefore, treatment for rashes is important to help you feel better physically as well as emotionally.

WHAT CAN YOU DO?

Treatment for rashes involves the use of different types of medications. Corticosteroid creams or ointments can help. In addition, whatever medication you are taking for the overall control of lupus will help the rash as well. In more extreme cases, antimalarial medications such as Plaquenil may be helpful. Different types of cosmetics or even medical makeup may be used to cover up the rash. This can reduce some of the embarrassment you might feel. A few of them also contain sunblock ingredients—two benefits for the price of one! Sometimes, just a basic skin cleansing routine may help reduce the rash and/or redness. Focus on the positive aspects of your appearance—

try not to dwell on the rash. And remind yourself that your rash can get better with treatment, and as your lupus improves.

Sun Sensitivity

Old Sol can create a lot of problems for people with lupus. People with lupus who have unusual reactions to sunlight are said to be photosensitive. It is estimated that up to two-thirds of all individuals with lupus experience adverse reactions to the ultraviolet rays that come from the sun and from fluorescent lighting. The other one-third or so may not need to be as concerned about the material covered in this section, but since lupus varies so much, everyone should be aware of the potential problems resulting from photosensitivity. What kind of reactions can be experienced? The degree of sensitivity varies from person to person. Even small amounts of exposure to the sun can aggravate symptoms and make them feel significantly worse.

If you experience photosensitivity, your skin may be affected. This may take the form of redness, hives, or other rashes, or you may feel a burning sensation. Your skin may itch. Not only can sun exposure cause a skin reaction, but it also may trigger a major flare, which could affect any part of your body. It may lead to arthritis-like joint pains, headaches, or general aches and pains. It may make you tired, weak, or nauseated.

During flares, sensitivity to the sun can increase, making the sun even more dangerous for you. During remissions, sun sensitivity may not be as much of a problem, but be careful: It is certainly very possible for the sun to trigger a flare even when you're in remission. So, if you want to stay in remission, do the smart thing. (Need I say more?)

WHAT CAN YOU DO?

What should you do if you are sun-sensitive? There are three ways you can protect yourself from the sun. Learn your ABCs: Stay *Away* from the most intense sun; reorganize your activities to have more control of when you're outside. *Block* the UV rays; protect yourself with sunblock preparations.

And *Cover* your skin and wear clothing that offers the most complete sun protection. Let's discuss the ABCs in more detail.

A = AWAY

The time you spend outdoors is important. As much as possible, try to avoid being out at all during the strongest hours of sunlight—the hours during the middle of the day. Early morning or late afternoon hours are not as potentially dangerous as the hours during the middle of the day (such as from 10:00 a.m. to 4:00 p.m.). So, if you can, try to arrange your schedule so you will be outside during the safer hours. If possible, remain indoors when the sun is at its strongest. In addition, be aware that even if the sun is not shining directly on you (for example, if you are wearing a wide-brimmed hat), reflected sun can also cause problems. Sun can be reflected off pavement, water, sand, snow, glass, and so on. Sun-sensitive reactions may occur even in the shade! Be aware that limited exposure to the sun (such as the time spent driving children to school, shopping, walking to and from work, and so on) is usually not dangerous if you adequately prepare yourself.

B = BLOCK

Protection from the sun can be improved by using sunscreens (transparent, once it has been applied to the skin) or sunblocks (opaque, rather than transparent; stronger than sunscreen; and blocks more of the ultraviolet rays). These creams or lotions have numbers on the container indicating how effective they are at blocking out the rays of the sun. The numbers (called sun protection factor, or SPF) range from 1 to 50 and up. (Recent FDA guidelines suggest capping the maximum SPF ratings at 50 or so, stating that there is not enough evidence that SPF ratings higher than that truly did a better job of protection.) The higher the number, the more protection is afforded from ultraviolet rays; preparations with higher numbers are more effective for sun-sensitive individuals. Make sure that the sunblock you use offers protection from both types of ultraviolet rays, UVA and UVB, and has an SPF of at least 15. (Some believe it should be 30 or higher. It depends on your sensitivity and age. For example, older individuals have more sensitive skin; they should use a higher SPF sunscreen.) Don't feel that you can go without sunscreen on cloudy days. The harmful rays still penetrate the clouds!

Don't assume that you're protected when you are driving in your car. For example, do you like to drive with your arm out the window? If you do, make sure it's protected. Even on a short drive, this exposure may be harmful. Being out for even a short period of time might cause problems, so always protect yourself. Wear sunblock even if you *don't* let your arm hang out. Remember: The UV rays can penetrate glass! Finally, don't forget your lips! Wear lip balm containing sunscreen to keep them sensual—and safe!

Physicians have different opinions as to whether everybody with lupus should use sunscreen. Some physicians believe that if you do not experience skin lesions or other specific systemic reactions to the sun, sunscreens are not necessary. However, others feel that even with no lesions, you should use sunblocks to protect yourself from the potential danger of a systemic reaction. The general consensus? Since it is easy to get into a normal routine of wearing these lotions whenever you go outside or whenever you have even limited exposure to the sun, use them. Keep them readily accessible in your bathroom, pocketbook, or briefcase, so that applying them will become second nature. They're an inexpensive insurance policy against further aggravation and flares. Note also that some moisturizers contain sunblock. If you are in the habit of using a moisturizer, consider using one with the added protection. The moral of the story: Apply sunscreen regularly, liberally, and frequently!

C = COVER

Make sure that you wear protective clothing anytime you are out in the sun. Long-sleeved shirts, jackets, gloves, and hats can help. Hats should have brims at least four inches wide, and should protect your neck, scalp, eyes, and ears from sun rays. Use sunglasses that offer UV protection (as opposed to those that just offer delightful colored lenses!). Look into clothing specifically designed to be UV-protective. The special fabrics of these items are comparable to an SPF of up to 30 or higher (as compared to regular clothing's SPF of 6 to 15 (or lower if wet). You may even want to cover up by carrying an umbrella to give yourself extra protection from the sun. (So what if everybody wonders why you think it's raining!)

WHAT IF YOU'RE NOT SUN-SENSITIVE?

If you have not experienced any sun-related reactions, you may be reluctant to restrict outdoor activities, especially if this means you can't participate in certain enjoyable activities such as swimming or going to the beach. Although your physician may not advise you against doing these things, be very careful anyway. Don't overdo, because you never know when you will experience a sun-sensitive reaction, even if you've never had one before. For example, some people have gone into a lupus flare after getting a sunburn, even though they had never been sun-sensitive before.

IS THE SUN THE ONLY VILLAIN?

If you are photosensitive, you may be sensitive to more than just the sun. Some individuals with lupus have reported that ultraviolet rays from certain unshielded fluorescent lights also cause reactions. Those reactions can be very severe, often as uncomfortable as those resulting from sun exposure. Lupus flares can result simply from exposure to ultraviolet rays in fluorescent lighting.

Therefore, if you are photosensitive, you might want to stop or minimize the use of ultraviolet or fluorescent light, get special UV-protective coverings for fluorescent lightbulbs, or use incandescent light instead. If you go somewhere where you can't pull out the lighting (imagine going to a friend's house and ripping out all of her fluorescent lights!), you may find it helpful to use sunscreens or sunblocks indoors. A little advance planning can help you feel better.

SUNNING UP

Don't feel that you should avoid stepping outside or become obsessed with the idea that you can't expose yourself to the sun. Don't put black tar paper on your windows, or join the Human Owl Society of America! By preparing for your jaunts outdoors, and by protecting yourself as much as possible, you can minimize any negative effects of being out in the sun. These precautions also apply to people without lupus. Plenty of people who don't have lupus also have to (or want to) be careful in the sun.

Neurological Involvement

Lupus can attack the nervous system. Estimates are that neurological problems occur in up to 80 percent of individuals with lupus. The statistics may be misleading, however, since something as common as a headache may be considered a type of neurological problem. So don't let the numbers get to you, and keep in mind that this section indicates different possible symptoms. By no means does it imply that you're going to experience them. But if you do, remember that treatment has improved many aspects of lupus, including this one.

TWO CATEGORIES OF NEUROLOGICAL INVOLVEMENT

There are two categories of nervous system involvement that may occur in lupus. One is central nervous system or brain involvement (also called CNS lupus). This may occur when the blood vessels that bring blood to the brain become inflamed (CNS vasculitis) due to lupus activity. The most common type of neurological problem experienced in lupus is cognitive dysfunction, which includes headaches, memory problems, and other cognitive difficulties (more on the next page, in the section on "Lupus Fog"). Other problems include focal seizures (trigger activity localized in one specific part of the brain), generalized seizures (trigger activity spread throughout different parts of the brain), visual problems (such as visual field defects, double or blurry vision, and droopy eyelid syndrome), dizziness, stroke, and psychotic-type behavior. There are times when central nervous system involvement may appear to be psychological, and sometimes it's hard to distinguish between a physiological and psychological cause to the symptom.

The other category of neurological problem is peripheral nervous system involvement, which may affect nerves throughout the rest of the body, potentially involving the five senses and movement. This category may include neurological problems such as tremors (where movements are uncontrolled), weakness (which may exist in arms or legs, or both, on either or both sides of the body), lack of coordination, and movement or balance problems.

TESTS FOR NEUROLOGICAL INVOLVEMENT

Among the laboratory tests that are performed to determine if neurological involvement is present, and to what extent, are the MRI (magnetic resonance imaging), EEG (electroencephalogram), CAT scan (computerized axial tomography), and spinal tap. X-rays may also be used, on occasion, to diagnose neurological damage.

LUPUS FOG

Janet was more and more frustrated by her inability to come up with the right words when she was talking to someone. There were times she forgot the name of the person she was talking to, or, in the middle of a sentence, she forgot what she was going to say next. Janet would apologize to the person, saying, "I'm having a lupus moment." Janet was experiencing a neurological manifestation called lupus fog or brain fog. Have you ever felt as though you couldn't think straight, as if you were all cloudy, overloaded, unable to think clearly, or had difficulty figuring out what to say or do? Well, then, you probably understand what Janet was going through. This lupus fog can come and go, as a reflection of your stress, symptoms you may be experiencing, medications you're on, or just having lupus!

Lupus fog is just one example of the most common type of neurological manifestation of lupus: cognitive dysfunction (an inability to think clearly). Examples of cognitive dysfunction include memory problems, difficulty speaking or finding the right words, cognitive fatigue, and confusion.

Cognitive dysfunction can be caused by lupus itself, or can be a manifestation of a number of symptoms of lupus (such as fatigue, headaches, or vasculitis), too much stimulation or multitasking, stress, not getting enough sleep, or some of the medications used to treat lupus.

WHAT CAN YOU DO?

Medication is often the primary treatment modality for neurological manifestations of lupus. It's hard to determine which treatments work best for the neurological complications of lupus because there are so many neurological symptoms that come and go quickly. However, because in so many cases neurological complications begin while you are not taking any medication or steroids, or when you're on a very low dosage, treatment for significant neurological problems in lupus primarily involves the use of steroids. Most individuals with neurological involvement improve rapidly after steroid therapy begins or after steroid dosages are increased.

Medication may also be used to deal with specific symptoms as they occur. Examples of this include anti-inflammatory medications for headaches, antiseizure medications for seizures, or psychotropic medications (such as antidepressants) for cognitive dysfunction, depression, or other emotional manifestations. Plaquenil has also shown some benefit in dealing with the fatigue that is common as a neurological manifestation.

Working with a mental health professional can also help you to deal with neurological manifestations, especially cognitive dysfunction. This may not lead to your symptoms going away, but by coping with them more effectively they will have less of an impact on you.

Other things you can do to deal specifically with lupus fog include pacing yourself, doing cognitively demanding tasks when you have more energy, simplifying your routines, avoiding multitasking or being overstimulated, and becoming better organized. Work on exercises to improve your cognitive abilities and your memory. And, of course, getting enough sleep is a no-brainer!

Finally, try to laugh at the fog! And work on accepting it. This will reduce the emotional reactions you may have to it, which can often make you foggier!

Infection

This can be a serious problem for people with lupus. Lupus affects the immune system. As a result, the body's ability to prevent and fight infection may be reduced. In addition, many of the more powerful medications prescribed for treatment of lupus (such as corticosteroids and immunosuppressants—see Chapter 10) may also affect the function of the immune system, adding to the problem. When a person's immune system is suppressed, because of either lupus or medication for the disease, he or she may be more vulnerable to unusual organisms that usually don't affect healthy people. This can lead to what are called *opportunistic* infections. Infections can be hard to diagnose, since it's sometimes difficult to distinguish between an infection and a lupus flare. Lupus treatment using corticosteroids can also camouflage the presence or symptoms of infection. Because of the potential dangers of infection, it is an important physical change to be aware of and to attempt to minimize.

WHAT CAN YOU DO?

Any symptoms suggesting the existence of an infection should be brought to the attention of your physician. There are two categories of symptoms: specific (burning on urination, frequency of urination, blood in the urine, cough, sputum, skin abscesses, etc.) and nonspecific (such as chills, fever, and sweats). As always, if in doubt, check it out. If an infection is a problem, you'll immediately begin a course of antibiotics to counteract it.

Because preventive steps are always the best, minimize exposure to others who have colds or infections. For the same reason, consult your doctor to find out if he or she wants you to use antibiotics preventively (antibiotic prophylaxis), such as before surgery or before having a dental procedure done. (This is not suggested as frequently as in the past.) Because infections can often cause, and be identified by, a fever, make sure you have a thermometer that works. An oral or rectal one is best—the digital ear thermometers are often not as accurate.

Antiphospholipid Syndrome (APS)

Many people with lupus have antiphospholipid antibodies. There are several kinds of antiphospholipid antibodies, including the lupus anticoagulant and the anticardiolipin antibody. Why is this important? Normally, blood clots form naturally after a cut or an injury, in order to stop bleeding. Antiphospholipid antibodies, resulting from an autoimmune reaction that forms antibodies toward phospholipid (a substance of the cell membrane), increase the body's natural response to clot formation and can increase the risk of developing blood clots. There is also a related autoimmune reaction against another component of cell membrane, called cardiolipin, forming what are called anticardiolipin antibodies that will have a similar effect—an increased risk of blood clots.

Some people with lupus who have these antibodies develop the clinical complication known as *antiphospholipid syndrome* (also called *APS*, or *antiphospholipid antibody syndrome*). This results in a higher risk of stroke, miscarriage, the formation of a pulmonary embolus (blood clot in the arteries of the lungs), or other dangerous complications. So it's important that your physician monitors you regularly to watch for the existence of these antibodies and determine if and when treatment is necessary.

Although here we are talking about people with lupus, antiphospholipid syndrome can occur in people who do not have lupus. In these situations, it is called *primary antiphospholipid syndrome*. A lot of research continues to investigate the reasons why these blood clots develop, why antiphospholipid antibodies can be present in some people with lupus without the formation of clots, and, of course, what can be done about it. The most exciting outcome of research into APS thus far is that awareness and treatment has led to a significant reduction both in the formation of clots and in miscarriages.

IDENTIFICATION OF APS

Despite the significant risks associated with the formation of clots (also called thrombosis), many clots may not even be clinically identified, nor a diagnosis of APS made, prior to the onset of a complication. Since preventing a complication is far more desirable than curing one, careful monitoring for APS is a necessary part of ongoing treatment for lupus. Fortunately, research has led to easier detection of the syndrome by using two blood tests, one that tests for the presence of anticardiolipin antibodies and another that tests for the presence of the lupus anticoagulant. Because these blood tests are so easy to administer, it is believed that their use should be more widespread, hopefully leading to a decrease in clot-related complications.

WHAT CAN YOU DO?

In an ideal world, treatment for antiphospholipid syndrome would stop the immune system from forming the antibodies that result in forming blood clots. Unfortunately, at the present time there is nothing that you can do to avoid developing antiphospholipid antibodies. Research is ongoing in this area. In the meanwhile, what you can do is work with your physician to try to avoid the complications of clinically significant blood clots (APS). Treatment for APS primarily involves the use of anticoagulants, medications that reduce the body's ability to form clots. Although there may be a risk of bleeding as a result of anticoagulation treatment (more on this shortly), it has to be weighed against the risk of clot formation in APS.

Medication treatment initially involves using aspirin. Low doses of aspirin (approximately 81 to 100 mg per day) have been effective in reducing the development of clots. (Aspirin's role here is similar to the way that baby aspirin is used in an attempt to prevent heart attacks.) But aspirin is not always sufficient. In cases when symptoms or complications of blood clotting have already been seen, treatment requires the use of more powerful anticoagulants, primarily warfarin or heparin.

Warfarin, best known as Coumadin, is a widely prescribed anticoagulant that is effective in the treatment of APS. (By the way, the popular name for this anticoagulant drug is "blood thinner," but that is actually incorrect. This drug does not affect the thickness or viscosity of the blood. Rather, it works by decreasing the production by the liver of a few important proteins in the blood that are associated with clotting.) The dose of warfarin needed to be effective is different for each person. Trial and error is necessary to come up with the exact dosage. Warfarin does not act immediately, taking up to several days before the number of these liver-produced proteins is reduced and the effect is seen in a key blood test, the INR (which stands for *international normalized ratio*, a lab test measure of blood coagulation). Too much warfarin can result in too much anticoagulation and bleeding. Careful monitoring of the INR is needed. The bleeding risk also is increased when warfarin is taken with other medications that decrease the body's natural clot formation, such as aspirin or other NSAIDs. It's also important to remember that there may be other substances, including certain foods, alcohol, or antibiotics that can interfere with the effectiveness of warfarin. For example, the proteins made by the liver for clotting are also found in green leafy vegetables. Temporarily increasing green leafy vegetables in your diet can decrease the effectiveness of your warfarin dose. It is important to maintain a steady, healthy diet when taking this anticoagulant.

Heparin, the other widely used anticoagulant, acts on a different part of the pathway of the body's clotting cascade. It is administered either intravenously or by subcutaneous (under the skin) injection, rather than in pill form. Warfarin should not be taken during pregnancy, so when a woman who has previously had miscarriages is attempting to conceive, her physician will often start her on aspirin and heparin even before conception is confirmed. Another time when heparin is used is immediately after a clot is discovered. We mentioned earlier that warfarin takes several days to have its full effect. Heparin, on the other hand, works within minutes. It is often used as a "bridge" for several days until the warfarin pills have gained their full effect. Unfortunately, heparin, if used over a prolonged period of time, can cause osteoporosis.

Pericarditis

"You gotta have heart." And you do. You also have a lining around your heart, called the pericardium. If this lining becomes inflamed, the resulting condition is called *pericarditis,* the most common cardiac problem in lupus. This symptom is being discussed because one of the most frightening feelings anyone can experience is a tightening, gnawing pain in the chest. "Uh-oh," you may panic, "heart attack!" So it's important to be aware that chest pains are not uncommon in lupus, and one of the causes may be pericarditis.

So what's the problem with pericarditis? Besides the pain associated with inflammation, fluid can also accumulate in the protective sac around the heart. This fluid accumulation in the pericardial sac prevents the heart from moving as freely as it should be able to. As a result, it cannot pump blood as well. When the heart doesn't pump efficiently, two things happen:

1. Blood does not return as easily to the heart nor does it pump out as quickly. This can result in a "backlog" of blood, similar to a traffic jam.
2. Blood supply throughout the body is diminished.

When there is a backup of blood, the result can be a pushing of fluid into the lungs. When this happens, people will often complain of difficulty breathing.

A major concern about pericarditis is that if it occurs repeatedly, scar tissue can form in the lining around the heart. This will permanently diminish the heart's ability to beat as efficiently as it used to.

WHAT CAN YOU DO?

Pericarditis is a major complication. Any symptom that you feel that might be evidence of pericarditis should be reported to your physician immediately!

Since this symptom is a type of inflammation, the primary medical treatment for pericarditis involves the same type of medications that are used for other inflammatory symptoms: anti-inflammatories or steroids.

In addition to medication, remember that chest pain is the most common symptom of pericarditis. When you inhale, your lungs expand, pressing the heart against the chest wall, increasing the pain. Try to breathe more shallowly. Smooth but more shallow breaths may not hurt as much as deep breaths.

The pain from pericarditis is not as severe when you are sitting up. That's because of the positioning of the different organs when you're in a sitting position. You might want to sit up or bend forward to try to diminish this discomfort. By the way, this is one way of distinguishing between pericarditis pain and other possible cardiac problems. An electrocardiogram and an echocardiogram are the ways your doctor will confirm pericarditis, after listening to your heart sounds for signs of pericardial inflammation.

Lupus can involve all parts of the heart. Other than pericarditis, possible heart complications to be aware of include *myocarditis* (inflammation of the heart muscle), *endocarditis* (infection on the inside of the heart), and *vasculitis* (inflammation of the blood vessels). People with lupus have a statistically greater chance of developing cardiovascular disease and *atherosclerosis* (hardening of the arteries). There is a higher risk of heart attacks in people with lupus. It is essential to reduce any risk factors for cardiac complications, including controlling weight, getting regular exercise, controlling high blood pressure, controlling cholesterol, not smoking, and reducing stress.

Raynaud's Phenomenon

Cold hands, warm heart! Have you ever heard that saying before? Unfortunately, it is a painful accuracy for people who have Raynaud's phenomenon.

All of our blood vessels are passageways designed to allow blood to flow smoothly. The walls of the blood vessels contain muscles. These muscles constrict or dilate the blood vessels, allowing for greater or lesser blood flow through the vessels. The muscles are regulated by nerve fibers that send signals causing the constriction or dilation. When more blood (oxygen and fuel) is needed by the tissues, or when the body temperature is getting too warm, the nerves send dilation signals to the skin blood vessel muscles. When it is necessary to preserve body temperature (such as on a cold day), the nerves send constriction signals to the skin blood vessels.

With Raynaud's phenomenon, you're probably ultra sensitive to changes in temperature. Your blood vessels are very sensitive to these changes in temperature—especially cool temperatures. Constriction signals are sent. Partial constriction of the tiny arterioles causes a bluish blood color as slower blood flow allows more extraction of oxygen by the tissues (higher oxygen levels in blood causes a redder blood color). More complete constriction of arterioles causes a whitish color because a minimal blood flow doesn't allow blood color to show up. When warming of skin occurs, dilation signals are sent, causing a red color of the skin as oxygenated blood flows to the previously oxygen-starved tissues. These changes in color are more likely to occur in some areas of skin (usually your fingers or toes and sometimes even your nose and ears). So the colors red, white, and blue are common for this condition. Does that mean Raynaud's is a patriotic symptom?

If you have Raynaud's, it's unusual to experience the phenomenon in one hand only, although one hand may be affected more than the other. Although Raynaud's can be very uncomfortable at times, it is usually mild and rarely results in any permanent damage. You may feel a tingling sensation when you are exposed to cold. You may sometimes feel this even when you experience stress.

You'll probably notice Raynaud's more frequently during the winter months than in the summer months. Cold, moist air is more likely to precipitate Raynaud's than cold, dry air. However, for some people, being exposed to air-conditioning, or even a gust of cool summer air, can bring about a Raynaud's-like response. Fortunately, Raynaud's phenomenon does not necessarily remain with you forever.

WHAT CAN YOU DO?

Try to minimize your exposure to extremely cold or widely varying temperatures. Since stress can cause physiological changes in your blood vessels, try to control stress more efficiently. Try to minimize caffeine, since it can exacerbate Raynaud's reactions. And, although it goes without saying, smokers should *stop* smoking! But try as you may, it is unlikely that you'll be able to control every possible trigger for Raynaud's phenomenon. So what can you do to feel more comfortable? Dress warmly. Keep your hands and feet warm: wear gloves and warm socks. If Raynaud's affects you, you may choose to wear gloves, or use oven mitts, when you're putting your hands into the freezer compartment of your refrigerator. Even a short exposure to cold can trigger a Raynaud's reaction. If sores or cuts at the fingertips are not healing, this is a sign that treatment should be seriously considered.

There are many medications that help to dilate the blood vessels. This facilitates an improved blood flow, offsetting the restrictions that constricted blood vessels can cause. However, these medications are not always effective. Psychological techniques such as relaxation, imagery, or biofeedback (see Chapter 9) may help to improve the flow of blood in your extremities without using drugs.

Sjögren's Syndrome

Do your eyes feel dry and burn frequently? Do they feel as though someone put sand or glue on your eyelids? Does your mouth feel dry, and do you frequently need liquid to "wet your whistle"? If you have experienced any of these or other symptoms of dryness, you may be experiencing the effects of Sjögren's (pronounced *show*-grins) syndrome.

Sjögren's syndrome can be a problem for some people with lupus. (It can also occur in people who do not have lupus or another disease, in which case it is called *primary Sjögren's syndrome*.) It is also known as the "dry eyes, dry mouth" syndrome. Why? In Sjögren's, the autoimmune response of the body destroys the glands that secrete mucus. This can affect, among other things, the production of tears and/or saliva, since both of these secretions are produced in glands. Other glandular areas also may become involved. The back of the throat and bronchi (leading to hard-to-treat bronchitis) can be affected by Sjögren's. The vagina could lose its lubricating ability and may develop sores or infections if artificial lubrication is not used during sexual intercourse.

WHAT CAN YOU DO?

Milder manifestations of Sjögren's may be treated with medications that increase saliva. Products called artificial saliva and artificial tears have been scientifically developed to increase comfort for people dealing with this problem. Reduced saliva will increase dental disease (affecting teeth and gums). You need regular visits to your dentist for proper preventive maintenance and treatment of damaged areas. In more pronounced cases of Sjögren's, systemic treatment may be necessary if your glands' ability to secrete mucus has been impaired or destroyed by Sjögren's syndrome. Medications such as Plaquenil, corticosteroids, or immunosuppressants may be considered if other systemic problems occur as well as the Sjögren's.

Kidney Problems

Up to one-third or more of all individuals with lupus will experience some kidney problems during the course of their illness. Kidney dysfunctions develop gradually over a period of time, ranging from months to even years, and they can be serious.

In lupus, some antibodies mix with the substances they are fighting and form immune complexes. These immune complexes remain in the blood until they reach the kidneys. They then become trapped in the kidney's filtering membranes that normally filter the wastes from the blood. When these complexes accumulate, inflammation occurs. This reduces the filtering processes, sometimes inhibiting them entirely. Waste materials that are normally filtered out of the blood continue to circulate in the blood. This is called *uremia*. Untreated uremia can result in increasingly dangerous physical and mental problems, in some cases even leading to death. Kidney tissues may scar, further restricting the ability of the kidneys to filter wastes from the blood. When this inflammation and tissue breakdown occurs in the kidneys, the condition is known as *lupus nephritis*.

How can you tell if you're having kidney problems? Certain symptoms may suggest it: headache, swelling in different parts of the body (including the arms, the legs, the face, and the area around the eyes or around the abdomen), a decrease in appetite, weakness and fatigue, changes in mental attitude and personality, and seizures. Since so many symptoms of lupus might indicate kidney problems, it's important that kidney functioning be carefully monitored through frequent checkups and tests.

TESTS FOR KIDNEY PROBLEMS

Your physician will check your urine for signs of kidney disease, such as cell casts or increased protein. To do this, you may be asked to collect all your urine for a twenty-four-hour period. Your kidney filtration rate and function can then be monitored by measuring the relative concentration of certain substances in the urine compared with their concentration in the blood. An example of the substances monitored is creatinine. Creatinine is the breakdown product of creatine—an important component of muscle—in your urine. Creatinine is eliminated from the body by the kidneys. An increase in the amount of creatinine in the blood suggests that kidney function is decreasing in effectiveness and can be indicative of kidney problems.

Depending on these results, your doctor may recommend that you have a renal biopsy, a procedure in which a thin needle is inserted into the kidney and a tiny piece of kidney tissue is removed for microscopic study to determine the degree and type of kidney involvement.

WHAT CAN YOU DO?

Certain medications such as prednisone, Imuran (azathioprine), Cytoxan (cyclophosphamide), and CellCept (mycophenolate mofetil) have been effective in controlling kidney involvement in lupus. The exact drug program for any one case has to be individually established, but most cases of lupus nephritis can be helped.

In addition to taking medications, it may be important to modify your diet (reduce salt intake and watch the amount of fat in your diet, for example) and work to prevent hypertension. Stress should also be controlled because effective stress management can lower blood pressure. Diuretics may be effective, as well as medications that stabilize the heart and circulation.

Thanks to modern medicine, in most cases, kidney problems need not become life-threatening. Treatment can usually enable normal functioning. However, in extreme cases, if kidney dysfunction becomes total and permanent, there are still two possible solutions: hemodialysis, in which the blood is filtered artificially through a machine, or a kidney transplant. Both of these procedures can be helpful for people with lupus.

Despite the dangers of lupus nephritis, it is at least reassuring to know that advances in medical science have improved the ability to diagnose and treat kidney involvement at virtually every stage.

Flares

Do you remember in Chapter 1 when we compared the cyclical pattern of flares and remissions to riding a roller coaster? Well, this is true for two reasons. First, the ups and downs of lupus can remind you of the up-and-down experience of your amusement park's roller-coaster ride. Sometimes it accelerates slowly, building to a point where you worry about soon being out of control. Sometimes it picks up speed and you wonder which twists and turns it's going to take. Sometimes you plummet, helplessly, into a scary feeling that it's never going to end. Many people hate the feeling of helplessness that occurs when they're going through a flare. They so desperately want to feel better, but don't know what they can do to make the ride come to an end!

So what do you go through when you're in a flare? Each person's experience of a flare is as unique as each person's experience in living with lupus. The symptoms that constitute a flare for one person may not be what constitute a flare for someone else. Do you know what indicates the beginning of a flare for you? The more experience you have in living with lupus, the more aware you will be when you're going into a flare.

WHAT TRIGGERS LUPUS FLARES?

Although it is still not known what causes lupus, more is being learned about what can trigger a lupus flare. Your body is changing all the time. The tissues of your body may change anytime you experience something very stressful. What might be stressful enough to cause a flare? Among the more frequent flare-provokers are fatigue, in which you wear yourself down and become more vulnerable to an increase of symptoms; and sunburn, in which your body reacts strongly to ultraviolet rays. Excessive exhaustion, emotional difficulties (such as severe stress), infections, certain environmental variables (such as UV rays), certain medications (such as sulfa drugs, penicillin, or female hormones such as estrogen), and even injury or surgery are among other factors that may trigger a lupus flare. Because you are unique, it may take experience in living with lupus to know what has the potential to cause you to go into a flare.

CAN YOU HELP JAM THE TRIGGER?

Although modern medicine is still unable to cure lupus, there are things you can do to help avoid or reduce the number of lupus flares you experience. Be careful of what you do. Try to avoid becoming overtired. Carefully protect yourself from overexposure to the sun. Try to minimize your exposure to highly stressful, anxiety-provoking situations. Don't overdo things. Keep any possible triggers in mind (especially ones that you have identified as culprits for you), and avoid them.

Pay attention to the early warning signs that may indicate that a flare is on its way. For example, one early warning sign is a low-grade afternoon fever (often ranging from 99.5°F to 100.5°F). Other early warning signs include feeling weaker and more fatigued, aching, noticing a loss of pep, and frequent chills. You may notice that you're experiencing more joint pain than normal, or in more parts of your body. You may feel that your medication seems to be less effective in controlling your symptoms. Of course, advise your doctor about any of these signs or the appearance of any new symptoms.

It goes without saying that if a specific drug has triggered your flare, your doctor should modify the dosage or eliminate it completely to attempt to stop the flare. However, the flare may not be controlled until you have stopped using the drug for a while.

Your doctor may choose to follow certain lab tests as a predictor that a flare is coming. Tests such as sed rate (a test for inflammation), CBC (complete blood count), complement levels, anti-DNA antibody levels, urinalysis abnormalities, and other tests may become abnormal prior to your going into a flare. The doctor may then raise medication doses to try to suppress the flare.

WHAT CAN YOU DO?

Once you sense that a flare is coming on, don't wait for your doctor to confirm what you already know. Start cutting back on your activities drastically. Minimize or eliminate any unnecessary activities. Do what is absolutely necessary. Pace yourself more attentively. Sit down rather than stand whenever you can. Get plenty of rest. Don't feel guilty if you're resting more than usual. Anticipate that the things you do may take you longer to complete. Feel good about the tasks that you accomplish, rather than dwelling on how long it may take you to accomplish them.

When you have energy to do something, try to engage in activities that are less physically draining. Catch up on those activities that require less energy. Examples include reading a book, watching a movie, calling a friend, doing some paperwork, engaging in a hobby (needlework? photography? bird-watching?) or other activities that you might not otherwise prioritize if you're feeling energized. At least you'll feel like you are doing something worthwhile, even during a flare.

Keep your stress and other emotions as calm and stable as you can. If they're making you feel worse, do what you need to do to get them in check!

If you are sun-sensitive, minimize your exposure to the sun and UV rays, and increase your use of sunscreen. Unless otherwise directed, drink plenty of fluids.

Don't hesitate to contact your doctor. And think about anything you may have done that contributed to the onset of this flare so you can be more in control in the future.

Remember: It may be too late to prevent this flare, but cutting back can reduce the seriousness of the flare, as well as its duration.

A Physical Finale

In this chapter, we have discussed a number of the more common physical symptoms and changes that you may experience with lupus. Although they are not pleasant to think about, it's important to learn as much as you can about them. You want to effectively cope with lupus, right? So you need to know what the possible symptoms of this illness are.

Although some of these symptoms can be serious (and scary), there's a lot you can do to prevent or reverse them or to minimize their effects. Learn as much as you can, make sure that you get up-to-date information about treatment for any symptoms that you may experience, work with your physician, and—most important—don't stick your head in the sand. Be aware of potential problems—and act on them. By marshaling all your forces to control these problems, you will not only improve your level of comfort, but also build the confidence you need to continue leading a happy, productive life.

8.

FATIGUE

Do you notice that you become tired more easily at certain times? Does your bed seem to be your favorite place in the whole world? If so, you're not alone. Fatigue is one of the most common and debilitating problems for individuals with lupus. Most experts believe that the hardest part of living with lupus is fatigue.

The fatigue experienced by people with lupus is not the same as the normal tiredness experienced by others. It makes you feel so tired that you just can't complete the things that you want to complete. People who are tired may be able to push themselves to do the things they really want to do. People with lupus fatigue may be unable to do even the most enjoyable activities because they simply can't move their bodies to do them. It encompasses the loss of that "get up and go" feeling, and is more of a debilitating exhaustion. Fatigue is such a common part of lupus that many people forget what it's like *not* to be exhausted!

One of the most upsetting things about fatigue is that you never know when it's going to hit you. You may be going along just fine, and then bang— all of a sudden it feels like somebody has just flicked your "off" switch! You may awaken in the morning feeling fine; however, fatigue may hit you unexpectedly during the day. On the other hand, you may awaken in the morning feeling very tired and find that your energy seems to build up during the day.

How might you feel when fatigue hits? You may feel like a rag doll, with arms and legs that are so floppy and limp that you just can't move them. You may feel like a string-controlled marionette after the strings are cut. You may feel like a balloon that has popped and just collapses in a *whoosh*. Or you may quiver and tremble uncontrollably, like a bowl of Jell-O. Whatever it feels like to you, fatigue is exhausting!

Unfortunately, the fatigue itself is not your only problem. The disbelief of the people around you will add to your frustration. They may not be able to understand how you can go from being active and on the ball to being tired and listless in such a short period of time. (And, of course, you may be too tired to even try to explain it!) They may think you're being lazy, or worry that you're depressed or just not motivated. You can try to have your loved ones read about fatigue, but don't be discouraged if they just don't understand it.

Louise was playing bridge with her friends. They were sitting and talking over the latest episode of their favorite television program when, seemingly all of a sudden, Louise asked to be excused so she could go and collapse on the couch. She couldn't get up, and she weakly asked her friends to help straighten up before they left. Lazy, no. Sleepy, no. Lupus fatigue, yes! People with lupus quickly learn to recognize the difference between normal fatigue (where you feel tired because of excessive energy expenditure) and lupus fatigue (where you feel like someone "pulled your plug").

WHAT CAUSES FATIGUE?

Why does fatigue occur? It is still not exactly known. Fatigue may, of course, be caused by the lupus itself—a common occurrence. It shows that the disease may be active. This is a physical kind of fatigue, and the best way to treat it is to treat the disease that is causing the fatigue (which may take some time). In addition, anemia, medications, infections, fever, pain, and other symptoms of lupus can cause fatigue. Sometimes, fatigue is totally unrelated to lupus or its treatment. You may simply be doing too much! In addition, emotions such as stress, tension, anxiety, and depression may also contribute to fatigue. Good nutrition is critical for a healthy body. Your nutritional status, poor dietary habits, and an insufficient intake of vitamins and other nutrients can make you feel more tired than you should be.

Sometimes fatigue can snowball. If you're chronically tired, you may reduce your day-to-day activities, and this may result in even more fatigue.

Unless something happens to break this chain, you may find that you have less and less energy.

Fatigue may also result from reducing or eliminating exercise, either because you don't want to exercise or because pain makes it too difficult. But the less you do, the more out of shape and tired you may become! (See Chapter 12 for more on this topic.)

Most people think of fatigue as negative, but this is not always the case. It can be positive. How? Usually, fatigue is your body's way of telling you that you need rest. If you never felt tired, you would push yourself too much! Then you'd certainly feel the effects, and might experience more serious symptoms. So, if you feel fatigue, listen to your body. If this happens to excess, make sure you discuss this with your doctor.

WHAT CAN YOU DO?

What's the best thing to do about fatigue? Rest. (Clever!) You see, fatigue can actually be a positive message—it's your body's way of telling you that you need to slow down and stop pushing yourself. So let's discuss some of the things you can try, to see if they make a difference.

IDENTIFY FATIGUE CAUSES

Fatigue can be caused by a single factor or a combination of different factors. Try to identify specific causes of your fatigue. Maybe you're pushing yourself too hard, trying to maintain the level of activity that was normal for you before your diagnosis of lupus. And, believe it or not, you may feel fatigued even if you haven't been very active. If you think that you may be tired and lethargic because of an emotional problem, try to pinpoint exactly what it is that's bothering you. Are you depressed because you've had to make some changes in your lifestyle? Are you fearful that you won't ever adjust to living with lupus?

Speak to your doctor to discuss whether or not there are any medical components of your lupus that may be causing fatigue. (This may include blood tests for anemia, hypothyroidism, or excessively high blood sugars.) Fatigue is one of the major diagnostic indicators of being in a lupus flare. If any of these medical factors are contributing to your fatigue, treatment for the factor may help the fatigue as well. But to confirm that these are the only main causes of your fatigue, make sure that you can rule out other factors such as depression, medication that you may be taking for pain, other emotional problems or syndromes, malnutrition, or excessive use of certain "substances."

GET PLENTY OF SLEEP

Allow yourself sufficient periods of time for sleep at night. It goes without saying that you should get enough sleep to help offset the fatigue of lupus. Not getting enough sleep weakens you and makes you less able to be as physical as you might like to be. On the other hand, too much sleep is not healthy either, because it can further weaken you, actually add to your fatigue. In addition to your nighttime sleep, try to arrange for at least one or two rest periods during the day, preferably in the late morning and late afternoon. This may help replenish some of your energy. Other strategies for dealing with fatigue depend on the nature and cause, of course, but you should always make sure that you get the proper amount of sleep so that your body can be nourished and heal.

GET PLENTY OF REST, AS WELL

Rest is important if you have lupus. Because you have lupus, occasional rest periods may help to keep you as strong as possible for the remainder of the day. It helps you to avoid wearing yourself down. It also helps you to maintain an alert, active state. However, if you feel very tired too often, your body may be telling you that you need additional rest periods. So pay attention!

Yes, rest is important. But too much rest can be as dangerous as too little rest. Although inflammation may decrease during rest, rest also allows muscles to become weaker and joints to get stiffer. Too much rest can make you feel more tired, leading to more rest, more fatigue, more rest . . . Well, you get the picture!

There are differing opinions regarding how long you should rest. Some people feel you should schedule several five-to-fifteen-minute rest periods a day. Others feel you should schedule two thirty-to-sixty-minute rest periods each day. You might want to do something, anything, for an hour or two, and then follow it with fifteen to twenty minutes of rest. Then do it again . . . and again . . . throughout the day. There are plenty of other opinions as well. Your physician, along with trial and error, will help you determine what length and frequency of rest periods are most appropriate for you. The severity of your disease, your lifestyle, and other aspects of day-to-day living will affect the amount of rest you'll need. For example, if your lupus is in a flare, you may need more bed rest (and less exercise) to give your body extra healing time. Hopefully, this additional rest will help to reduce your pain and inflammation as well. Just remember: Each person is different, so each person's need for (and pattern of getting) rest is different. Keep experimenting and you'll figure out what's best for you.

It's important to have an efficient balance between activity and rest. Not only will this be healthy for your body, but it will help your emotional state, and you'll be surprised at how much more productive you are. This may fly in the face of older beliefs that you should always "put in a day's work," in which you would feel like you accomplished something only if you worked from morning till night to complete a task or job. By being active in shorter, more efficient spurts, followed by a rest period, you'll get a lot more done, and feel better about it, all the while helping your body to be healthier.

Finally, keep in mind that although rest breaks are important for people with lupus, they may not relieve your intense fatigue. If fatigue is a message that your body is unable to do as much as you want it to do, though, rest is certainly an important way to gain more control.

PLAN AND PACE

You can also reduce fatigue with efficient planning and pacing. Determine your exact responsibilities and schedule activities so that you won't do too many strenuous things at one time. Make sure you intersperse rest periods with any energy-expending activities you need to do. And be flexible. Be ready to change course if fatigue hits you out of the blue or if you have a sudden burst of energy!

Learn how to pace yourself during your normal routines. Clara Gottaclean was obsessed with the feeling that if she did not do all her household chores on Monday, the world would fall apart! However, this was more likely to force her to remain in bed on Tuesday and Wednesday. It might be helpful for Clara to learn to spread out her chores: do the laundry on Monday, shop on Tuesday, and so on. Be more organized, and you may reduce your chances of being fatigued. Expend your energy productively. Things you used to do that took extended periods of time may have to be shortened or eliminated. If, for example, you were a professional shopper, one who normally spent six hours in the shopping center, you may have to reduce your shopping time, shop in smaller stores, or shop where there is less walking to get from one place to another. Be careful that you don't fatigue yourself to the extent that you will be bedridden for days!

Other techniques that you can learn in becoming an "efficiency expert," such as reorganizing your house and making things more convenient (see Chapter 13), will also help you to do more and to feel less fatigued. Betty, a thirty-six-year-old mother of three, generally made one day a week a "no errands" day. No running around; no outside activities. She would focus on doing things around the house and on catching up on rest and projects that required less energy. It helped her to keep her pacing under control and to compensate for those days when she may have inadvertently done too much. Don't feel obligated to figure out what changes to make by yourself. Getting advice from professionals or others who have had lupus for a while can help you improve the quality of your day-to-day functioning.

MAKE CHANGES WHEN NECESSARY

You may have to change your general lifestyle in order to maximize your energy level. Obviously, when you have more energy, you'll keep busy doing things that result in a greater expenditure of energy. Know your priorities. Focus on the top priorities while you still have the energy. In this way, if fatigue sets in, it will be the less significant activities that need to be delayed. Set a schedule for yourself—try to avoid taking on too many strenuous activities in a row, and intersperse rest periods with any strenuous activities that you must follow through on. You may choose to hire someone to do some of the more strenuous necessary tasks, such as heavy house cleaning, or you may choose to have your groceries delivered by ordering them by phone or online.

If you're fatigued, try to keep busy doing things that require low expenditure of energy. Examples? Catch up on phone calls, correspondence, paying bills, or even doing simple puzzles. Of course this assumes that you have enough energy even to do these things. If you don't, don't be upset with your-self. Recognize that this is the lupus fatigue that affects countless thousands of people . . . and it will pass.

EAT PROPERLY

Eating a proper diet is as critical as rest and proper pacing. Try to eat regu-lar, well-balanced meals. Also, speak to your doctor about supplements, as they can ensure that you're getting the nutrients, vitamins, and minerals that are vital for a healthy body. (For more information on diet, see Chapter 11.)

EXERCISE APPROPRIATELY

Make sure you're getting the proper amounts and types of exercise, based on your physical capabilities. Exercise helps to break the cycle of fatigue and out-of-shape deconditioning. Exercise helps circulation, and better cir-culation clears waste products from the body. It strengthens muscles and helps injured cells to heal because they get more oxygen. Another benefit of exercise is that it helps to reduce other potential causes of fatigue like depression, anxiety, and insomnia. It also helps psychologically, improving your state of mind and your sense of well-being. The best aerobic exercise, of course, is walking. (Find more about exercise in Chapter 12.)

KEEP YOUR EMOTIONS STABLE

Consider that your fatigue may be caused or worsened by emotions. Try to determine which feelings are contributing to your fatigue. (Are you depressed? Stressed? Tense? Bored? Anxious?) Then work on improving your outlook. Part Three should help you pinpoint and control any emotional problems you may be having.

Ride out the storm. There are times when the fatigue that you experi-ence is so overwhelming that not only can't you do anything, but you worry that you'll never again feel energized. Just as with other symptoms of lupus, fatigue can pass. Ride it out. Hold your head up high (at least, as high as your fatigue lets you!). Don't be down on yourself because you're going through this. Remind yourself that this is because of lupus. By keeping your emotions stable and positive, you're actually going to help yourself to get through this more quickly—and comfortably.

Speak to Your Doctor

Finally, consult your physician. It is important that your health care specialists are aware of the fatigue that you are experiencing. In some cases, they will simply suggest that you get more rest or cut back on your activities. In other cases, they may want to reevaluate the medications that you're on and consider changes or additions. Or they may want to consider whether your fatigue is an indication of more active lupus, possibly requiring appropriate treatment.

Your physician may recommend medication for your fatigue. Although taking medication for fatigue may not seem like the ideal solution, if your fatigue is debilitating, it may be as important to take medication for this symptom as for any other symptom. Among the medications that have been helpful for fatigue include antimalarials (Plaquenil) and corticosteroids (prednisone). In addition, antidepressants, such as Paxil or Zoloft, or tricyclic antidepressants, such as Elavil or Pamelor, have also been useful for some people.

A Sleepy Sign-offffffff

Certainly, you may feel more fatigued at certain times. Don't let that get to you. Just remind yourself that you're doing everything you can, both physically and emotionally, to enable yourself to return to a more normal routine. Are you exhausted from reading all of this? If so, maybe it's time to put the book down for a little while and rest!

9.

PAIN

Ouch! (Just getting you ready for this chapter!) Is lupus painful? Are you kidding?! Many individuals with lupus believe that, other than fatigue, pain is the hardest thing to deal with. It's hard to deal with because it just hurts, you feel as though there's this big, black (painful) cloud constantly hanging over you, and because it stops you from doing so many of the things you'd like to do. It's also hard to deal with because you feel like you're suffering alone; other people, even the most important people in your life, just don't get it! And they can't see it! But regardless of the location, intensity, and duration of pain you experience in living with lupus, there's a lot you can do about it. Let's get right to it.

When and Why Does Pain Occur?

Pain is a message sent from your body to your brain saying that something is wrong. This painful signal begins when tissue is damaged or hurt. An electrical impulse is sent through the spinal cord to the sensory center of the brain, called the thalamus. The signal then goes to the brain's outer layer, or cortex. Once the message is received in the cortex, you're able to determine the location of the pain and its intensity. Signals are then sent from the brain back through the spinal cord, triggering the release of natural painkillers such as *endorphins*—the body's own "morphine." This often diminishes the pain.

So where does it hurt? You can feel pain in virtually any part of your body, but most typically in your joints or muscles, or in the form of headaches. Some people experience intense muscle pain that may be diagnosed as fibromyalgia, a condition that affect up to 30 percent of people with lupus. Making matters worse, your emotions can exacerbate any pain you're feeling. Anxiety or boredom, for example, can cause pain to appear more pronounced. Stress can cause muscles to tense, also increasing the degree of pain. Depression, too, may cause you to feel more pain, since it increases the tendency to focus on this sensation. And, of course, any pain you feel may increase the degree to which you experience anxiety, stress, or depression, which, in turn, can lead to more pain, creating a vicious cycle.

Other factors, too, may exacerbate the pain. For instance, fatigue may worsen pain. Your perception of pain may also vary based on your own tolerance or threshold, as well as the degree to which you think the pain can be controlled. So, you see, the experience of pain is highly subjective and is affected by many factors. You'll want to try to improve some or all of these factors in order to manage your pain more successfully.

What can you do about your discomfort? How can you cope with it? The best way to cope with pain is to get rid of it! (You think?) To see if you can do this, it's first necessary to identify the cause of the pain. Once this is done, treatment can be aimed at eliminating the cause. But there's a problem. In some cases, it may be impossible to do anything about the underlying source of the pain. So pain itself, rather than the cause of the pain, is the most important concern. What does treatment aim to accomplish, then? Relief from pain!

Treatment for Pain

How can you start to deal with pain? First, you need to be aware of it! Keep track of when the pain occurs, how often it occurs, how long it lasts, and how intense it is. (You may want to keep a pain diary to maintain these records.) This information will help you decide if the pain is something you can handle yourself or if it's serious enough to be brought to your doctor's attention. Together you can work out the best way of dealing with it. Remember that health care professionals have no way of knowing how severe your pain is unless you tell them, so don't be afraid to let them know exactly how you feel. (You may want to do this by using the pain scale described a little later in this chapter.)

Despite the effectiveness of the pain control techniques mentioned in this chapter, it's important to consult your physician to determine which techniques are appropriate for you. Make sure that any techniques that you're thinking of using will not be dangerous for you, considering your condition.

Three general categories of treatment are used in the control of lupus-related pain: medical treatment, physical therapy, and psychological strategies. All three types of treatment work by interrupting the transmission of pain messages before the brain receives and interprets them. Let's see how these three approaches can help you to control—or, ideally, eliminate—pain.

MEDICAL TREATMENT

Medical treatment for pain generally involves medication. This can effectively control a lot of problems, which can decrease or eliminate the pain. Your doctor will recommend medical treatment based on the nature and location of the pain and, of course, partly on your previous responses to pain-control techniques. In the case of mild pain, analgesics (painkillers) or anti-inflammatory drugs may prove helpful. (Because of their use as an important treatment modality for lupus, however, information on anti-inflammatory drugs will be presented in the next chapter on medications.)

Two of the simplest nonnarcotic pain relievers are aspirin (acetylsalicylic acid) and Tylenol (acetaminophen). These medications can be very effective in relieving mild to moderate pain. Aspirin can also reduce swelling and inflammation, but may affect the stomach (more information about aspirin in the next chapter). Tylenol, on the other hand, is useful in countering pain and fever, but doesn't act against inflammation. If you experience stomach upsets or are sensitive to aspirin, try coated aspirin (although recent studies do not show these to do all that much more than regular aspirin) or any of the drugs in the Tylenol category to see if they help.

When pain is more severe, however, stronger drugs may be prescribed to decrease or eliminate the pain. Narcotic pain relievers are much more powerful than nonnarcotic analgesics. Narcotics, which are derived from opium or synthetically produced to act like drugs derived from opium, work by changing your perception of pain and creating a heightened sense of well-being. Unfortunately, these drugs can also be habit-forming and frequently cause side effects, including nausea, vomiting, and drowsiness. Examples of narcotic painkillers include codeine, Demerol (meperidine), morphine sulfate, Percodan (oxycodone/aspirin), Percocet (oxycodone/acetaminophen), and many others. These medications may be used by themselves or in combination with over-the-counter pain relievers.

Analgesics can be administered orally, in pill or liquid form; by medication-imbedded skin patch; by injection; through rectal suppository; or intravenously. Pain medication can also be delivered using a pump, which can be either implanted or worn next to the body. The pain pump is commonly used to allow the self-administration of prescribed doses of powerful, fast-acting painkillers.

Whenever you deal with painkillers—as well as many other types of drugs—you have to be concerned about addiction. In fact, some people who have pain are reluctant to use painkillers because they are so afraid of becoming addicted or because they worry that other people will think less of them for using these drugs.

When any of these medications work for you, pain may be controlled. Unfortunately, with lupus, there are cases in which not all pain can be eliminated, such as if a dull, throbbing discomfort continues, despite the use of medication. In extreme cases, surgery may be helpful in treating the cause of pain. For example, joint replacement surgery may be necessary, more often involving the hips or the knees, but other joints may be targeted as well. But not all pain conditions lend themselves to, or would even benefit from, surgical treatment. So it may be necessary for you to learn other techniques for dealing with pain.

PHYSICAL THERAPY

The pain of lupus can often be effectively relieved with one or more types of physical modalities, such as heat, cold, massage, energy medicine devices, acupuncture, and magnetic field therapy. In addition, getting a proper balance of rest and exercise is very important. By pinpointing the location, frequency, and intensity of the pain, a knowledgeable health care professional can determine which type of physical modality is most likely to help your specific circumstances.

HEAT

Heat can be a very beneficial way of relaxing and soothing your muscles to relieve soreness and pain. This is called thermotherapy. It's considered to be the oldest form of pain reliever or analgesic. If you are going to use heat, be careful about how intense (hot) it is and how long you apply it. Too much heat for too long a period of time is not advisable. Don't assume that if a little bit of heat is good, a lot of heat can be better. This is a good way to get burned (pun intended)!

Some professionals recommend applying heat with a hot water bottle, an electric heating pad, a hydrocollator pack, a microwavable gel pad, or a wet towel. Very warm baths or showers may also be helpful. Just be sure to take any precautions necessary to avoid burns. For instance, do not use a heating pad on "High" for a long period of time or apply it directly to the skin, and do not allow yourself to fall asleep while using any type of heating pad (although an electric blanket might help!).

Whirlpool baths, although seemingly beneficial, may be set at too high a temperature. If set above your body temperature, you should not immerse yourself for more than a few minutes at a time. Physical therapy in a heated pool (hydrotherapy or aquatic therapy) may be the best method of treating arthritic symptoms.

COLD

Although there are many benefits to using heat, some people with lupus respond better to cold treatment. Some people don't like cold treatments, saying that they're good only for polar bears. Others, however, find that cold can provide even more effective pain relief than heat. Cold treatment, also known as cryotherapy, can help by numbing the nerve endings in the affected areas. It also decreases the activity of the body cells.

One common method of cold treatment involves soaking a cloth or towel in ice water, wringing it out, and applying it to the painful area. Gel packs, which can be obtained from pharmacies and medical supply stores, are an excellent means of applying cold and, because of their pliable consistency, are often more comfortable than ice packs. These gel packs are kept in the freezer, removed for use, and then refrozen. Of course, if you don't have a gel pack, ice cubes, a bag of frozen peas, or a frozen wet cloth placed in a plastic bag can be just as effective. As with hot compresses, be sure to wrap these applications in a towel before holding it against the skin. If you have Raynaud's phenomenon, protect your hands when handling these applications. And make sure you follow professional recommendations regarding how to use any of these techniques or procedures.

MASSAGE

Massage is another useful physical modality for reducing pain. For centuries, the therapeutic use of touch has been applied to heal the body and reduce stress and tension. Practitioners often use a combination of bodyworks techniques (such as acupressure, reflexology, polarity therapy, and therapeutic touch) to help balance energy in the body and bring about enhanced well-being. Prolonged tension can often cause pain. Massage helps to release tension and promote relaxation. It also helps break up the waste deposits concentrated in muscles and other tissues, and stimulates circulation.

Massage can be performed by a professional, your partner, or you can perform it yourself, provided that the uncomfortable area is accessible to you and that you can use the technique effectively. To maximize both safety and effectiveness, be sure to check with a physician, physical therapist, or massage professional before attempting to use it as a means of controlling your pain.

ENERGY MEDICINE DEVICES

Energy medicine refers to therapies that manipulate a healing energy—electrical, magnetic, sonic, acoustic, microwave, or infrared—to treat health conditions. Energy medicine uses diagnostic screening devices to measure the various electromagnetic frequencies emitted by the body to detect imbalances in the body's energy fields and then correct them. Most energy medicine devices are based on the acupuncture meridian system (the network of energy channels throughout the body). An example of a commonly used treatment device is the TENS unit.

TENS stands for transcutaneous electrical nerve stimulation. These devices have been used in doctors' offices and physiotherapy clinics, and can be used at home. The TENS unit is a little box about the size of a deck of cards. It contains a generator that has wire leads with electrodes at the ends of them. The unit may have anywhere from two to forty electrode wire leads. A little gel is attached to the electrodes, which are then placed on your skin, on or near the area to be treated. When you turn on the unit, a low level of electricity flows into the area from the TENS unit. This stimulates the nerve fibers and blocks the transmission of pain messages to the brain. Shocking, right? Don't worry. You probably won't even feel anything, or you may just experience a mild tingling sensation.

One problem with TENS is that its effectiveness seems to decrease over time. The effectiveness of this type of therapy is also dependent on your diligence, the knowledge of your therapist, and the placement of the electrodes.

If you want to get a TENS unit, you usually need a prescription from your physician. A nurse or physical therapist will then teach you how to place the electrodes to provide maximum pain relief. But it's probably a good idea to rent a TENS unit before buying one, to see if it works for you.

ACUPUNCTURE

Another pain-relief technique—one that has gained increasing acceptance by professionals in the last few years—is acupuncture. This ancient Chinese technique is based on the belief that health is determined by a balanced flow of *qi* (also known as *chi*), the vital energy present in all living organisms. An acupuncturist inserts very thin needles at various depths and angles at specific points predetermined to bring about pain relief. The needles suppress pain perception and may also trigger the release of endorphins and enkephalins, the body's natural painkilling chemicals. In fact, in China, acupuncture is often used as an anesthetic during surgery, indicating a high degree of effectiveness in many cases.

Although the insertion of needles may sound painful, they are not inserted like injections, but just sit on the top of the skin, and patients rarely experience anything more than a little "pinch." If you are interested in trying acupuncture, speak to your physician or other health care professional, who should be able to refer you to a qualified professional.

MAGNETIC FIELD THERAPY

Recently, scientists have been exploring the concept that external magnetic fields can affect the body's functioning. The healing potential of magnets is possible because the body's nervous system is governed in part by varying patterns of currents and electromagnetic fields. Magnetic fields can stimulate metabolism and increase the amount of oxygen available to cells.

Magnetic therapy is applied in many ways and may be used to alleviate pain and other symptoms. Treatment times and duration vary. To better understand the therapeutic use of magnets, consult a practitioner for guidance.

TRADITIONAL CHINESE MEDICINE

Traditional Chinese medicine (TCM) is an ancient method of health care that combines the use of medicinal herbs, acupuncture, food therapy, massage, and therapeutic exercise. Its approach to health and healing is very different from traditional or modern Western medicine. TCM looks for the underlying causes of imbalances in the body. It focuses more on the response of the patient to the disease than on the disease itself. Traditional Chinese medicine has become more appealing to people who want to assume more responsibility for their own healing.

HERBAL REMEDIES AND DIETARY SUPPLEMENTS

Herbs and certain dietary supplements can be effective when used over an extended period of time to help reduce pain (and other symptoms). Some people with lupus have found them to be beneficial secondary therapeutic agents to help with pain relief. Vitamins and minerals also play a role in pain relief. Vitamin C with bioflavonoids, vitamin E, and B-complex vitamins (B_1, B_6, and B_{12}) and minerals, including zinc and magnesium, may help to reduce pain and inflammation. However, you should take herbs, nutritional supplements, vitamins, and minerals only under the supervision of a nutritionally oriented doctor. You will find more information on these and other important dietary considerations in Chapter 11.

Be aware that many of these alternative therapies are controversial and have not been tested in scientific studies. Make sure that you know what you're doing, and consult with your physician. You don't want to waste money and time, and potentially allow your disease to progress, as you use "remedies" that may be ineffective and unproven.

As you can see, there are several physical modalities that can be used for pain relief—most of which can be used at home. These can be helpful by themselves or in combination with medication, surgery, other alternative therapies, or psychological strategies. You can further enhance the effectiveness of these techniques by being sure to get the proper balance of rest and exercise. (See Chapter 12 for details on how exercise can help you better cope with lupus.)

You can learn how to employ techniques for controlling pain by consulting physicians, physical therapists, occupational therapists, and mental health professionals (such as psychologists who may specialize in certain pain control techniques). Or you may want to learn more about these strategies in some of the many books on pain that can be found in bookstores and libraries, or online.

Despite the effectiveness of many pain control techniques available today, it's important to consult your physician to check that any and all of the techniques are appropriate for you. Make sure that any techniques you're thinking of using are not dangerous for you, considering your condition. And make sure that you don't stop using your medications without close supervision by your doctor.

PSYCHOLOGICAL STRATEGIES

As we discussed earlier in the chapter, there are many factors that may influence your experience of pain, including anxiety, depression, and stress. Once you learn to control these factors, you're sure to feel a lot better. This is not to say that the pain is "all in your head." But pain is usually a combination of physiological and psychological factors. So although you may be experiencing true physiological pain, your mind is very much involved in determining exactly how much it hurts.

Lisa was limping around her house for hours because of severe joint pain in her ankle. The pain overwhelmed her every time she tried to move faster. Even when she was doing something she enjoyed, her movements were restricted. Suddenly, she heard her nine-year-old son cry out for help. Without a thought about her ankle, she went flying across the room to help him. Does this mean her pain is all in her head? Of course not! Sure, Lisa's ankle did hurt (and the pain was real), but her mind had probably magnified the amount of pain she felt. When she realized that her son was in trouble, the pain temporarily took on secondary importance.

What does all this mean? If medication and various physical therapies don't alleviate your pain, you can still relieve some—if not all—of it by working on your mind's perception of the pain. Many people have found effective pain control through the use of relaxation techniques, imagery, hypnosis, and biofeedback. These techniques work by separating you from your sensations of pain, enabling you to feel better. Some of these techniques may be learned at home. Others must be taught by professionals. The following discussions should help you decide which of the psychological pain-control techniques may best help you as you learn to cope with lupus.

RELAXATION TECHNIQUES

As discussed earlier, tension can actually increase your pain. So it makes sense that relaxation—the opposite of tension—can help you reduce your overall level of pain. As an added benefit, relaxation techniques may increase your general sense of well-being and help you to better deal with many day-to-day problems—not just those related to lupus. A number of procedures may be effective, including progressive relaxation, meditation, autogenics, deep breathing, and a method called the Quick Release. Let's look briefly at each of these techniques.

Progressive relaxation is based on the premise that when you experience anything stressful, the body responds with muscle tension—which, of course, can increase pain. In this procedure, which is usually performed for fifteen to twenty minutes once or twice daily, you sequentially tense and then relax the different muscle groups in your body, one group at a time. If you wish to learn more about this popular and effective technique, don't hesitate to consult books at your local library or bookstore, check online, or speak to a professional.

Meditation can allow you to achieve a deep level of relaxation in a short period of time. It really is a name for any activity that keeps the attention pleasantly anchored in the present moment. When the mind is calm and focused in the present, it is neither reacting to memories from the past nor being preoccupied with plans for the future, two major sources of stress. During meditation, you focus your mind, uncritically, on one object, sound, activity, or experience, and "clear out" any extraneous thoughts. This technique usually works best when taught by a professional or learned from a reliable book, tape, or video, depending on the type of meditation you choose.

Autogenics is a systematic program that helps you train your body and mind to respond to your own verbal commands to relax. With this procedure, which can be used for short periods of time and repeated as frequently as needed, you give yourself verbal suggestions of heaviness, warmth, and calmness. Again, information online, a book on relaxation techniques, or a qualified professional can guide you in the use of this procedure.

Many people find that *deep breathing* can significantly increase their relaxation and, as a result, decrease their pain. Deep breathing can be used in a number of different ways. Let's try one simple deep-breathing exercise together. First, assume a comfortable position on your bed or on the floor. Then put one hand on your abdomen and the other on your chest. Inhale slowly and deeply through your nose, so that the hand on your abdomen moves higher. Hold your breath as long as you're comfortable doing so; then exhale slowly through your mouth, making a peaceful *whoosh*ing sound. Feel the hand on your abdomen sink slowly, and allow a growing feeling of relaxation to deepen inside you. Repeat this sequence for five to ten minutes. Then give yourself a few minutes to become aware of your surroundings before getting up. Practice this technique at least twice a day, extending its duration if you wish.

Another simple but effective relaxation technique is the *Quick Release*. Try this now: Close your eyes, take a deep breath, and hold it as you tighten the muscles in every part of your body that you can think of—your fists, arms, legs, stomach, neck, buttocks, etc. Continue to hold your breath and to keep your muscles tense for about six seconds. Then let your breath out in a *whoosh*, and allow the tension to drain out of your muscles. Let your body go limp. Keep your eyes closed, and breathe rhythmically and comfortably for about twenty seconds. Repeat this tension-relaxation cycle three times. By the end of the third repetition, you'll probably feel a lot more relaxed. Keep on practicing this technique, as continuous practice will condition your body to respond quickly and completely.

Many other relaxation techniques may also prove helpful. Remember that your ability to increase relaxation and decrease pain by means of the mind-body connection are limited only by your imagination. Don't overlook this valuable way of improving your well-being.

IMAGERY

Much research has indicated that bodily functions previously thought to be totally beyond conscious control can be modified using psychological techniques. Imagery, a technique that has grown in popularity over recent years, uses this mind-body connection to help you cope with disease.

Imagery, also called *guided visualization*, is the process of conjuring up mental pictures or scenes in order to harness your body's energy. In practice, imagery has been beneficial in helping people deal with a host of physiological and psychological problems. In addition to reducing stress, imagery has been successful in the control of headaches, hypertension, depression, pain, and a variety of other symptoms. Sometimes used alone, imagery can also be used in combination with prescribed medical treatment.

How can you use imagery to control your pain? Get into a relaxed position in a comfortable chair or in bed. The lights should be dimmed, and outside sounds or noises should be minimized. Try to avoid interruptions. Breathe smoothly and rhythmically, allowing your body to release tension and relax. Then imagine a scene of your own choosing, trying to make the image as vivid and real as possible. This scene can be used therapeutically to help you feel better.

Anita was suffering from sharp pains in her knees. She was instructed to relax and then develop an image of what this joint pain looked like. She imagined it as very sharp knives jabbed into her knees. Others may feel as if their knees are being hit by a hammer or have dozens of pins stuck into them. Whatever imagery you develop, it should be as vivid and detailed as possible. Anita was then instructed to slowly reverse what was happening in the image. So she imagined the knives slowly being removed from her knees, and a soothing, healing cream being applied. Finally, the knives were completely out. She was then able to deepen her relaxation, greatly reducing her discomfort.

There are other images you could use to reduce joint pain. For example, you could imagine oil or a soothing lotion being gently massaged into the painful joint to allow smoother motion, or you could picture yourself taking a warm bath. Imagery is restricted only by your creativity and can be used anywhere. (Have you ever taken a bath on a bus?!) With regular use, imagery can truly help you feel better. Two good books on the subject are *Guided Imagery for Self-Healing* by Martin Rossman and *Visualization for Change* by Patrick Fanning. See if your public library or local bookstore has them.

HYPNOSIS

Hypnosis involves a calm repetition of words and statements designed to induce a state of deep relaxation in which there is a heightened receptivity to suggestion. During this state, verbal suggestions help the mind to block the awareness of pain and replace it with a more positive feeling. Recent studies show that 94 percent of people can benefit from hypnotherapy, even if the only benefit is relaxation. While hypnosis is often quite effective in the area of pain control, it may not be as effective in dealing with severe pain.

You can learn how to hypnotize yourself so that you can use this technique whenever you need it. However, the technique must first be learned from a professional—a licensed psychologist, social worker, or certified hypnotherapist, for instance. Many good books on clinical hypnosis can give you further information about this valuable tool. Organizations such as the American Institute of Hypnotherapy, the American Society of Clinical Hypnosis, the International Medical and Dental Hypnotherapy Association, or the National Guild of Hypnotists can refer you to a legitimate practitioner in your area.

BIOFEEDBACK

Biofeedback combines the techniques of relaxation and imagery, already discussed, with the use of electronic measuring instruments. These machines give you feedback in the form of sounds or images, letting you know what's going on inside your body. Biofeedback provides moment-by-moment information about the effect that your imagery and relaxation techniques are having on your physiological responses. What responses can be measured? Most frequently, the biofeedback units measure skin temperature, pulse, blood pressure, the electrical activity resulting from muscular tension, or the electrical activity coming from the brain.

How, exactly, can biofeedback help you control pain? Electrodes connected to the biofeedback unit are taped or otherwise attached to your skin. These electrodes monitor one or more of the physiological responses mentioned above, and transmit the information they pick up to the biofeedback unit in the form of electrical impulses. The unit then translates this feedback into sounds, lights, or pictures that you can see or hear. Using this information, you can experiment and find the types of imagery and other relaxation techniques that will allow you to best control your internal responses, and thus induce relaxation and reduce muscular pain.

Gayle was experiencing a lot of abdominal pain, so her physician suggested she try biofeedback. A machine measuring muscle tension was attached to her abdomen in much the same way that electrodes from an EKG machine are connected. (There is no pain, and you won't get jolted!) As Gayle attempted to relax her abdominal muscles, the machine gave her instant feedback as to whether she was really relaxing, and also how well she was relaxing. As she became aware of her lessening tension, Gayle learned what mental images worked best for her. Eventually, she was able to use these images on her own, without the machine, to help her relax and control her pain. She then began using biofeedback to successfully control her Raynaud's symptoms by learning how to warm her hands. Gayle was convinced!

Certified biofeedback professionals can be found throughout the country. Check with your physician or local hospital or clinic for names of certified biofeedback professionals in your area. Good resources for names of local practitioners include your physician, local hospital or clinic, the Association for Applied Psychophysiology and Biofeedback, and the Biofeedback Certification International Alliance.

PSYCHOLOGICAL COPING STRATEGIES

By now you probably understand the connection between emotions and pain, and want to do everything you can to decrease your fear, stress, tension, and other negative emotions—emotions that may make you more aware of pain or even increase it. Part Three should help you pinpoint the source of your emotional distress, and then find ways of better coping with your feelings. Never underestimate the effect that emotions can have on your physical health!

Of course, the more time you have to think about your pain, the worse it will seem. So try to divert your attention. Develop interests that require concentration—computer games, crafts, crossword puzzles, or whatever suits your fancy. Volunteer your time someplace where your skills are needed. Read a good book, rent a movie, or create something. You can always come up with activities that will entertain your mind while increasing your feeling of physical well-being.

EXPLAINING PAIN TO OTHERS

Do you get frustrated trying to explain the way you feel to others? Since one of the most difficult parts of living with lupus is being in pain, you want the people around you, the significant people in your life, to understand your pain and be sympathetic. Here's the problem. Sure, they may have an idea what pain is all about. But they probably think about it as something localized or short term, such as the pain of a burn, cut, childbirth, puncture, migraine, or intense headache. It's much more difficult for others to understand the pain of lupus. The fact that it may be long-lasting, a type of pain others may not be able to relate to, can lead people to start questioning you. You certainly don't want to be in a defensive mode. You don't want to have to convince others of the way you feel, especially when you're unable to get your point across.

An effective strategy to try to get others to understand your pain is to use a number scale. Describe your pain on a rating scale from 0 to 10. This may help others more readily understand what you're referring to than if you use adjectives such as "pretty bad," "not bad," "terrible," "excruciating," or other terms that are more subjective. For example, if someone asks how you're feeling and you say, "I'm at a 9," they may not know exactly what kind of pain you're feeling, but they can imagine how they would feel if *they* were at a 9, and may be more supportive.

There are many other ways to improve your communication with others, discussed elsewhere in the book, about pain or other aspects of lupus (see Part Four, for example). But don't get frustrated, or feel as though you're banging your head against the wall trying to explain your pain. After all, that would create an additional type of pain!

Pain-Control Resources

You can learn and gain access to many pain-control techniques from your own physician; from mental health professionals, including psychologists and social workers who specialize in certain pain-control techniques; and from other health care professionals. You may want to read some of the books on pain control that are available in libraries and bookstores. Or you may want to research many of these methods online. Certainly, many techniques can be used at home—although, in some cases, they may work better if you learn them from clinics or centers. In fact, certain clinics specialize in the control of pain.

If you decide to consult a pain-management specialist, there are both diagnostic and therapeutic types. Various tests can be administered at a diagnostic center to determine more about the causes of your pain and the pathways involved. These include thermography (mapping the body's surface temperature), spinogram (measures the involvement of the spinal pathways), selected blind nerve blocks (injections to identify the nerves or nerve bundles involved in the pain), and neurological assessments. The results from these tests may help you and your doctor make decisions about treatment. A therapeutic pain clinic or center will identify a combination of medication, adjunctive treatments (such as biofeedback, physiotherapy, and others), exercise programs, and group counseling that can help relieve pain, improve your general health, and strengthen coping skills. Be sure to seek out a pain-management center or specialist who is up to date on the complexities of lupus-associated pain. And, of course, make sure any specialists you see consult with your primary physician.

You may want to read some of the many books on pain that can be found in bookstores and libraries. (See some suggestions for books on this topic in the Appendix.) Or you might want to get involved in a support group specifically for people living with pain. Examples of organizations that provide information about support groups are the American Chronic Pain Association (www.theacpa.org) and the U.S. Pain Foundation (www.uspain foundation.org). Refer to the Appendix for additional listings. It can be comforting to know that you're not alone in trying to cope with pain. You may even learn some new pain-control strategies.

Despite the effectiveness of the many pain-control techniques available today, it's important to consult your physician to make sure that any or all of the techniques you're considering are appropriate for you and will pose no danger to your health. And, of course, your physician may make you aware of further coping techniques, one of which might be just what you need!

Additional Pain-Controlling Ideas

There are a number of additional things you can do to relieve the pain of lupus:

- Employ a take-charge approach to lupus.
- Get plenty of rest.
- Take control of your medical treatment. Become a partner with your doctor or other health care professional. Learn as much as you can to enable you to make the best possible decisions for yourself.
- Eat healthy foods (see Chapter 11).
- Take nutritional supplements that are known to reduce inflammation.
- Evaluate the benefits and actions of certain herbs that may help. Check with a nutritionist or an expert at your local health food store for additional information in this area. (Make sure you discuss anything that you're considering with your doctor—certain supplements may be contraindicated for lupus. See Chapter 11, on diet and nutrition, for further details.)
- Keep a daily pain diary. It will give you a clearer picture of your pain and help you to anticipate it and determine if it has a regular pattern. You can learn how long the pain usually will last, enabling you to more easily handle it, with less element of surprise.

- Be as active as you possibly can, despite the pain, without going too far.
- Maximize your use of stress reduction techniques.
- Cry—it is a surprisingly helpful way of ridding the body of toxins and reducing pain.
- Do things that bring you a sense of fulfillment, joy, and purpose.
- Visualize and emulate the coping strategies of healthy people—or people with lupus (or other illnesses) whose coping styles you admire.
- Maintain a positive attitude. Hang up inspirational sayings. Talk to yourself in a positive manner.
- Pay close attention to yourself, tuning in to all your needs.
- Release all negative emotions—constructively. Express your feelings—constructively.
- Accept yourself and everything in your life as an opportunity for growth and learning.
- Develop images that make you feel peaceful or happy to offset fear of, or experiencing of pain.
- Keep a sense of humor.
- Take care of yourself by supporting and encouraging yourself.
- Hold positive images and goals in your mind.
- Create fun, loving, honest relationships. Try to heal wounds in past relationships.
- Make a positive contribution to society.

An Unagonizing Conclusion

Unfortunately, pain is one of the most common symptoms of lupus, and it is likely that you will have *some* pain because of the disease. But don't throw in the heating pad! Realize that the pain need not last forever. A lot can be done, both medically and psychologically, to increase your level of comfort and help you to more fully enjoy each and every day.

10.

MEDICATIONS

Other than changes in lifestyle, the main treatment for lupus is the use of medication. The value of medication as a treatment varies, depending on its therapeutic goal. Different medications are prescribed for different reasons.

Believe it or not, some people welcome drugs as a powerful way to control physical or emotional symptoms. Other people are afraid of their power and the possibility of becoming dependent on them. Still other people resent the presence of any artificial substances in their bodies. Where do your feelings fit in?

Regardless of what your attitudes are about using medication, your physician has probably made it perfectly clear that you don't have much choice in the matter. Taking medication is not enough, though. You must take it properly: the right drug, the right dose, at the right time, for the right length of time. Otherwise it can be ineffective—or very dangerous.

So let's talk about medication, since you must adjust to taking it for lupus. In this way, you'll be informed and able to maximize safety and effectiveness, while minimizing potential side effects.

Why Drugs?

Because lupus both creates and is created by physiological problems in your body, medications designed to deal with these problems can be helpful in

controlling the disease. There are various kinds of drugs that are very helpful in the treatment of lupus. Some may be used to control flares, reduce
inflammation, or suppress symptoms, among other things. Because of the
chemical natures of these drugs and the way they may interact with your
body, it is extremely important that you follow your doctor's instructions in
taking the drugs prescribed for you. Do not play with medications that you
don't have a prescription for (or even with the ones that have been prescribed for you, for that matter)!

Choosing the Appropriate Medication

How does your physician determine which medication will work best for
you? In prescribing a drug program, your physician will take many factors
into account, including your age and overall health, the severity of your
lupus at the time, the amount of pain you're experiencing, and any other
lupus-related symptoms you're experiencing. If, in the past, you have shown
sensitivities or allergies to any drugs, you should certainly let your doctor
know—even if you think this information is already part of your medical
record. Of course, it's important for you to inform your doctor about any
other medications—prescription or over-the-counter (OTC)—that you are
currently taking or considering taking. Some prescription and OTC drugs
can interact with other medications—and some drug interactions may even
be dangerous (more about this later).

Even when all of these factors are taken into consideration, doctors may
still not be sure exactly how certain medications will affect you. So some
amount of trial and error may be necessary to determine the medication and
proper dosage that will be suited to your needs. This may be very frustrating,
but the results are worthwhile. Make sure you understand exactly why you're
taking the medication and what it's supposed to do.

Knowing How and
When to Take Your Medication

Whenever your doctor prescribes a medication, be sure you understand exactly what the drug is supposed to do, how and when it should be taken, how long you are expected to take it, and what potential side effects you may experience. For example, certain medications should be taken only after meals, while others must be taken on an empty stomach. Some medications should be taken with water, some with food, and some in other ways. Be sure to obtain and read a copy of the package insert for each medication that you take. This will explain how the drug works in the body, list indications for use, possible side effects, contraindications, and other valuable information. As we'll discuss later, your pharmacist is another good resource for this information.

Each person has different needs as far as dosage and frequency of drugs are concerned. Even if somebody you know has the same symptoms that are troubling you and is taking the same medication, that person's dosage may not necessarily be appropriate for you. And once you start taking any drug, the dosage may have to be adjusted based on any side effects you're experiencing, how well the medication is managing your symptoms, and the severity of the problem that is being treated.

Once you begin taking medication in certain dosages, don't attempt to change these dosages on your own. While some medications may be necessary for only a short time, you may always need other types of medication. However long you must take a medication, recognize that it is being prescribed specifically to help you live as healthy a life as possible. It's extremely important that you follow your doctor's orders as carefully as possible when taking the drugs prescribed for you. *Never* mix drugs without knowing if the combination is safe. If you need to take many different pills, make sure that you don't play with your dosage or with the times you take them, or move around the number of pills you take at a particular time. If you miss a pill, try to take it as soon as you can, but do *not* "double dip" to make up for this. Try to use the same pharmacy so all of your records are in the same place and the pharmacist will know that the drug combination is acceptable.

You probably want to take as little medication as possible. Very few physicians will keep you on high doses of any medication unless they feel it's absolutely essential. Still, if you're taking a substantial amount of any drug and question the need for it, don't be afraid to discuss your concerns with your doctor or pharmacist. Every physician should be willing and able to explain your prescribed medication and why you need it. If you're feeling good and would like to reduce your dosage—or stop taking the drug altogether—by all means, speak to your doctor. If it is reasonable and appropriate, together you will be able to plan a schedule for reducing your dosage and, if possible, ending treatment.

They Might Not Get Along!

Never take any medications other than those prescribed for you without first checking with your doctor or pharmacist. If you see physicians other than those who are treating your lupus, be aware that they may prescribe medications that absolutely should not be taken with your lupus medications. Some mixes can make your symptoms worse, interfere with the action of the prescribed medication, or cause additional problems. (This can also apply to something seemingly as "innocent" as over-the-counter medications.)

It makes sense to have one primary physician in charge of your care. Any other doctor you see can then consult with your primary physician to verify that the treatment strategies will work together. Because certain medications are chemically incompatible, you should never mix drugs without first knowing that the combination is safe. Don't take the chance. Check it out. And always make sure that *each* physician you're working with knows about all the medications you're taking.

Side Effects

Most people with lupus require medication, often for months or years. But that doesn't mean you're thrilled with the idea. Not too many people are. What might bother you? Well, you're probably concerned about what the medication may be doing to your body, or what the side effects may be. Clearly, side effects are one of the biggest concerns about taking medication, and they may occur whenever a drug is taken. Side effects, as you know, are the less-than-pleasant effects a drug may have on your body. They indicate that a drug is interacting with your body in a way other than the way it was intended. Because medication causes chemical changes within the body, side effects may occur whenever medication is taken. Unfortunately, the more powerful the drug, the more potent its side effects may be.

If the side effects you experience are slight, they probably won't upset you—especially if the medication you're taking is having the desired effect. Even if the side effects are disturbing, you may want (or need) to continue the medication if its benefits outweigh any discomforts you're experiencing. Physicians are aware of possible side effects; they won't prescribe any medication that isn't necessary nor will they prescribe higher dosages than are necessary. However, if side effects are causing you excessive discomfort, you should discuss this with your physician, and the two of you should weigh the disadvantages against the advantages. You want to balance the side effects of the drug with the potential side effects of the disease! And, of course, never stop any medication without discussing it with your physician. Some need to be tapered off; if you stop too abruptly, it can be dangerous.

With any drug, it's important to find the lowest effective dose. The goal is to find the dosage level that will maximize the therapeutic value and minimize any side effects. Taking any medication exactly as it is prescribed is also important in lessening the incidence of side effects. (Again, if there are any problems, call your doctor!)

There are many different drugs involved in the treatment of lupus, and each specific medication has its own unique side effects (more about specific drugs and their side effects later in the chapter). However, it is unlikely that you will experience all, or even some, of them.

Getting Down to Specifics

Let's talk about some of the medications for lupus. The goal? You want to cope with any medicine you have to take as part of your life.

Other than analgesics (medications for pain control that were discussed in the previous chapter), the medications that generally have been helpful in treating lupus can be divided into four categories:

- Anti-inflammatories
- Antimalarials
- Corticosteroids
- Immunosuppressants

Anti-inflammatories are prescribed to control lupus symptoms, including pain. However, they don't do anything about the disease itself. The other three categories contain drugs that can actually have an impact on lupus itself and, as such, can be called *disease-modifying drugs*. Let's discuss these four categories.

ANTI-INFLAMMATORIES

As you know, lupus is an inflammatory disease. The inflammation and its effects bring about most of the damage caused by lupus. So it is understandable that the most prescribed drugs for lupus are anti-inflammatories—drugs that have as their primary function controlling and reducing existing inflammation in the body. Two main types of drugs fall into this category: aspirin and nonsteroidal anti-inflammatory drugs (NSAIDs).

ASPIRIN AND ASPIRIN DERIVATIVES

Aspirin, part of the family of salicylates, is a common, relatively safe, and effective drug. Aspirin can be helpful in reducing the low-grade fevers that frequently occur in lupus. It can also help lessen pain and discomfort. For example, aspirin has been shown to be very helpful in controlling joint pain and joint aches, as well as the chest pain that accompanies both pericarditis and pleuritis.

But aspirin is more than just a painkiller. Aspirin can also be helpful in controlling lupus-related inflammation. How does aspirin "know" if it will simply be an analgesic to control pain, or whether it will also act as an anti-inflammatory? The answer is in the dosage! At low dosages, aspirin can help reduce pain. How? It acts on the central nervous system and reduces your ability to feel pain. But if aspirin is going to be effective in reducing inflammation, a higher dosage is needed. Why? Higher levels of aspirin are necessary to block the production of prostaglandins. These are the chemicals that help to trigger and prolong the inflammatory process. Prostaglandins are substances that are released in inflamed areas. These prostaglandins seem to increase the pain you experience because they sensitize nerve endings. By interfering with the production of prostaglandins, aspirin blocks pain and reduces inflammation.

Even though aspirin is available over the counter, if it is going to be part of your treatment for lupus, it should *not* be taken on a self-prescribed basis. It can be very harmful if not taken carefully, especially if taken with other medications that are described below.

Side Effects

Aspirin does have its side effects, including stomach upset, nausea, or indigestion. Vomiting may occur. It is recommended to take aspirin with food, milk, or an antacid to alleviate some of these side effects. Liquid aspirin or time-release aspirin may also help to avoid an upset stomach, as may buffered aspirin or aspirin mixed with antacids.

Another side effect from high doses of aspirin is tinnitus, a ringing or buzzing in the ears. Dizziness, slight losses of hearing, or slight changes in vision may also result from high levels of aspirin. Aspirin can also cause irritation of the walls of the esophagus and/or the stomach, which results in bleeding. While not indicating that an ulcer is definitely present, these surface "erosions" from aspirin can lead to a low red blood cell count (anemia). Black stool may be a sign of blood loss. Sometimes, light-headedness, increased fatigue, and pallor may indicate that significant anemia is present. It is critical that you tell your doctor if any of these symptoms occur.

There are some people who should not take aspirin. Some asthma sufferers may not be able to tolerate it. People with gastrointestinal problems should always use great caution if told to take aspirin. People who are taking other types of medication, such as blood thinners, may also be advised to avoid aspirin. Aspirin may cause serious bleeding and, on rare occasions, may even lead to hemorrhaging.

People who are allergic to aspirin (although this does not occur very often) must avoid it. There is a difference between side effects and allergies. Ask your doctor to explain the difference so you know what to watch out for. If you are allergic to aspirin, you must eliminate it from your treatment program; however, if you are experiencing side effects, you may still be able to use it by adjusting the dosage. Symptoms that indicate an allergic reaction include a rash, a runny nose, and wheezing. On the other hand, symptoms such as ringing in the ears, headache, nausea, abdominal pain, and stomach upset are simply side effects.

Why is it so important for you to be able to recognize aspirin's side effects? Like many other people, you may experience side effects from aspirin if your physician has been prescribing it at high doses. If this occurs, talk to your doctor. You may be advised to reduce your dosage slightly in order to determine exactly what the best dosage is for you.

Don't give up on aspirin too quickly. Using different brands may reduce the side effects. However, if you experience any of the allergic symptoms mentioned above, these can be more serious. You should then stop taking aspirin and notify your physician immediately.

NONSTEROIDAL ANTI-INFLAMMATORY DRUGS (NSAIDs)

Nonsteroidal anti-inflammatory drugs (NSAIDs) are prescribed for lupus because they reduce both inflammation and pain. NSAIDs were cleverly named, because they reduce inflammation but don't contain steroids! NSAIDs are slightly more powerful than aspirin, and most require a doctor's prescription. (Even though some lower-strength NSAIDs can be obtained over the counter, make sure you don't take them without discussing this with your physician.) They usually cost more than aspirin, too. But NSAIDs may be easier to take since you don't have to swallow as many tablets or take them as often as aspirin.

Nonsteroidal anti-inflammatories are used in lupus for general feelings of discomfort, as well as for pain in the joints or muscles. They are usually the medications of choice when there is little or no lupus-related organ involvement. As with aspirin, NSAIDs work to inhibit prostaglandin, the chemicals that produce inflammation. Although the variety of available NSAIDs seems to work in the same way, different people experience different effects from these drugs. That's why what works for one person with lupus may not work for another.

Examples of NSAIDs

There are many different types of NSAIDs. The main difference between them is their chemical molecular structure. Some of the more common NSAIDs include over-the-counter, nonprescription-strength Motrin (ibuprofen), Advil (ibuprofen), Nuprin (ibuprofen), and Aleve (naproxen sodium); and there are many of prescription strength, including Motrin (ibuprofen), Naprosyn (naproxen), and Indocin (indomethacin).

Side Effects

Many of the side effects of NSAIDs have already been mentioned above in the discussion of aspirin side effects, including stomach pains and cramps, nausea, vomiting, diarrhea, constipation, bleeding from the stomach, and ulcers. Headaches, ringing in the ears, and blurred vision may also occur. Just as certain people may develop aspirin allergies, some may also experience these symptoms when taking NSAIDs. If this occurs, the medication should be stopped and your physician notified immediately. You can also ask your doctor about other stomach protective medications to help you tolerate NSAIDs.

SELECTIVE COX-2 NSAIDs

COX-2 inhibitors have been getting some attention as effective pain relievers with fewer side effects than NSAIDs. "COX" is actually an abbreviation for cyclooxygenase; there are two cyclooxygenase enzymes produced in the body, COX-1 and COX-2. All currently available "standard" anti-inflammatories inhibit both COX-1 and COX-2. Why is this a problem? Without going into too much detail, COX-2 is part of the inflammatory response, so it's responsible for pain and inflammation. On the other hand, COX-1 produces healthy stomach barrier mucus. As a result, when an anti-inflammatory drug inhibits both COX-1 and COX-2, you might experience side effects such as stomach pain and bleeding. So the next step was for scientists to find a drug that would selectively block the effects of COX-2, but would leave COX-1 (the good one) alone. That's basically what's been developed in COX-2 inhibitors, an example of which is Celebrex (celecoxib). They work in the same way as other anti-inflammatory drugs, but studies have documented an improved gastrointestinal safety profile. Rates of gastric ulceration and gastrointestinal bleeding were significantly reduced (but not eliminated) using these drugs as compared to conventional NSAIDs. So they may help you, but caution needs to be used in dealing with these drugs, as with any other type of medication.

ANTIMALARIALS

Another group of medications that often play a role in treatment programs for lupus are the antimalarials. Antimalarial or quinine-related drugs also are appropriate in treating lupus without organ involvement, primarily to help control the skin lesions that may occur with either discoid or systemic lupus, to reduce the painful arthritic symptoms of the disease, and to improve fatigue and fever. An added plus for their use is that in some cases, taking antimalarials enables your physician to reduce the amount of corticosteroids that might otherwise be necessary. It is not completely understood how antimalarial drugs work in helping people with lupus. The primary antimalarial drug used in the treatment of lupus is Plaquenil (hydroxychloroquine).

Side Effects

Side effects are not as common from hydroxychloroquine as they are from other antimalarials. Achiness, headaches, queasiness, or other gastrointestinal problems, including nausea and vomiting, may occur with antimalarial drugs. Other side effects may range from mild ones such as premature graying of the hair to severe effects such as convulsive seizures. Some people have noticed discoloration of patches of skin. However, the most significant potential problem involves the eyes.

With certain antimalarials, such as Plaquenil, changes may infrequently occur in the eyes. The most serious side effect of Plaquenil is gradual damage to the retina of the eye, leading to loss of vision in extreme cases. Because it has been known to occur with the use of some antimalarials, it is very important to see your eye doctor before medication is even started. Antimalarials should be stopped if the slightest change occurs, and you should have your eyes checked regularly (at least once every six months is recommended). In addition, because your eyes will be more sensitive to light when you are taking antimalarials, you should wear protective sunglasses. Wear them in daylight, regardless of whether there appears to be strong sun. You may want to wear them under fluorescent lights as well.

CORTICOSTEROIDS

Many people with lupus are, have been, or may be treated with this category of medication. Corticosteroids (called steroids, for short) have been shown to be effective in treating lupus. However, they must be taken carefully because there can be severe side effects. This is unfortunate because corticosteroids are among the most effective anti-inflammatory drugs known.

Corticosteroids are hormones that are produced by the cortex of the adrenal glands. Nowadays, all corticosteroids used in the treatment of disease are produced synthetically. They are not the same as the anabolic steroids that are used (illegally) by some athletes.

Steroids are very potent anti-inflammatory drugs. They can quickly reduce pain and inflammation, allergic reactions, asthma attacks, many types of eye inflammation, and colitis attacks. There are occasions when steroids are used for short periods of time if an individual is experiencing a severe flare-up of symptoms.

There are many different generic steroids available, including cortisone, prednisone, prednisolone, methylprednisolone, and hydrocortisone, among others. There also are many different brand names (including Meticorten, Drasone, and Deltasone). Each physician usually has a preference. Prednisone is the most commonly prescribed steroid.

Corticosteroids are used when drugs stronger than NSAIDs are necessary to control inflammation and minimize damage to internal organs, as well as when medication is necessary to control potentially dangerous symptoms. As with NSAIDs, corticosteroid reductions in inflammation can also reduce the pain (such as joint pain) and discomfort you may have with lupus.

Steroids are one of the major components of treatment responsible for so much of the dramatic improvement in the prognosis for lupus. Steroids have saved many lives—those of people with lupus and those of people with a number of other serious illnesses or conditions for which other treatments were ineffective or unknown.

Steroids can be given by mouth (orally) as well as intravenously. If given to you to take at home, they will be given in the form of tablets. Because they may make your stomach feel like the inside of an erupting volcano, taking steroids with food or other stomach-protecting medications can help.

The dosage of steroids prescribed for you will depend on many factors, including the severity of your condition, the organs and systems affected, and your weight, habits, and age (among other things). Under more stable conditions, such as when symptoms are milder, low to moderate dosages will be prescribed. Occasionally, steroids may be prescribed for shorter periods of time, lasting for a few weeks or months. In more serious cases, such as if you're in a severe flare, higher dosages of steroids may be given. If your lupus flare is serious enough to require hospitalization, your doctor may decide to try "pulse therapy," intravenous administration of as much as a gram (1,000 milligrams) a day for three days of methylprednisolone (the soluble form of prednisone used for intravenous treatment). This is only a short-term measure that often "jolts" your body into an improved condition. Then the dosage is rapidly dropped to a safer, more manageable level.

Obviously, your physician will advise you of how much medication to take and when to take it. Don't decide on your own to modify your dosage, because that could be downright dangerous.

YOUR ADRENAL GLANDS MAY GO ON STRIKE!

All right, you're taking steroids. They're replacing the hormones your adrenal glands produced. What if these glands no longer find it necessary to produce their own hormones? They may become less and less active. In fact, if you use steroids for a long period of time, your adrenal glands may stop producing these hormones altogether. You'll then need the synthetic drugs to stay alive. This is one of the main reasons you shouldn't stop your medication suddenly if you are taking steroids. If you do, your body will not be getting any corticosteroids—either natural or artificial. It may take months for your adrenal glands to begin their own natural production of cortisone once again. So a gradual tapering down of the dose is the only healthy way to stop taking steroids. This should be done only when your symptoms seem to be under control (and only under a doctor's supervision). Hopefully, your adrenal glands will increase their production of cortisone as you cut back your medication.

Also remember that the hormones produced by your adrenal glands help your body handle sudden, extreme stress. So if your use of steroids causes your glands to cut back on hormone production, steroids must be administered in high dosages at times of extreme physiological stress, such as if you experience a serious injury or if you need surgery. Because of the possibility of your needing greater amounts of corticosteroids during stressful situations, remember to tell all of your physicians, dentists, and other health care providers before, during, or after a major stressful situation that higher dosages of the steroid medication may be necessary.

Side Effects

It might seem as if steroids are the answer to your problems, if you discount the complications that can occur with the adrenal glands. If they're so great, how come everyone isn't taking them? It isn't that simple.

Although they are extremely important in treating lupus, steroids do have side effects, some of which can be significant. Potential side effects vary from person to person (just as lupus does!). For example, some people experience the "moon face" syndrome, in which your abdomen or cheeks may swell if you have been on steroids for a long time. Not everyone using steroids experiences this swelling. Some don't experience it at all. Others may experience very noticeable changes even with small dosages. This can be depressing, especially if you're sensitive about your looks or weight. Another side effect may be weight gain. This can be of great concern to you, and it's why many people with lupus object to the prescription of steroids. Weight gain can occur because of fluid retention (try to minimize salt in your diet) or changes in appetite (follow a healthy, nutritious, low-fat, low-carbohydrate diet), and make sure you're getting all the nutrients you need.

Other side effects include changes in hair growth (slow growth, loss of hair, or increased hair growth on your face and body), an increase in injuries (easier bruising) and slower healing, thinning of the skin, and a weakening of the bones (osteoporosis). Discuss the use of calcium and vitamins with your doctor, to deal with this. There can also be an increased chance of infection (eat healthy and stay away from sick people!), cataracts, avascular necrosis of bone (mentioned earlier), depression, mood changes, and, in some uncommon cases, stomach bleeding (among others). Extensive use of steroids has, on occasion, led to cases of diabetes mellitus, and may cause ulcers or aggravate already existing ones. (As a note, if you have an ulcer condition or any known active infection, steroids are usually not prescribed.) Your blood pressure may rise from steroid use, so keep monitoring it. Occasionally, emotional problems or other highly individual reactions may occur with steroid use.

Another problem is that steroids may mask symptoms, not only ones related to lupus, but also those that may indicate the presence of other chronic or acute conditions.

Nobody develops all of these side effects, and usually they will occur only if you have used steroids for a long period of time. Unfortunately, little can be done to prevent most of these side effects. You'll have to bear with them until steroid dosages can safely be reduced. This takes time. There are medications, however, to prevent osteoporosis, ulcers, and other side effects. And, of course, you can work on your thinking—reminding yourself that these drugs are necessary to treat your disease and that eventually they will diminish.

One strategy that is occasionally used to lessen the chances of unpleasant side effects (usually if you are experiencing mild symptoms of lupus) is to take your steroid medication every other day. In addition, this *alternate-day* strategy may also lessen the chances of developing adrenal insufficiency, where the adrenals stop producing hormones. A problem with this technique is that it is not usually as effective in controlling more active, serious symptoms of lupus. Don't even consider this technique unless your physician has approved it. And if your doctor implements this strategy, make sure that you let your doctor know if your symptoms seem to get worse toward the end of the day that you are off the medication.

So remember: Even though steroids are extremely beneficial in many treatment programs for lupus, they are hardly ideal drugs. Despite their advantages, they are used only in such dosages and for such duration as is absolutely necessary.

IMMUNOSUPPRESSANTS

Immunosuppressants (also called cytotoxic, anticancer drugs, or chemotherapy) are very powerful, but also far from ideal. They are extremely potent, have considerable risks of unpleasant side effects, and, in some cases, can be dangerous. The drugs in this group, which have been used for many years to decrease the chances of rejection of transplanted organs, have been found to be effective in treating some individuals with serious organic symptoms of lupus. Because they are so powerful and potentially dangerous, they are usually used if other milder drugs are not effective or if the disease appears to be aggressive. Some doctors feel that using immunosuppressants can reduce the need for steroids. Examples of immunosuppressants used for lupus include Imuran (azathioprine), Cytoxan (cyclophosphamide), and Rheumatrex (methotrexate). CellCept (mycophenolate mofetil) is a more recent addition to the arsenal of immunosuppressive drugs used with lupus. It has shown benefit primarily in dealing with symptoms such as lupus nephritis (kidney problems), is comparable to Cytoxan in effectiveness, and may be less toxic.

Immunosuppressants are used to suppress the effectiveness of the body's immune system. For example, if Kenny Kidneyfailure needed an organ transplant, his immune system normally would reject the new organ because it was foreign to his body. That wouldn't help poor old Kenny, so he would receive dosages of immunosuppressants designed to decrease the chances that his immune system would reject the transplant. What does Kenny's situation have to do with lupus? The rejection process seems to be very similar to what happens in lupus, where the antibodies are fighting or rejecting healthy cells. So, if these drugs slow down the rejection process, they may reduce the harmful immune system activity that occurs in lupus. They may also fight some of the rebelling white blood cells that are the villains in lupus.

Side Effects

There are inherent dangers in taking immunosuppressants. Since the immune system is being suppressed, it is less able to fight off infection or to protect your body from other possible problems. There may be a decreased production of cells by the bone marrow. As a result, there could be a drop in the platelet, red blood cell, or white blood cell counts. This can significantly lower your body's ability to resist infection. As you know, infections are very common in lupus, and potentially dangerous—physicians certainly don't want to make you even more vulnerable!

Other side effects of immunosuppressants include vomiting, nausea, diarrhea, and heartburn. Skin rashes, easy bruising and bleeding, hair loss, blood in the urine or stool, damage to the lungs, kidneys, and liver, and ulcers can also be a problem. Because birth defects are a risk, immunosuppressants must not be used immediately before or during pregnancy; your doctor will tell you when to stop immunosuppressants if you're trying to conceive. Both men and women with lupus are discouraged from using immunosuppressants prior to attempt at conception. If an unplanned pregnancy occurs while on immunosuppressants, speak to your doctor about discontinuing the medication as soon as is realistically possible. Finally, using immunosuppressive drugs may slightly increase your chances of developing certain cancers.

In addition, these drugs have been known to interact dangerously with many other drugs. Because of this, some physicians are still very wary about recommending immunosuppressants for people with lupus. However, other physicians feel they are justified in using immunosuppressants in life-threatening cases when steroids are just not doing the job.

THE BLISS OF BENLYSTA

Benlysta (belimumab) was approved with great fanfare in 2011. Why all the excitement? It was the first new medication approved specifically for the treatment of lupus in more than fifty years. (The last drugs approved by the FDA for use in treating lupus were aspirin in 1948, and corticosteroids and Plaquenil in 1955.)

How does Benlysta work? For people with lupus, a protein called BLys (which stands for B-lymphocyte stimulator) is naturally produced in the body and stimulates the immune system to produce antibodies that attack the body. Benlysta binds to BLys to prevent these antibodies from being produced. As a result, it was hoped that Benlysta will be effective in improving symptoms of lupus without adversely affecting the immune system in general. Benlysta was the first drug in a new category called *BLys-specific inhibitors*.

Researchers found that the drug can reduce the chances of lupus flares, reduce fatigue, reduce disease activity and lupus symptoms, reduce dependence on steroids, and improve quality of life for some people with moderate symptoms. The most common side effects experienced with Benlysta include headaches, infections (such as urinary tract and upper respiratory infections), and joint pain.

Here's the most important caution about Benlysta. It's brand-new! It is now in Phase 4 of clinical trials, meaning that results are still being accumulated even though the drug has been approved. So it's important to be realistic about the potential benefits of Benlysta, since it is not yet in widespread use and no long-term results have yet been accumulated. In addition, it has not shown improvement for all people with lupus, especially those with more severe symptoms of the disease, and may not work with all ethnic groups. Another potential problem is the cost. Initially, Benlysta is administered as an intravenous infusion every twenty-eight days. First estimates were that Benlysta might cost about $35,000 per year. As you can imagine, insurance companies may not be thrilled about that, and may make it more difficult for patients to get reimbursed for it. Therefore, at least at this point, Benlysta should not be looked at as a miracle, just something to watch and be hopeful about. Keep this in mind when discussing it with your doctor.

Caution!

There is always the chance that certain drugs, including over-the-counter ones, may not be appropriate in your lupus treatment program—even if they are good for others with different health problems. There are certain drugs you should not use because of the possibility of aggravating the symptoms of lupus or causing flares.

There are two types of medications that should *not* be taken by people with lupus:

1. Sulfa drugs or drugs that are related to this group
2. Drugs that you have had an allergic reaction to in the past

Other drugs, such as penicillin derivatives, or some of the drugs that are used to control epilepsy, may present problems (possibly causing what is called drug-induced lupus). You've heard this a lot already, but it's important: Check with your doctor! Question, learn, and help yourself. Consult with your physician before taking even the most innocent over-the-counter drug. You never know when you might have an adverse reaction.

In addition, be careful about bad mixes. This is so important that it bears repeating. For example, provolone cheese and medication for high blood pressure may not mix! Tranquilizers and alcohol should never be taken at the same time. Do not consume alcohol with acetaminophen or narcotics. There are plenty of other such cautions. Many of these incompatibilities could have extremely dangerous outcomes: by making your symptoms worse, interfering with the action of the prescribed medication, or causing additional problems. By working closely with your physician, you will be helping to make sure that all the medications you take are appropriate for you. Again, don't hesitate to ask questions!

Work with Your Pharmacist

It is almost impossible for any physician to keep up with all the thousands of different types of prescription drugs on the market. However, this is the pharmacist's specialty. Frequently, pharmacists know even more than physicians as far as what drugs can go together and what drugs interact dangerously. So it can be very helpful for you to have a good working relationship with your local pharmacist. Not only will your pharmacist be able to tell you about the medication that has been prescribed for you, but he may also be able to help you reduce costs. Occasionally, generic products that cost less than their brand-name counterparts may be available. There may be nothing wrong with this, but make sure you consult your physician before making such a substitution. In some individuals, generic drugs may not work as well as the brand-name medication. If you have a good relationship with your pharmacist, you will find it a lot easier to get the medication you need.

You may find that dealing with the same drugstore and pharmacist is very comforting. The more time you spend there, the better the pharmacist will get to know you and your specific case. You'll have somebody else looking out for your welfare in addition to your physician!

Additional Medication 'Minders

Once you've begun a medication program, make sure you let your physician know how effective the drugs are in helping you with your condition. Any significant changes in your health, whether good or bad, should be reported to your physician. In this way, your doctor will be best able to decide whether to keep prescribing the medication you're taking.

Keep track of everything you're taking—in detail. Put together a list of all the medications you are taking, and keep it with you at all times (well, maybe not when you take a shower). Keep it on your computer as well. This will make it much easier to access for future reference. You will then be able to show the list to your doctor, your pharmacist, or anyone else who needs to know what drugs you're taking. As previously mentioned, certain drugs are chemically incompatible with one another or may be incompatible with other aspects of your treatment. This is another reason that it is essential to have a comprehensive list of everything you take.

If you find that you're having trouble remembering to take your medication—or if you're sometimes unsure if you've already taken a dose—find ways to keep track of your medication schedule. For instance, you might be able to use your list of medications to prepare a daily chart that lists each dose separately, allowing you to check off each one as you take it. You might also purchase a multicompartment pill box, which can store a week's worth of drugs, divided into appropriate days and times. Some sophisticated devices even sound an alarm when the time comes for you to pop your pill! Use the alarm on your cell phone (since you usually keep it with you, right?) to remind you to take your medications—as well as which ones. Many cell phone alarms can be programmed to signal you on a daily basis, in fact several times each day if necessary. Shut the alarm off after you have taken each medication.

Make sure you take care of your medications. Store them properly (for example, don't keep them in the refrigerator unless indicated), and keep them away from children and pets. Keep them in a comfortable environment. For example, if it's too warm for you, it's probably not good for your pills, either! Watch those expiration dates, and renew your prescriptions far enough in advance that you don't go through days (or more) without them.

You may experience certain emotional reactions from some medications, such as depression or anger. Remember to learn how to cope with these responses before they adversely influence your physical and emotional well-being. Mention any emotional reactions to your doctor, who may suggest the need to change medications or dosages. If necessary, refer to the chapters in this book on coping with emotions. If the suggested strategies don't provide relief, by all means seek out a qualified professional who can help you become more comfortable with any side effects you may be experiencing as a result of your treatment plan.

A Final Prescription

This chapter doesn't include all medications used by people with lupus. Instead, it emphasizes the more common ones. And by the time you read this book, there may be additional drugs on the market that are far superior to the ones you've been taking. But at least this information will help you become more familiar with the ones you may hear about. There is nothing wrong with discussing your medication with your physician, asking if new drugs are available. But remember, this doesn't mean that these drugs will necessarily be better for you. And if your doctor prescribes something new, ask about it. Then, if your new medication makes you feel better, you'll know why!

Hopefully, the information presented in this chapter has given you a good idea of what you must know in order to use medication as safely and effectively as possible.

11.

DIET AND NUTRITION

Food, glorious food! Or is it, "Food, who needs food?" Are you eating less now and enjoying it less? Proper diet is an important part of a comprehensive treatment program for lupus. It is necessary to nourish your body and maintain as much strength and vitality as you can. It is especially important if you have any nutritional needs related to some of the symptoms or problems that may develop during your life with lupus (such as kidney problems, osteoporosis, or high blood pressure). Good nutrition is a powerful way to improve health.

Some people with lupus experience a reduction in appetite. Along with this may come a desired (or undesired) weight loss. However, not everybody with lupus experiences this. Some people with lupus find themselves eating more and, of course, gaining more weight. Steroids may also increase appetite. In addition, steroids used to control symptoms of lupus may frequently result in a bloating side effect with swelling of the face and body.

But don't put all of the blame on lupus or your medication! Your weight may increase or decrease, and your appetite may change, but these fluctuations may have nothing to do with lupus. It's easy to blame anything that is happening on lupus. Some people, physicians included, tend to do this. But perhaps your weight is fluctuating because of binges over the weekend! Maybe you've gone to some food orgies! You may reason that you're probably just retaining water (an abused excuse!). Maybe emotional crises have caused you to overeat. One of the most important things you can do to help stay as healthy as possible is to eat properly and keep your weight at a proper level.

Why is nutrition so important, and what exactly is a good diet? Let's learn more about the role that diet plays in helping you to maximize your health.

Can a Particular Diet Help Lupus?

Is there any particular diet that is most appropriate for lupus? The answer is a resounding no! At this time, there is no specific "lupus cure diet." Most people with lupus do not require special diets; however, it's important to maintain a nutritionally sound and well-balanced diet. A proper diet ensures that we consume all of the necessary vitamins, minerals, and supplements. However, if your doctor feels it would be helpful for you, it may be suggested that you try a reducing diet, salt-free diet, or low-protein diet, or combination of the three. If you have kidney involvement, a salt-free, low-protein diet may be helpful in minimizing water retention and controlling your blood pressure.

It is best to avoid high-fat diets, not because they'll cause lupus flares (they probably won't), but because they're just not nutritionally sound. You need a nutritionally balanced diet to maintain proper health. Lupus causes you enough problems already without your adding an unbalanced diet to the picture!

Determine any foods that make you feel drained of energy, bloated, or that give you some other unpleasant side effects, and limit the amount you eat. The most common ones are cow's milk products, food preservatives and artificial colors, wheat, chocolate, eggs, citrus fruits, and foods containing salicylates (such as apples, cherries, grapes, peaches, eggplant, broccoli, tea, and coffee). But that doesn't mean you *can't* have any of these foods. Discuss it with your doctor. Eating healthfully, and eating in moderation, is always a good goal.

One type of food that has received some favorable reviews is fish. Fish oil has been found to be helpful as an anti-inflammatory. But it's healthier to have several fish meals each week than to just take fish oil capsules, because of the number of capsules necessary and the possibility of some stomach irritation resulting from them. Be aware, however, that fish oil may interfere with the function of blood thinners. So make sure you discuss this with your doctor. One type of food to avoid is alfalfa sprouts, which have been known to trigger lupus flares! Avoid natural supplements containing alfalfa, as well.

If you have lupus, you may occasionally experience certain nutritional deficiencies. During a flare-up, your body may use up certain nutrients at a faster rate than it normally would. This may lead to your feeling more fatigued and tired than usual. Therefore, your physician may suggest that you supplement your diet in order to make up for these deficiencies. However, this does not mean that dietary changes or nutritional supplements are going to eliminate or cure your lupus! Lupus is not caused by dietary deficiencies; nonetheless, eating a well-balanced diet is an important part of a complete treatment program.

There are some important dietary recommendations that all people should follow. Consider those of the United States Department of Agriculture (USDA). If you remember the original "four basic food groups," which heavily emphasized the importance of meat, poultry, and dairy, note that the USDA now recommends a complex-carbohydrate, low-fat, high-fiber diet. The government has made it clear that whole grains, fruits, and vegetables are the basics of a good diet. Of lesser importance is the dairy group and the meat, poultry, and fish group. Fats, oils, and sweets, the USDA states, should be used only sparingly.

Why Is Nutrition So Important?

Nutrition is the process of eating appropriate amounts of nutrients and using them to meet energy needs, to accomplish body-sustaining healing, and to satisfy maintenance requirements. The human body is very complex, but it can heal itself if you provide it with proper nourishment and care. If you do not give your body the proper nutrients, you can actually impair its normal functions and cause yourself harm. Here are just some of the benefits a sound diet may provide for the person with lupus:

- A body that is well-nourished is stronger than a poorly nourished one. So proper nourishment helps the body fight infection, heal itself, and thrive.
- A good diet actually helps people respond better to lupus treatment and makes them more resistant to treatment side effects.
- Good nutrition provides good energy, so important because of the potential energy-zapping effects of lupus.
- A balanced diet increases the speed at which body tissues heal themselves.
- Without proper nutrition, the body's stores of protein, fat, vitamins, and other nutrients may be depleted. A good diet ensures continuous healthy stores of these nutrients.
- Eating healthy foods actually reduces food cravings and the urge to binge.

It may never have been your desire to become a lay nutritionist. But now that you know how a sound diet may be beneficial, let's discuss some of the basics of nutrition, with the goal of understanding how what you eat can help your health.

Nutrition Basics

There are six types of nutrients that your body needs for survival. The first four basic nutrients—water, carbohydrates, fats, and proteins—are called *macronutrients*, because your body requires them daily in large amounts in order to function properly. Water is the most essential macronutrient in maintaining life, even though it contains no energy in the form of calories. Carbohydrates (which supply the energy that your body needs to function each day), fats, and proteins supply your body with energy and serve as the building blocks for growth and repair.

The final two—vitamins and minerals—are known as *micronutrients*, because they are needed in relatively small amounts in the body when compared with the macronutrients. Although micronutrients are not considered a source of energy, they are necessary for normal body growth, maintenance, and tissue repair.

It's always better to eat a variety of whole foods so that you get all of the macro- and micronutrients that you need naturally through dietary sources, instead of having to depend on nutritional supplements to make up the difference. Food processing—including refining, enriching, hydrogenating, preserving, and irradiating—can destroy a percentage of the nutrient content of foods. None of these processes enhances the food nutritionally. And, because these processes actually result in considerable loss of nutrients, diets that include too much of these foods supply only the bare minimum of nutrients necessary for survival. So you're better off choosing foods that have undergone minimal—if any—food processing.

Let's discuss the main nutrients in more detail.

CARBOHYDRATES

The primary role of carbohydrates is to supply the energy that your body needs to function each day. Carbohydrates are divided into two groups— simple carbohydrates and complex carbohydrates. Simple carbohydrates, sometimes called simple sugars, consist mainly of single sugar molecules, and are found mainly in sugar and in fruits. Complex carbohydrates are contained in vegetables, as well as whole grains, beans, and legumes. These carbohydrates are made up of long, complex chains of sugars. Therefore, complex carbohydrates take longer to break down than simple sugars. They have to be digested in the stomach and intestine, where they are broken down into single sugar molecules that are more easily absorbed.

Fiber is a complex carbohydrate that your body cannot digest and absorb for energy. However, dietary fiber helps the intestines to function efficiently and aids absorption of sugars into the bloodstream. It also binds bile acids, cholesterol, carcinogens, and other harmful substances. In other words, fiber is good for removing certain toxins from the body. Fiber-rich diets also promote a feeling of fullness by adding bulk to meals—without adding calories. Because the refining process removes much of the natural fiber from our foods, our diet lacks this important substance. Fortunately, it's easy—and delicious—to add more fiber to your diet every day. High-fiber cereals are one of the best sources. Also good are brown rice, whole-grain breads and pasta, bran, most fresh fruit, dried prunes, nuts, seeds, beans, unbuttered popcorn, and lentils. Raw vegetables, Brussels sprouts, broccoli, kale, and cabbage are also fiber-rich.

FATS

Lately, there has been a great deal of confusion concerning the place that fats have in the diet. Reports linking high-fat diets to illnesses such as heart disease, certain cancers, and diabetes have driven some people to reduce the fat in their diets to very low levels. However, the fact is that some amount of dietary fat is needed for your body to function properly. Besides being your body's most concentrated source of energy, with nine calories per gram, fat provides insulation, helps the cells in your body send signals to communicate with other cells, and acts as a protective padding for your bones and internal organs. Fats are also components of all cell membranes.

Fat is stored and used as a reserve for energy, so the body always has a backup source of "fuel" when other nutrients, such as carbohydrates, are running low. For example, when insulin levels drop or if carbohydrate intake drops, fat becomes the main source of energy. Unfortunately, the typical American diet includes too much total fat, so that excess fat is stored in the adipose (fat) tissues of the body. A high intake of the wrong kinds of fats can cause blood vessels to become clogged, increasing the risk of heart disease and stroke. And a high-fat diet can lead to obesity.

How, exactly, can you reduce the fat in your diet? Limit your consumption of red meat to about once every ten days, and eat only lean cuts. Any dairy products that you consume should be nonfat, or lactose-free if necessary. And, as much as possible, eliminate saturated oils and fats, including butter, margarine, lard, and vegetable oils. When oils can't be totally avoided, use only small amounts of polyunsaturated oils, such as corn oil and safflower oil or use olive oil, peanut oil, or canola oil, which are monounsaturated. Get to know the good fats—such as omega-6 fatty acids found in foods such as pumpkin seeds, pistachio nuts, wheat germ, primrose oil, and borage oil; omega-3 oils found in food such as flaxseed oil, walnuts, salmon, and mackerel; and omega-9 oils (a *nonessential fatty acid* as opposed to omega-3 and omega-6, which are essential fatty acids) found in food such as extra virgin olive oil. Speak to your physician or nutritionist to learn more about how to include this in your diet, and in what amounts.

Let's take a closer look at two kinds of fat found in the diet and in the body: triglycerides and cholesterol.

TRIGLYCERIDES

There are three major types of triglycerides found in the diet and in the body—saturated, polyunsaturated, and monounsaturated.

Saturated fats tend to be solid at room temperature. They are found mainly in animal products, including butter, lard, whole milk, cream, sour cream, cheese, and fatty meats. A diet high in saturated fat can significantly raise blood cholesterol levels, so these fats are considered to be the "bad" fats.

Polyunsaturated fats are generally liquid at room temperature and are found in corn, soybean, safflower, and sunflower oils. Although these fats have been shown to reduce total blood cholesterol, they may also lower the level of the "good" high-density lipoprotein (HDL) cholesterol (see Cholesterol, below). Polyunsaturated fats are healthier than saturated fats, but not as healthy as monounsaturated fats, which lower the "bad" low-density lipo-protein (LDL) cholesterol without affecting HDL cholesterol. Olive, peanut, and canola oils have high amounts of monounsaturates, and so do almonds, cashews, peanuts, and pistachios.

CHOLESTEROL

Cholesterol is a fatty substance that has many important functions through-out the body, especially in the creation, maintenance, and repair of cell membranes. It is also used in the formation of hormones such as estrogen, testosterone, progesterone, and cortisol. In the brain and spinal cord, cho-lesterol serves as part of the insulation that covers nerve cells and keeps nerve signals going to the right locations. Most of the cholesterol in the human body is produced by its own cells, particularly the cells of the liver.

Unfortunately, too many people eat diets overloaded with fat and calories and, as a result, get far more of these substances than their bodies can pos-sibly use. Simply put, too much dietary cholesterol in the blood can create some serious problems. And eating too many foods that contain saturated fats compounds this problem, since these types of fats can increase over-all blood cholesterol. Excess cholesterol can clog and harden the arteries, increasing the likelihood of heart disease and stroke.

There are two different types of cholesterol—high-density lipoprotein (HDL) cholesterol and low-density lipoprotein (LDL) cholesterol. HDL cho-lesterol is often called "good" cholesterol, because it is believed to protect the body by transporting fats, or lipids, through the body. LDL cholesterol, on the other hand, is referred to as "bad" cholesterol, since it tends to deposit fats in the body, increasing the risk of atherosclerosis and other cardiovascular diseases.

PROTEINS

Protein is necessary for growth and development, and is essential in the repair of cells. All proteins are made up of structural units called amino acids. Of the more than twenty amino acids that have been identified, nine are considered essential amino acids, which cannot be manufactured by the body. Essen-tial amino acids, therefore, must be obtained from dietary sources. Complete proteins are proteins that contain all of the nine essential amino acids in suf-ficient amounts for adequate growth, development, and cellular repair.

To some extent, amino acids are converted to glucose and may increase blood glucose levels—but not by much and not quickly. The body tends to spare protein as a source of energy because of the nutrient's importance in growth and development, and its role in the production of hormones, anti-bodies, enzymes, and body tissues. As such, the body uses mostly carbo-hydrates and fats for energy, and relies more on protein as the other energy sources are depleted.

Many experts believe that there is more than enough protein in the aver-age American diet, so it's not essential to increase protein intake. In fact, too much protein may be unhealthy, because a high-protein diet tends to put added strain on the kidneys. However, it is important to remember that adequate protein intake is important for a balanced diet.

Good sources of proteins include milk products, poultry, seafood, beef, pork, eggs, peanut butter, and legumes. Smaller amounts of the nutrient are contained in nuts, vegetables, grains, and whole-grain bread.

VITAMINS, MINERALS, AND NATURAL FOOD SUPPLEMENTS

Vitamins are essential to life. They help regulate metabolism and assist the biochemical processes that release energy from digested food. Vitamins are organic (carbon-containing) substances that occur naturally in plants and animals. Generally speaking, our bodies cannot manufacture vitamins, so we must obtain most of these nutrients from the foods we eat or from vitamin supplements.

Every living cell depends on minerals for proper function and structure. Minerals are needed to properly compose body fluids, form blood and bone, maintain healthy nerve function, and regulate muscle tone. Whereas vitamins are organic substances, minerals are inorganic substances, meaning that they are not bound to carbon. Minerals originate in soil and water, and they are absorbed by the plants that are eaten by the animals that make up the human diet.

Both vitamins and minerals can function as coenzymes in the body—that is, they "help" the enzymes that promote all of the body's biochemical processes, including nerve transmission, muscle contraction, blood formation, protein metabolism, and energy production. In addition, they help build strong bones and teeth and are necessary for the manufacture of hemoglobin, the oxygen-carrying component of blood.

Antioxidants are micronutrients that may help protect against a variety of diseases, including heart disease and cancer. Some well-known antioxidants include vitamins C and E, and the mineral selenium. These nutrients seem to work by protecting body cells from damage that can be caused by factors such as cigarette smoke, toxic chemicals, and environmental pollution. There is still much to learn about antioxidants and how they function in the body, and scientists are continuing to study the effects of these potentially beneficial nutrients.

A healthy intake of vitamins and minerals is important for everybody. If you eat a good variety of nutritious foods—including fresh fruits and vegetables, fiber-rich cereals and grains, and lean cuts of meat—then you're probably getting all of the vitamins and minerals you need to be healthy. There's little scientific evidence to prove that taking in extra amounts of micronutrients, such as through supplementation, can help improve your lupus. In fact, as important as vitamins and minerals are for health, you need to be prudent about your intake, since some nutrients—such as vitamin A and iron—can actually *cause* health problems when taken in high doses.

If you think that you may not be getting all of the micronutrients you need from dietary sources alone, make an appointment with a dietitian. He or she will be able to educate you about the benefits and possible risks of taking nutritional supplements. Always let your dietitian know what you are already taking; some nutritional supplements can interact with certain drugs and can cause potentially dangerous adverse effects. Also, make sure that your supplement plan is customized to fit your age, sex, and medical needs.

Let's discuss a few specifics. The vitamin B complex is particularly important. This nutrient group helps prevent fluid retention. The B complex, as well as vitamin E and vitamin C with bioflavonoids, helps to reduce the severity of internal inflammation and inhibit prostaglandin production. Some believe that taking a multivitamin supplement or individual doses of these vitamins can be helpful, even if you do follow a healthy diet. Minerals such as iron, calcium, magnesium, and zinc are also important. For example, your doctor may recommend iron supplements if you have been diagnosed with anemia. However, you should take iron only under a health care professional's supervision. If you are taking medication that contributes to loss of bone density, you should ask your doctor about taking a calcium, magnesium, and vitamin D formulation. You should also ask about minerals, such as magnesium and zinc, that may help to reduce inflammation and pain.

If you have high blood pressure, you've probably heard a lot about sodium. Our bodies need some amount of this essential mineral. Sodium helps transport nutrients into cells, so they can be used for energy production, as well as for tissue growth and repair. In addition, it helps maintain the volume and balance of all fluids outside the body's cells, including blood. Unfortunately, too many people include too much sodium in their diets every day. Because high blood pressure can exacerbate certain lupus complications (such as lupus nephritis), it's prudent to keep your sodium intake to a minimum. This is not as simple as limiting your intake of table salt, however.

There are many foods that naturally contain salt or sodium, and many foods use salt in their preparation, including frankfurters, luncheon meats, and canned vegetables.

Some studies have shown that diets rich in calcium, potassium, and magnesium can help reduce blood pressure. So you can see how a healthy, balanced diet—in combination with exercise and moderate weight loss—can be very beneficial in lowering blood pressure and keeping your cardiovascular system strong.

Remember, some physicians are not knowledgeable about vitamins, minerals, and dietary supplements that may help with lupus symptoms. Some people prefer to find a practitioner who specializes in these areas. Be sure to keep your physician informed of whatever alternative therapies you decide to use.

HERBS

What about taking herbs if you have lupus? Some people believe that certain herbs, used in conjunction with diet, can promote health and well-being for people with lupus. For example, black currant oil, ginger, feverfew, and turmeric are known to have anti-inflammatory results. There may be some incompatibilities, though, so make sure you discuss any herbs you're considering with your doctor. Echinacea is another example of an herb that should be avoided because of its tendency to boost the activity of the immune system. So if you are considering including herbs in your program, make sure you clear this with your physician. You may also want to work with a certified nutritionist who has worked with people with lupus. (You can find more about herbs in Chapter 21.)

AVOID HARMFUL "NONFOODS"

In addition to some of the foods you may be eating, a number of nonfoods—additives, pesticides, hormones and steroids, alcohol, caffeine, and tobacco—can also be hazardous to your health. Let's take a brief look at each of these and why they should be eliminated from your diet.

ARTIFICIAL ADDITIVES

Believe it or not, the average American diet includes 5,000 or more artificial additives used to maintain freshness and to preserve the attractive look or taste of food. While some of these additives are safe, we don't yet know if any may be linked to lupus. Other additives have not yet undergone sufficient studies to determine their safety. For example, monosodium glutamate (MSG) and aspartame are used without warnings, but have been known to cause a wide range of problems, including gastrointestinal upset, bloating, and diarrhea. Cyclamate and saccharine are examples of additives once deemed safe but later banned or allowed to be used only if accompanied by warnings.

What can you do to eliminate all—or, at least, many—of these chemicals from your diet? Obviously, additives are most common in processed foods—canned, frozen, and prepackaged. Avoid these foods whenever you can. Instead, eat whole foods that are as close as possible to their natural state. When you do buy prepared items, choose those that have been made without additives. In addition, don't eat smoked foods (such as bacon or lunchmeats), which contain some of the most harmful processing chemicals used.

PESTICIDES AND OTHER HARMFUL SUBSTANCES

Like additives, the pesticides used to control weeds and pests are abundant in your diet. These chemicals are found in meat, poultry, fish, dairy products, vegetables, fruits, coffee—virtually all of your foods. Many pesticides are banned in the United States, but reach us through produce grown in other countries.

How can you avoid these harmful additives? Well, unless you eat only organic food that has been grown in pesticide-free soil, you consume these potentially harmful substances every day. Scrub or peel all fruits and vegetables, particularly waxed fruit. You can also clean produce with nontoxic rinsing preparations, available in health food stores. If possible, buy organically grown foods, and avoid imported produce. Animals raised for human consumption are often fed steroids and hormones to induce growth. To reduce their effect, buy meats that are certified drug-free and eat less meat, eggs, and dairy products. Finally, be aware that a diet high in fiber and antioxidants can help eliminate pesticides and other harmful substances from your body.

ALCOHOL

Excessive alcohol consumption can exacerbate some of the problems associated with any illness. For example, if you are taking medications that may lead to loss of bone density, you should avoid alcohol because it can add to this loss. Alcohol is also contraindicated with many medications, especially the ones taken by many people for pain, such as aspirin, NSAIDs, and narcotics. If you have problems sleeping, you should also avoid alcohol in the evening and before bed.

Is it necessary to avoid all alcohol? There's no simple answer to this question. However, it does seem wise to reduce your consumption of alcohol as much as possible. Many experts believe that one drink a day is a safe amount. Less is better. After all, you want to do all you can to make your body strong and healthy!

CAFFEINE

Like alcohol, caffeine—found in coffee, tea, cola, chocolate, and other foods—can affect people with lupus. For example, caffeine can contribute to loss of bone density. And it stands to reason that you should cut out caffeine if you have sleep problems.

Again, if you want to do everything possible to strengthen yourself, it makes sense to significantly reduce or eliminate consumption of products that contain this chemical. If you wish to drink coffee, make sure it is decaffeinated. And what should you drink in place of your coffee, tea, and caffeinated beverages? Your best bets are skim or soymilk, mineral water, unsweetened fruit juices, and vegetable juices. Besides eliminating harmful caffeine, most of these drinks take a further step toward improving your health by supplying valuable nutrients.

TOBACCO

Finally, we come to tobacco. By now you know that tobacco and secondhand smoke have been implicated in several life-threatening conditions, including cancer, heart disease, and stroke. Smoking also causes great damage to the immune system, and it, too, contributes to loss of bone density. For people with lupus, smoking can increase the effects of the disease on the heart and blood vessels. Chewing tobacco and snuff have been found to be just as harmful as cigars and cigarettes. Tobacco is also a stimulant and will cause sleep problems in many individuals. The list of reasons for you not to smoke is extensive. But you shouldn't need to read the list to know that you just should not smoke!

So in the case of tobacco, the best course of action is clear. By avoiding all tobacco—including secondhand smoke—you'll strengthen your body against not only lupus but also a number of other diseases. Look for ways to kick the habit, set a timetable, and do it!

Losing Weight

Weight control is very important for people with lupus. You'll certainly want to lose weight if you are overweight. Why? Added weight can put more pressure on joints such as the knees and hips (which bear much of the body's weight), worsening pain and increasing stiffness and inflammation.

"WEIGHS" TO LOSE WEIGHT

There are practically as many programs to lose weight as there are people needing to lose weight. Some of them are very healthy and can be implemented into your routine (with the approval of your health care team). Others, however, should be avoided because they may simply not be healthy. No matter what program you use, it is essential to work on modifying your eating routine. And make sure that your health care team approves any program that you are considering.

Some people just need to maintain their weight by adjusting their caloric intake and including moderate exercise in their routines. Others need to lose weight and want to reduce calories and increase exercise.

You may choose to work with a dietitian to set up weight loss goals and an eating plan that will best help you to achieve your goals, especially if you have a lot of weight to lose. But any plan should take time. In many cases,

a strict weight loss program is not necessary (and sometimes is more difficult to follow for the duration). A well-balanced, nutritional, common-sense
approach to eating is the best way to do this. Don't try to lose weight too
quickly. You want to develop an eating plan that you can comfortably live
with for the rest of your life.

Getting Started

Now you know why a good diet, although it won't cure your disease, is such
a valuable part of a comprehensive treatment program. So it's time to get
started to make the changes necessary to create the healthiest diet possible!
Here are some suggestions:

- Keep a food diary and record everything you eat. This will give you a
  realistic look at your present diet and will suggest ways in which you can
  make improvements.
- Decrease the amount of fat you eat by limiting meat intake and increasing
  fresh fruits, vegetables, and whole grains.
- Decrease your consumption of dairy foods, and make sure that the ones
  you do eat are nonfat.
- Eat all foods in a form that is as close as possible to their natural state.
  This will maximize their vitamin, mineral, and fiber content, and minimize
  additives.
- When possible, eat organically grown produce. When this isn't available,
  be sure to scrub or peel fruits and vegetables to eliminate some of the
  pesticides. Always peel waxed produce.
- Do what you can to avoid harmful nonfoods—including additives, pesticides, hormones, caffeine, alcohol, and tobacco. While you may not be
  able to avoid all of these substances all the time, by cutting down on them
  as much as possible, you'll be doing a great deal to improve your overall
  health.
- Avoid "empty" calorie or "junk" foods. Cookies, potato chips, and candy,
  for instance, have little or no nutritional value, and may keep you from

eating vitamin- and fiber-rich foods. In addition, many of these foods are laden with fat.

- To help ensure an adequate intake of vitamins and minerals—especially the antioxidants—add certain ones to your dietary program. Speak to your doctor or a nutritionist about the ones that would be best for you.

- Discuss with your health care professionals the possibility of taking herbs and natural nutritional supplements to correct imbalances or deficiencies, alleviate some of your symptoms, or ease certain medication side effects.

- Eat regularly. If digestion is regular and frequent, your blood sugars won't fluctuate wildly and you'll enjoy greater energy and fewer mood swings. Frequent smaller meals may be the answer.

- Drink plenty of fluids. Aim for eight to ten glasses of water each day. It will help flush out your system, assist in absorption of nutrients, and improve your overall nutritional balance and skin tone. It will also help you to feel full.

- Include physical activity in any dietary program. Besides toning your body, exercise before a meal can help stimulate your appetite. (See Chapter 12 for more about exercise.)

- If you're suffering from nausea or loss of appetite, try eating frequent, smaller meals.

- Eat when you are hungry and stop when you are full, knowing that you can eat whenever you need to.

- Eat slowly and enjoy your food fully.

- Consider the fact that your appetite may vary based on how you feel on any given day. During times when you're feeling better, make sure that you eat all the nutrient-packed foods you can to compensate for those times when you don't feel well.

- Stay informed! Knowing more about any discovered connections between diet and lupus will help you to make healthy dietary changes.

Before modifying your diet, be sure to speak to your physician or a qualified nutritionist who can offer guidance on what changes are right for you. A good nutritionist understands the biochemistry of your body and will recommend ways to balance it through the use of foods as well as vitamins, minerals, and other dietary supplements. Be sure to ask if your lupus treatment has any effect on the body's supply of vitamins and minerals. Also keep in mind that, although proper diet is an important part of any treatment program—and is almost totally within your control—it is one of the most frequently ignored adjuncts to treatment. Nutrition should not be an alternative therapy. It is fundamental to everything else you do for your body. While it is sometimes difficult to eat the right foods, isn't it encouraging to know that when you do, your cells can change? Don't think that you have to completely change all at once. Start by eating more whole grains, beans, and vegetables for a month. Try to reduce meat, dairy products, caffeine, and refined foods. Or eliminate all dairy products for at least one month. Then evaluate how you feel and how your body responds.

It may be difficult for you to change your eating habits, but once you begin to eliminate any harmful products and increase your intake of nutrient-rich foods, you're sure to feel healthier and more energetic. And you'll benefit from the peace of mind that comes from doing everything you can to help yourself.

A Culinary Conclusion

Because diet is on everybody's mind these days, it garners a lot of attention in the media. You may hear of miracle remedies involving certain types of dietary modifications that are "destined" to cure your physical symptoms. Unfortunately, no diet has yet been invented that can do any such thing. Be wary of any diet, pushed by an "expert," that claims that the diet, all by itself, will cure your lupus. Even though research is constantly exploring the possible effects of dietary factors on lupus (as well as other diseases), not enough information has yet been obtained to know whether certain diets can really help, or how to best implement any such diet.

So what's the moral? By understanding basics about nutrition and meal plans, not only will you eat a well-balanced healthy diet, but you'll be doing more to help yourself cope with lupus. Accordingly, eat healthy, eat properly, eat in moderation, and enjoy!

12.

EXERCISE

A very important component in your effort to live more comfortably with lupus is exercise. The proper type and amount of exercise is something to discuss with your physician, since no two people have the same needs. But let's discuss exercise and how it can help you in your life with lupus.

Exercise is an important component of your treatment program for lupus. It is essential for improving your emotional and physical well-being. The right types and amounts of exercise can help you break the fatigue-rest-fatigue cycle and make you feel better in countless other ways. But remember the importance of maintaining a proper balance between rest and exercise. Too much exercise may increase the amount of pain and inflammation in your joints, doing more harm than good. This proper balance varies from person to person and can best be determined by your physician or physical therapist. However, only by trial and error can you really determine whether you are exercising or resting in the proper amounts.

Try to participate in activities that emphasize good muscle tone, rather than build muscle bulk. For example, walking or swimming is better exercise than weightlifting! It's also a good idea to have a regular exercise program, rather than exercising whenever "the spirit moves you"! (After all, what if the spirit just disappears?) All it takes is commitment and motivation to adopt a regular exercise program. Whatever your exercise choice, be sure it's something you enjoy doing. There are many different kinds of exercise that you can try, so it should be easy to find an activity that you like and that is comfortable for you.

Maybe you've been motivated to start exercising, only to find that your motivation quickly dissipated. Or maybe you've put off starting a workout program altogether. It's easy to find excuses not to exercise. How many times have you talked yourself out of exercising by falling back on the old stand-bys: "I'm too tired," or "I don't have time today," or even "It probably won't work, anyway"? That's not uncommon. However, it's important to realize that regular physical activity is an important part of your treatment program, and it's an aspect that you can't afford to neglect—for your health's sake.

Next, you'll learn about the many benefits of exercise, and see how you—with the help of your physician or other health care professional—can design your own personal exercise program.

BENEFITS OF EXERCISE

Exercise is important for everyone, but can be very helpful for people who have lupus. Some of the benefits of exercise include:

- Better muscle tone
- Stronger and more stabilized joints
- Improved mobility
- Improved cardiorespiratory fitness
- Improved weight control
- Improved body image
- Reduced stress
- Less depression and anxiety
- Better mental efficiency
- More relaxation
- Less fatigue
- Stronger bones—increased bone thickness and mass
- Stronger muscles
- Improved flexibility and coordination
- Reduced chance of injury
- More restful sleep
- Higher self-esteem

Don't you wish it did all this instantly? If you don't already exercise regularly, now's the time to start! Exercise can keep your body trim. And for best health, you should keep your muscles firm, firm, firm, which is better than flabby, flabby, flabby! Exercise benefits your cardiovascular and digestive systems by helping them work more efficiently. As a result, someone who participates in regular exercise usually has more energy, has fewer physical complaints, and sleeps better than a more sedentary person. Is that all? Nope! Exercise can also reduce pain and make you feel less fatigued. Some people actually find that exercise can help them to recover from a lupus flare. (Make sure you speak to your doctor for guidance in this area.) It has even been named as the closest thing to a "magic bullet" for maintaining youth and optimal health when used in combination with proper nutrition.

Exercise is as important for your state of mind as it is for your body. Sure, you'll feel better physically—and you'll like what you see, too! Your self-esteem is sure to get a boost when you start to notice the results of your commitment to exercise. And working out can help relieve stress and tension, and ease feelings of depression, anger, fear, and frustration. (For many people, exercise is more calming than a tranquilizer, and it has no untoward side effects.) Through exercise, you can let off steam, relieve any boredom and frustration, and clear your mind. In fact, all of the emotions that may be troubling you—depression, anger, fear, and anxiety among them—can be controlled, either wholly or partially, through exercise. Exercise can also help you to enjoy deep sleep, so you'll be able to face each day fully rested. And if that's not enough of a lure, unless you exercise alone, your exercise program will lead to some healthy social interactions—which are always good for the mind!

SO, WHY AREN'T YOU EXERCISING?

Considering all the good things that exercise does, you may wonder why everybody isn't out there doing it. Well, many people feel that exercise is, at best, extremely boring and, at worst, very unpleasant. Only a small percentage of people really and truly enjoy regular exercise. (Are you one of them?) So the best approach is to focus on exercises—and environments—that are as pleasant as possible! This will enable you to more easily keep your commitment to your exercise program.

Then again, some people may avoid exercise not because of a lack of desire, but because they find it so tiring. Or they're in so much pain that they either can't exercise or fear that it will increase their pain. Or perhaps they are afraid that exercise may cause additional problems. While these feelings are understandable, as we've mentioned before, as you become less and less active, your fatigue will only increase. Why? Because of deconditioning. Deconditioning—the result of inactivity—causes your muscles to grow weaker and weaker over time, giving you less and less energy. What are the symptoms of deconditioning? Shortness of breath, rapid heartbeat, and increased fatigue are the most common signs.

Guess what? Deconditioning can gradually be reduced. How? Through exercise! By embarking on a gradually building exercise program, you can slowly increase your ability to participate in these activities.

TYPES OF EXERCISE

Exercise can be divided into two categories—*aerobic* and *anaerobic.* Aerobic exercises are vigorous exercises that require the body to use increased amounts of oxygen, which makes your heart and lungs work harder and keeps your cardiovascular system in peak operating condition. Fast walking, running, swimming, dancing, step aerobics, and bicycling are examples of aerobic exercise. When you engage in these types of activities, your muscles become more attuned to burning fat, and they will increase their fat-burning activity at rest.

Anaerobic exercise requires shorter bursts of activity that can build strength, increase flexibility, and improve muscle tone and coordination. One good example of anaerobic activity is strength training, which makes the muscles work against resistance. Strength training—for example, weightlifting or pushups—is the most effective type of exercise you can do to build and maintain muscle mass.

Another way of classifying exercises is into the following categories: range of motion, muscle strengthening, positioning or stretching, or endurance (or functional) exercises. Let's discuss these briefly.

RANGE-OF-MOTION EXERCISES

Range-of-motion exercises help maintain or increase a joint's complete movement by moving a body part as far as possible in every direction. Has lupus reduced the range of motion possible in any of your joints? If so, exercise may be able to stop that reduction. Just as important, it may be able to gradually increase the range of motion that is possible. Range-of-motion exercises stretch joints in various directions by manipulating the muscles attached to them. These exercises may be very helpful in preventing loss of motion, restoring lost movement, and reducing stiffness. They also help you to maintain normal movement in your joints. Like all types of exercises, range-of-motion routines can be learned through books and video, from health care professionals, or from the staff of your local gym.

MUSCLE-STRENGTHENING EXERCISES

Some exercises are important because they build up strength in the muscles or other tissues that support the joints and keep them stable. These exercises also help maintain the strength that you already have.

There are two types of strengthening (or muscle-tightening) exercises that may be helpful for you: isometric exercises and resistive exercises. Isometrics are strengthening exercises that do not involve any movement within the joints. In these exercises, you strongly tighten the muscle but do not move the joint. These involve pushing one immovable force against another. As a result, strength can be improved without further stressing the joints. Trying to pull your hands apart after firmly clasping them together and pushing the palm of one hand against the palm of the other are both isometrics. Isometric exercises are convenient in that they can be done anywhere—in the car, in a chair, even in bed. And although you won't be moving around, you'll still be giving your muscles a great workout.

Resistive exercises actively move the joint against a resistance such as a weight or against another object. Because there is less chance of stressing an already fragile joint, isometric exercises are usually considered safer than resistive exercises.

Where can you learn some appropriate muscle-strengthening exercises? Again, libraries, bookstores, video stores, websites, health care professionals, and your local gym are likely to be your best resources.

Positioning or Stretching Exercises

Positioning exercises can also be helpful, especially for the hips, knees, hands, shoulders, and back. By stretching your body into certain positions, you may be able to help keep these joints limber. Examples of positioning exercises include reaching a high spot on the door and stretching out your body.

If you are inactive and do not use your joints properly, you become less flexible and can even experience muscle spasms, cramps, and decreased flexibility. In fact, when joints are stiff, even the smallest motion can cause pain. If pain immobilizes a joint, the muscles controlling that joint are not doing anything. Stretching exercises help to eliminate any stiffness or tightness in the muscles, tendons, and ligaments surrounding the joints, relieving pain and preventing injury. Stretching exercises are a great way to begin any exercise routine because they strengthen muscles, improve circulation, and increase flexibility.

Where can you learn stretching exercises? If you belong to an exercise club, the instructors will certainly be able to show you some gentle, effective ones. Just make sure that they know about lupus, and how it's affecting you, or any other problems you're experiencing. Make sure that they are competent to advise you. And, of course, numerous exercise books and videos are available for all levels of proficiency.

Endurance Exercises

Endurance exercises are also referred to as aerobic exercises. By definition, an aerobic exercise is one that involves or improves oxygen consumption by requiring increased amounts of oxygen for prolonged periods of time. These are less beneficial for specific joints, but are more helpful for overall fitness.

Doing aerobics for at least twenty minutes per session, a minimum of three times a week, can strengthen your heart, improve circulation, reduce blood pressure, and relieve tension. So aerobics can give you more energy, improve your endurance, and make you feel a whole lot happier, too.

However, when beginning your exercise program, be careful not to overdo. Depending on your treatment and your current level of fitness, consider starting with a sustained five- or ten-minute effort. Then gradually increase this time as you feel stronger and have more confidence.

What are some examples of aerobic activities? Aerobics include brisk walking, step exercises, jogging, riding a regular or stationary bicycle, climbing stairs, using a treadmill, aerobic dancing, and swimming. (Of course, the aerobic exercises you select will depend on your physical condition.) So you see, you don't have to belong to a gym or buy a video to enjoy aerobics!

Is aerobic exercise for you? Everybody can certainly benefit from the many advantages aerobics has to offer. And aerobic activities are a good complement to stretching, strengthening, and range-of-motion exercises.

ACTIVE VERSUS PASSIVE EXERCISES

You can also categorize an exercise as either active or passive. If you're moving your body without anybody else helping you, you're doing active exercises. If you're moving it and someone is helping you, you're doing active assistive exercises. If you "relax" while a physical therapist, family member, or friend moves your joints (for example, if you're in a severe flare), then you're doing passive exercises.

GETTING STARTED

The kinds of exercise you do will depend on a number of factors, including the severity of your pain and inflammation, your overall physical condition, and the joints affected.

If your medical condition has kept you from being active, be prepared for a little frustration. When you first begin to exercise again, *wow*, will you be out of shape! That's not a put-down. For your exercise program to be successful, you'll need to start slowly and gradually build up your endurance and intensity over several weeks or months. The idea is to give your body time to become accustomed to physical activity so that you won't overexert yourself. The longer it's been since you've done any exercising, the slower your return should be. And again, to benefit most from an exercise program, you have to do it regularly.

Before you begin any exercise program, you should schedule a complete physical to make sure that exercising (and the type of exercise that you'd like to do) is appropriate for you. Your physician (or another health care professional) will help you develop an appropriate exercise regimen based on the types of activities you enjoy and your overall physical condition. Depending on your symptoms, some exercises may be contraindicated, so your program will also take into account your physical limitations. When you are ready to get started, you should begin slowly and gradually build up your endurance and intensity over several weeks or months.

How often must you exercise in order to reap the many benefits? Usually, experts say that three or four times a week, for a minimum of twenty minutes each time, is needed to recondition your body. But each case is different (just like each person is different). Give yourself a chance, and you'll find out what works for you.

Work on your motivation. Set goals for yourself (such as: "I'm going to start walking five minutes a day and build from there"). Work on your self-discipline. Find the best time of the day to exercise. Some people may prefer or benefit more from morning exercise, other people may be better able to exercise in the afternoon or evening. Make exercise part of your daily routine. If you're not feeling great, even a little bit of exercise, moving slowly, is better than no exercise at all.

EXERCISING CAUTION

There are a number of measures you should take that will ensure your safety when you exercise. For example, we discussed earlier that you should expect to feel more aches and pains as you begin your program. But it's important to learn the difference between muscle soreness, which is probably a normal response to exercise, and acute pain. Acute pain may mean that you're overdoing it or that you're participating in an exercise that's not appropriate for you. The old adage "no pain, no gain" is not necessarily accurate if you have lupus. So if the discomfort you feel is extreme, by all means stop exercising and consult with a professional. You may have to choose a different form of exercise or otherwise modify your routine. What you really want to do is enough exercise to comfortably improve both muscle tone and strength.

CONSULT WITH A PROFESSIONAL

We've already mentioned the importance of working with a physician, a physical therapist, or another health care professional when starting an exercise program. This will not only ensure that the program you've chosen is safe, but also give you a "partner" in your program—someone who will help you keep track of what you're doing and of how it's helping you. If you're working with a health spa or club, you should, of course, inform the staff of your condition. But remember that they are not health care professionals or experts in lupus! So be sure to okay any exercise program recommended by the club with your doctor.

INCLUDE A WARM-UP

You should always warm up before beginning any type of exercise. A good warm-up should include a variety of stretches and a few minutes of gradually increasing, low-intensity activity. Stretching increases blood flow to the muscles and will increase the temperature of the tendons the muscles are attached to, making it less likely the muscles will be pulled to the point of injury during exercise. Then you'll be ready to participate in twenty to thirty minutes or more of aerobic activity to get your heart pumping and your blood flowing.

Exercise at a rate at which you can comfortably carry on a conversation. If you feel weak, become short of breath, or have any pain, stop immediately. When you have finished your exercise routine, take another five to ten minutes for a cool-down period. Light stretching during this time will reduce soreness and increase flexibility.

Be careful to avoid exercising certain parts of your body for too long. If you exercise an inflamed joint, the inflammation may temporarily worsen. Therefore, although exercise doesn't necessarily have to stop if your joints are inflamed, it should focus either on joints that aren't affected, or very carefully (and minimally) on joints that are.

DRINK PLENTY OF WATER

Water is involved in almost every function of the body. When you exercise, your body loses water through sweating and evaporation. Sweat is your body's coolant and is therefore an essential mechanism for regulating body temperature. As such, replacing water that is continuously lost through sweating is very important.

Dehydration can put you at risk of overheating, especially if you're exercising in hot weather. Although it may be impossible to offset all of the water lost through sweating, even partial replacement can minimize the risk of overheating. To be safe, make sure you're well hydrated before you exercise. If you will be exercising for a long duration, make sure you have water with you so you can replenish lost fluids during your workout. And don't wait until you're thirsty to take a drink—thirst is often a sign that you're already dehydrated.

LISTEN TO YOUR BODY

If you're just starting an exercise program, you should expect to feel some minor discomfort from exercising. This is only natural, since your body is not used to regular physical activity. Bending a joint and stretching the surrounding muscles, tendons, and ligaments may cause some pain. Remember, you're moving joints that may not want to be moved! Despite the fact that some amount of muscle soreness is a normal result of exercise, you shouldn't ignore this discomfort. Some professionals recommend pushing a joint just a little beyond the level at which pain first occurs, because this may help to increase joint mobility. But if you experience too much discomfort or pain, or if it lasts for a long time (an hour is too long), cut back. Listen to your body. If the pain is moderate or severe, or if your aches and pains aren't going away, your body's telling you that you're overdoing it, so you should take a day or two off. Also, take a break from your exercise program if you have an injury, such as a sprain or muscle strain. You need to give your body time to heal. And skip your workout if you're feeling ill, because you don't want to make the situation worse. Rest as long as necessary, and be assured that you will eventually be able to exercise.

STAYING WITH THE PROGRAM: A REVIEW

Once you begin your exercise program, you want to stick with it. But it's not always easy. To be sure you derive the most benefits from your exercise program and find that it's not so difficult to make exercise a regular part of your life, consider some of the following suggestions:

- Don't feel that you have to wait until your lupus symptoms disappear before starting an exercise program. Starting sooner may even help you to feel better more quickly. Just make sure you get professional advice and supervision.

- Try to build up your tolerance to exercises slowly. You'll want to follow a concept in exercise known as the "progression principle," which states that exercise should be started slowly and, as time goes by, increased in intensity. You can improve the way your joints and muscles function by gradually and regularly increasing the amount of exercise you do. Too rapid an increase, or too intense an exercise program, may only increase the pain that you're experiencing. It may also damage the very joint that you want to protect and improve.

- If you experience a lot of pain or inflammation in your joints, exercise must be done with much more caution. Isometric exercises may be helpful. Very gentle range-of-motion exercises may also be suggested.

- Aim to do as much exercise as possible on your own, although you should initially get help in selecting your exercises from either your physician or a physical therapist.

- Don't compare your exercise program to somebody else's. You wouldn't compare your doses or types of medication to somebody else's, would you?

- Set up a workout schedule and stick with it. Remind yourself that exercise is a priority and is just as important as any other activity or appointment you may have during the day.

- Add variety to your exercise program. Ideally, exercise should be fun. Choose activities that you enjoy, and alternate exercises daily. This will keep you from getting bored with your exercise program and ensure that you don't overwork a particular part of your body.

- Set specific, short-term goals to keep yourself motivated, and stay focused on achieving these goals. Long-term goals are good, too, but if they seem too distant and unachievable, you might get discouraged when you don't see immediate progress.

- Reward yourself for sticking with your exercise program. Sometimes we all need artificial incentives to do things that we may not otherwise want to do. Every so often, buy yourself a desired book, CD, or other goodie that will serve as a reinforcement for your hard work . . . and a motivator to continue.

- Keep track of your progress. Write down what kind of exercise you did, at what intensity, and for how long. Keeping an exercise journal will enable you to see the progress you've made, and this will help you stay motivated.
- Exercise with a buddy. Make a commitment with each other to stick with the exercise program. Also, a training partner who is aware of your lupus can help ensure your safety when you work out. Your friend can help you (or get help for you) should you be unable to help yourself.
- If you experience muscle cramps, tightness, or discomfort after exercise, treat yourself to a hot bath or a massage. And make sure you're not doing too much.

A Final Exertion

Because every person is different, there is no one set of exercises that can be recommended for everyone. But everybody is capable of doing some exercises, and everybody can benefit from them. Just don't jump in feetfirst! Use your head. Work with your physician or exercise therapist to choose an exercise regimen that will help you achieve your fitness goals. Make sure you work rest into your routine. Then start slowly, build up your stamina, and enjoy your improved health!

Exercise should be a pleasant experience. If it really becomes a chore or drudgery, look for other ways to exercise that can be more enjoyable. Ask others what they do, or what suggestions they may have for you. Start moving!

13.

ACTIVITIES

What to do, what to do? Sure you have lupus, but what does this mean in terms of the basic activities in your life? What can you do and what can't you do? Each person is different. The kinds of things you did before being diagnosed with lupus will influence what you can or want to do now. Your current physical condition is also an important factor. If you're in the middle of a flare, for example, you may not want to expend a lot of energy until your doctor has given you the green light (or even a cautious yellow) to resume activity. And even if you feel wonderful, you'll probably want to curtail any vigorous activities. You don't want to put any strain on your body. In fact, you may not even have the strength! So let's discuss some of the activities that may concern you, and see how you can make various kinds of changes that will enable you to be as active as you want to be.

Working

Working can be very important for you. Besides being a primary source of income (can't overlook that!), working will make you feel like your life is proceeding as usual. You may be concerned (an understatement!) that your lupus might interfere with your ability to work, which may threaten your financial security.

Even though you have lupus, you'll probably want to do as much as possible of what you used to do. Are you afraid that you'll feel like less of a person if you have to stop working? Work is important. It helps you to feel independent. It gives you a sense of self-fulfillment and self-worth. It provides more financial strength than not working, of course. And it is an important component of your social life.

Understandably, you are probably quite concerned that your lupus may interfere with your work. Perhaps you feel too tired to shoulder your usual workload. Many people question whether they should even continue to work. If you want to and you need to, and you can, then it's a good idea. You may have to make some modifications because you don't want to chance running yourself down. Let's look at some specific job-related concerns and learn a little bit more about the ways in which lupus can affect your work, and what you can do about it.

SHOULD YOU CONTINUE WORKING?

Five basic points may help you when you are thinking about working. First of all, ask yourself if you feel comfortable doing the job. Do you feel physically and emotionally capable? It's fine to continue working if you're not wearing yourself down or compromising your health. Is it something you want to do? Your condition may have made you more determined that you want to start doing something you really want to do! Second, does your employer still want you to work there? Or will a new employer hire you, given your present physical condition? Should you even say anything about it? (More about this later.) A third very important matter is whether your colleagues will accept you. This, of course, does not necessarily mean that they will even notice your condition. Fourth, will your condition and its treatment affect your performance, attendance, or punctuality at work? If so, will this cause any difficulties on the job? A fifth factor that may relate to your choice of employment is the amount of stress involved. Because of the negative impact of stress on your physical condition, this is certainly something you'll want to minimize. If you find that working is creating a stress that is counterproductive, you may need to consider a job change, reducing hours, or at the very least a change in responsibilities within your job. As you might suspect, it would be best to consult with your doctor regarding any job-specific limitations or restrictions that you should heed.

WHAT IF FATIGUE OR OTHER DISCOMFORTS ARE A PROBLEM?

You may be concerned that symptoms or side effects will prevent you from adequately performing on the job. Certainly, lupus may cause you to experience fatigue and other discomforts, and this may affect your productivity. You may get tired easily and feel that you just don't have the stamina necessary to complete your job satisfactorily. Your work rate may have slowed down, and you may be absent or late more than usual. If your employer is aware of any of these problems, you may be afraid that your value to the company will be questioned—that your job may be in jeopardy.

What should you do? Pace yourself. Take rest breaks whenever necessary—and possible—to get reenergized. Build your stamina slowly. Don't expect too much all at once. Try to reduce the time involved in nonessential activities. For example, if there's a way you can work closer to home, you will find that it will be less stressful to have a shorter commute. If you can adjust your work hours, you'll find that it will be less stressful to avoid the traffic you might otherwise encounter going to or from work. If you're not sure how much you can do, do what you can, and let your body be your guide.

Will your employer make any special provisions for you because you have lupus? You may be able to continue working at a particular job with only a few modifications. For the most part, if your employer is satisfied with the work you're doing, there shouldn't be a problem. But remember: You still have to do what you're supposed to do.

Of course, you may be uncomfortable about approaching your employer to find out if these changes can be made. It may bother you to seek "special treatment." But consider that any necessary modifications may be small in comparison to the ones your company would face if they had to hire a new employee to replace you!

Maria had been working in the same office for eighteen years. Lately, though, because of lupus, she had been having more difficulty completing her responsibilities and getting to work on time. Unfortunately, her supervisor was a perfectionist who apparently was not willing to bend to accommodate Maria's needs. She called her in for review and made it perfectly clear that unless her performance and attendance improved, she would be out of a job. As if that wasn't bad enough, the supervisor frequently reminded Maria that she was watching her. The pressure became so hard to bear that it began to affect Maria's emotional and physical health.

What if your employer refuses to bend the rules? What if an ultimatum is given, stating that if productivity does not improve, you will be discharged? If this happens, simply do the best you can. If your employer doesn't understand enough about lupus to know that you must pace yourself and shows little or no willingness to cooperate, then you're probably better off not continuing employment there. You don't want to look for trouble, but you do want to fight for your rights.

What if another employee resents any special treatment you've been given? Find time to sit down, one-on-one, and have a conversation with your unhappy colleague. Explain your situation as much as necessary. Often, this is all that's needed to bring about greater understanding and cooperation. If your co-worker still doesn't understand, content yourself with knowing that you tried. It's not your problem anymore. (For more information on dealing with colleagues, see Chapter 31.)

SHOULD YOU DISCUSS YOUR CONDITION WITH YOUR EMPLOYER?

How appropriate is it to discuss your medical condition with your employer? How much should you share? You're not looking for sympathy, but you are looking for understanding. And unfortunately, there are times that it's absolutely necessary to inform others as to what you're experiencing. Each case is different. Each situation is different. You want to make decisions about how much and what to say that are most comfortable for you.

Some employers will be very supportive and understanding, while others will be somewhat apprehensive about retaining—or hiring—an individual who has any kind of physical problem. Remember that your employer's primary responsibility is to keep productivity at its highest possible level. So it may be helpful to reassure your employer that you'll work to keep your condition from interfering with your own productivity. If, at some point, modifications do have to be made, you'll deal with them—and your employer—at that time.

WHAT IF EMPLOYERS REFUSE TO RETAIN OR HIRE YOU?

If you are applying for a job, it's important to know which questions your interviewer is legally allowed to ask, and which questions must not be asked. For example, a potential employer can ask if you have any health or medical problem that would interfere with your ability to do the work involved in the position for which you're applying. Keep in mind, however, that this question cannot be asked in more general terms—an interviewer cannot ask whether you have a health problem. Also, by law, an interviewer is not permitted to list a series of medical problems and ask you if you have any of them.

It is not recommended that you lie about your condition during an interview. However, you can be circumspect about how much information you provide and respond with only the bare minimum necessary. The best way to prepare for an interview is to rehearse. Ask a close friend or family member to bombard you with difficult questions. Practice your answers so that you can confidently and smoothly respond to these kinds of questions during your interview.

Once you have begun work, your employer can ask medical questions only if they are asked with the intent to find reasons why you aren't able to handle the responsibilities of your position. Be aware that your employer is required by law to accommodate your special needs (within reason, of course).

Employers may be hesitant to retain or hire someone with lupus for a number of reasons. For instance, an employer may feel that health insurance premiums will be that much higher if you are listed on the plan. But don't accept this argument. The Americans with Disabilities Act (ADA), most recently amended in 1997, clearly states that any employer with fifteen or more employees must not refuse you appropriate work or discriminate against you because of any disability. So if you are denied a job or dismissed from your present one because of lupus, don't take it sitting down. Instead, call someone! For example, you can contact the Equal Employment Opportunity Commission (EEOC). Or check into resources such as your local bar association, which can direct you to an attorney who can help enforce the terms of the ADA.

WHAT ABOUT RETURNING TO WORK?

If you have gone through a period of time when you could not work because of lupus, your return to work will be a very important step, not only for you, but for your family members as well. All of you will hope that life is about to return to a more normal state.

When should you return to work? Some people are ready to return as soon as they feel better. What you choose to do should depend on you, your doctor, your employer, and the nature of your work. If you are apprehensive about your return, have confidence in yourself. The more positive your attitude and the better you present yourself, the more quickly you'll adjust.

EMPLOYER ACCEPTANCE OR HARASSMENT?

What if you've been out of work for a while and are ready to reenter the job market? You might worry about whether you should go back to your old job, or whether anyone else would even consider hiring you. The decision to hire you or not to hire you is based on a number of factors. Among them are your prior sickness or absentee record, your present state of health, and the possibility of prolonged absences in the future. The employer will certainly want to consider whether you and your medical condition will create any problems on the job. Concerns about morale, sick benefits, and liability usually top the list.

The most upsetting cases involve employers who are unwilling to hire you simply because they know about your condition. At this point, you're faced with two choices. You can either give up and look for something else, or try to educate the employer (not with your fists!). This can be done through discussions or reading materials, or you can put your employer in contact with a physician or a nurse. If necessary, your physician can probably reassure your prospective employer that you are fit for the job and should be able to handle it in more or less the same way as someone without lupus.

All this groundwork is frequently worth the effort! If you get the job, your relationship will already be a good one. Greater understanding will exist. In addition, it's nice to know that your employer has at least some insight into your condition.

WHAT IF YOU HAVE TO CHANGE JOBS?

Because of new limitations, your old job may no longer be right for you. If this is the case, you should certainly consider changing to another job, even if it means getting additional training.

Lenny, a thirty-nine-year-old father of two, had been working in construction. But Lenny's doctors felt that he shouldn't continue doing this type of work because it was too strenuous for him. Lenny became very depressed. He didn't know what else he could do. Rather than face the prospect of being unable to work, he shut down emotionally.

Certainly the prospect of having to look for work is more daunting to some than it is to others. But if you are unable to continue working at your present job, don't despair. There are many ways in which you can get the training you need to move into a different type of position. Your first step might be to check with any of the government services that offer vocational counseling. Counselors in these offices will work with you to determine exactly what your aptitude is for different jobs. You will then be able to get the training and support you need to obtain employment in the desired field. If you need help finding jobs that are appropriate for you, your state employment services may be a good place to start. These services are available free of charge and may guide you in locating jobs that will match your abilities and limitations. In addition, the Federal Rehabilitation Act of 1973 requires states to include individuals in vocational rehabilitation programs if their previous jobs are no longer appropriate for them. These programs vary, so it's important to check with your state to find out what's available. Any financial advisor you're working with should also be able to help you in this regard.

Some people feel that, for financial reasons, you should postpone looking for new employment until your old employment has been terminated. This tactic has its pros and cons. If you receive unemployment benefits for losing your job, this could ease your financial burden. But if subsequent employers are reluctant to hire you because of your grounds for dismissal, this tactic may explode in your face. Only you, with your unique knowledge of your own situation, can decide which course of action is best.

IS WORKING YOUR ONLY OPTION?

As you know, there are many benefits to working, including satisfaction, pride, and money. But what if you can't work? Or what if you're between jobs? But a paying job is not the only type of satisfying work that's available. Many meaningful, productive activities can be pursued on a voluntary basis. Check with nonprofit charities, religious organizations, political groups, hospitals, schools, senior citizen centers, and the like. These types of organizations can always use some extra help. Volunteer work may even allow you to explore an area of interest that you've never been able to participate in before, due to work commitments. And this work will help you feel good about yourself in the bargain.

What if you just don't want to work? If this is your preference, and you're able to manage without a job, that's great. But don't use your condition as an excuse for not working. Instead, try to find out what's really bothering you, and explore ways of eliminating the problem.

School

Teenagers and young adults with lupus may have problems in school that are similar to those experienced by people who work. There may be times when your condition just doesn't allow you to feel comfortable enough to attend classes. Or you may be concerned because pain or other physical restrictions prevent you from participating in your usual activities. When necessary, you should inform your teachers about your condition so that they can help whenever possible. For example, a child with lupus may be concerned about the comments of other students while in school. Having teachers who are aware of lupus may help to minimize this potential problem.

(More information on children or adolescents with lupus can be found in chapters 19 and 20.)

Recreation

As we've mentioned in earlier chapters, it's vital to continue involving yourself in the activities you've always enjoyed. Why? Depending on their nature, of course, these activities may help keep you limber and vigorous. Just as important, they will provide a welcome diversion from any worries, prevent boredom and depression, and, very likely, put you in contact with other people.

Fortunately, most people with lupus may be able to participate in a number of recreational activities, including boating, skating, golf, tennis, dancing—the list goes on and on. What you do or don't do will depend on your physical condition, your physician's recommendations, and your personal preferences. As long as your doctor has given approval, you should let your body be your guide.

Activities of Daily Living

Among the things you do each day are numerous routine tasks—the activities of daily living (ADL). Of course, any restrictions you're experiencing because of lupus may now be limiting these activities. If so, you're probably experiencing a lot of frustration. Why? Because before your diagnosis, you most likely took the accomplishment of these simple tasks for granted. And the way you're feeling now, you may be just too tired, depressed, or upset to look for a creative solution to these day-to-day problems.

What should you do? Well, you may not want to ask for help. You may feel that it takes away from your dignity. So you're stuck, right? Absolutely not! In a very short period of time, you can reorganize your lifestyle, your house, and your ADL in a way that will lessen your difficulties and salvage a lot of your dignity. Remember: Not all people with lupus experience these problems. (And if you do, doesn't it make sense to see what you can do to improve the situation?)

Modifying your lifestyle or your home is not the same as giving in to lupus; rather, these changes will help you learn how to live most effectively and cope most successfully with your condition. How? Read on!

SIMPLIFY YOUR TASKS

Your goal is to make daily living as easy as possible. Why? One of the most important components in your treatment program for lupus is energy conservation. So you'll want to eliminate those activities that aren't necessary and simplify those that are! Conserving your energy can be very important in helping you to avoid much of the excessive fatigue that can be a negative factor in living with lupus.

In many cases, problems with daily living can be conquered without professional help. It can be very satisfying for you to develop your own solutions to these problems. This can be one of the most important ways of coping with lupus. Of course, any questions you have can be bounced off physicians, physical therapists, other therapists, or other experts who are in a position to help you.

How can you start? Well, begin by evaluating everything you do on a day-to-day basis. Then see how you can make every single thing you do easier. Is this taking the lazy way out? Of course not! You're simply recognizing that every bit of energy you save in the performance of one activity will give you more energy with which to do something else.

Any specific suggestions? There are lots of things you can do to help yourself with daily living. For example, you may want to reorganize your home and your habits in such a way that makes movement easier and puts things within easy reach. You can replace small handles on drawers with bigger ones. You can lubricate drawers so that they open and close more easily. You can wear clothing that is easier to get on and off—especially if you often have to spend a lot of time fiddling with buttons or zippers. There are a number of different types of gadgets that may make life easier for you.

Try to reduce the amount of energy you expend in performing any activities. If necessary, modify the method that you use. Eliminate any unnecessary activity. Rest intermittently, frequently, and whenever needed. You'll then be able to do more of what you want or need to do. And you'll accomplish it in a healthier way.

Any activities that cause you pain should be modified as much as possible. And you certainly don't want to do anything that causes severe pain, even if it is very short-lived. If you've already reduced a task to the bare minimum and absolutely can't do anything more about it, put a limit on how much pain you're going to let yourself endure. An ache that lasts five to ten minutes may be bearable if it is not severe, but severe pain may be a problem.

PLAN AND ORGANIZE YOUR ACTIVITIES

In addition to eliminating unnecessary activities and making the remaining tasks easier to accomplish, you'll want to learn how to use planning and pacing to conserve energy.

Try charting your activities, including your required tasks and your optional social and leisure activities. This may help you better organize your time. The more advanced the planning, the better—especially when big projects are involved—as this will give you time to figure out exactly how you're going to perform a given task, what equipment you'll need, and how the task might be broken up, if necessary, to allow for rest periods. Your local library and bookstores should have some excellent books on time management. Many of the tips in these books make such good sense that you'll probably wonder why you didn't think of them yourself! And every bit of time you save will be a big plus.

TIPS FOR CONSERVING ENERGY

Let's summarize some of the things that you can do to conserve energy and maximize your abilities:

- Pace yourself appropriately.
- Include sufficient amount of rest.
- Work, move, and play—with moderation.
- Include relaxation regularly in your routine.

- Reduce the chances of stiffening up. Move or stretch as needed.
- Keep things interesting, but don't overdo.
- Try to prioritize your activities that are necessary, and eliminate the unnecessary ones from your routine.
- Reduce the amount of time you spend standing.
- Build in short rest periods frequently, and longer rest periods occasionally.
- Distinguish between activities that are light on energy, and those that are energy drains. Balance what you do and when you do it.
- Organize your day to do the more energy-involved activities when you have more energy.
- Think about reorganizing certain critical areas of your home to reduce the amount of stretching, reaching, and bending that would normally be required.
- Improve your ability to delegate tasks to others when necessary and/or desirable. This can include delegating to children as well.

An Activation Summation

By now, you've learned a lot about coping with lupus, and you know that staying active is just as important as any other coping strategy. You want to feel productive and enjoy life. You don't want to let lupus confine you to your bed or chair. Certainly you should modify any activities that are causing you discomfort, and you should do only what you physically can do, but *do* . . . !

14.

FINANCIAL CONCERNS

Having lupus can be a pain in the pocketbook! Why? The cost of treatment, doctor visits, and other medical costs, as well as the cost of medication, hospitalization (if needed), and laboratory tests, all add up. In addition, money is lost from the number of work days that are missed because of symptoms. The cost varies considerably for each person with lupus. It doesn't take long for financial security to drain into a financial problem.

Decreased Work, Increased Costs at Home

Financial problems arise from lost earnings or income. You may not be able to work at all, or perhaps you can hold down only a part-time job. Your condition may affect your ability to work. This may cause problems with your job. So it's possible that your "employability" will be reduced because of your lupus.

Lupus can also be costly because of changes at home. You may need to have other people help you, or you may need to make renovations in your home. You may need help around the house, such as a baby-sitter or a cleaning person. All of these things cost money, adding to your financial burden. As your medical costs rise, your budget will become tighter and tighter. If costs continue to skyrocket, you may feel as if you're being strangled!

Although lupus can be an expensive disease, it need not be alarmingly so if you're careful. If you take proper care of yourself and follow your treatment program correctly, hopefully you'll be able to prevent the more serious (and expensive) problems that can occur. Let's take a look at the many ways in which you can prevent or ease financial problems as you cope with lupus.

Talk to Others

If mounting medical costs threaten to engulf you, perhaps the first thing you should do is speak to other people. Through a support group, for instance, you may meet others in similar situations. Find out what they have done to control and meet the costs of their own care. Even though you may initially be embarrassed to bring up this subject, the common bond that exists among people with medically induced financial problems should quickly put you at ease. You'll be glad you brought it up!

For more ideas, you might contact your physician, hospital administrators, and other health professionals; social workers; and various organizations, such as the Lupus Foundation of America. Speak to financial experts or advisors for their suggestions. Through these contacts, you can learn how other people have dealt with these problems.

Lower Medication Costs

Since most treatment for lupus includes medications, the use of generic drugs may save you money. Generic medication is sold by its chemical name rather than the more common brand name and is usually less expensive than the brand-name product. However, generics do not always work as well as their brand-name counterparts. Ask your physician if it would be acceptable to take the generic versions of any drugs you're currently using.

Some people try to cut costs by ordering their medications through the mail. This can be a legitimate way to save some money—but only if you deal with a reputable mail-order supplier. It's important to discuss this option with your doctor before you make *any* purchases. Ask your doctor, or your local lupus organization, which companies—if any—they recommend.

Some pharmaceutical manufacturers have programs to help make some drugs available free of charge to needy patients. These are known as "indigent patient drug programs" and are available through your physician. To qualify you must have low income and no health insurance. Your doctor or nurse will contact the pharmaceutical company and request an application that you must complete and then have your doctor authorize.

Attend a Clinic

If medical costs are overwhelming you, consider attending a clinic. Because clinics usually operate on a sliding-scale fee schedule, you may be able to receive quality medical care and equipment at a reduced cost. In some cases, you may even be able to continue seeing the physician who's treating you now; many physicians donate their time to clinics.

How can you locate a good clinic in your area? Your local hospital or your physician should be able to guide you to a local clinic that has the resources you need.

Insurance Can Be Assurance

Health insurance is essential, and a good health insurance plan is even more valuable. Fortunately, many people with lupus have at least some of their medical costs defrayed by insurance. Even if you have health insurance, lupus can be a costly disease. That's all the more reason to get the best insurance coverage possible.

GETTING THE MOST FROM YOUR INSURANCE POLICY

If you have a health insurance policy, contact your agent as soon as possible and find out as much as you can about your policy. (The policy itself will provide this information, too, of course.) Ask your agent the amount of your deductible; how many hospital days are covered, and how much is paid per day; how much coverage you have for surgery and anesthesia; whether second opinions are covered; and what your maximum lifetime coverage is. Also, make sure you know all of the procedures necessary to file a claim or submit an appeal.

How can you help ensure that the process of claim filing and reimbursement runs smoothly? If you are responsible for the payment of your insurance premiums, make sure you pay them on time. Don't allow your insurance policy to lapse. And be sure to keep track of paperwork. Every time you send in a claim, keep copies of the claim form and of any attached doctors' bills for your own files. These may prove invaluable if a problem arises when your claim is processed. If, in fact, you do not receive a reimbursement on a claim, follow up by phone or letter, and request an explanation of the denial. If no satisfactory response is received, contact the insurance commissioner of your state, requesting an investigation.

Also keep records of the amount your insurance company pays on each claim, as well as the amount you pay on each claim. Your own payments may prove to be deductible on your next income tax return. (Your accountant should be able to provide more information on this.)

WHAT IF YOU LEAVE YOUR JOB?

In the past, when people left jobs (either voluntarily or involuntarily) they also lost the health insurance that was included with that job. However, a federal law called the Consolidated Omnibus Budget Reconciliation Act (COBRA) changed that. Under this plan, your employer has to allow you to keep your existing health insurance policy with the same coverage for up to eighteen months after you leave. You will have to pay for this coverage, and it may cost you more than when you were working, but it's better than not having any insurance.

WHAT IF YOUR INSURANCE IS INADEQUATE?

What happens if your health coverage is exhausted, or if your insurance is not good enough? Well, you may be able to increase the ceiling for your coverage. Additional insurance may also be available for "catastrophic" medical expenses. Be aware, though, that people with chronic illnesses may have difficulty obtaining additional health or disability insurance. For example, a disability plan may exclude you from coverage for a period of two or more years if you have surgery or any event related to this condition. However, a good insurance agent can work with you to get this exclusion time reduced if you have supporting medical documentation. Don't give up, though! It's important to fight any insurance discrimination. This can take the form of canceled coverage, reduced benefits, increased premiums, or loss of insurance due to employment termination.

WHAT IF YOU HAVE NO HEALTH INSURANCE?

If you are not presently covered by health insurance, you'll want to immediately contact all your resources—your accountant, your lawyer, your financial advisor, and health organizations such as the Lupus Foundation of America, for instance—to learn about available options. The more individuals you contact, the more likely it is that you'll find the information you need. Of course, if you are unable to obtain coverage and can't afford to pay your medical costs, you may be able to obtain assistance from government programs.

Government Programs May Help

Government insurance programs are an important source of financial support for many people. You may be covered (at least to some degree) by Social Security Disability Insurance, Medicaid, or Medicare. Each of these plans has its own specific criteria for eligibility, and the criteria are often complicated, so you'll probably need to work with a professional to see if you qualify.

Let's take a closer look at these three programs.

SOCIAL SECURITY DISABILITY INSURANCE

If you are unable to work because of your lupus, you may be eligible for disability benefits. The Social Security disability program is a federal government program. It is administered and run by the Social Security Administration. Disability benefits were added to the Social Security Act in 1956. An individual is considered to be "disabled" if he or she is unable to do any substantial gainful work due to a physical or mental impairment; and if the physical or mental condition is expected to last, or has lasted, for at least twelve months, or is expected to result in death.

The Social Security benefit plan is funded by workers and their employers. You must have worked five out of the ten years prior to your disability in order to qualify. This requirement may be reduced to one and a half years if the individual becomes disabled before reaching thirty-one years of age.

Benefits are available from the Social Security disability plan if you fit into any of the following categories:

1. Individuals under the age of sixty-five who are disabled (and their families).
2. Single individuals under the age of twenty-two who were disabled before that age and are still disabled.
3. Widows who are disabled.
4. Widowers who are disabled and also dependent.

There are also other specific cases that may entitle you to benefits.

There is one very rigid rule that the Social Security Administration enforces in order for benefits to be approved. Remember this guideline: "The physical or mental impairment must prevent you from doing any substantial, gainful work, and is expected to last (or has lasted) for at least twelve months, or is expected to result in death." This *must* be the case if you are applying for disability.

Even if you meet eligibility criteria for disability insurance, there are other steps that must be taken before you can collect any money. You will have to provide the names and addresses of people involved in treating you, including any physicians involved in your care. Additionally, you'll need to list hospitals and clinics where you receive treatment. The Social Security Administration will need to see copies of your medical records, substantiating the dates you were treated and the treatments prescribed. Then, a Social

Security team, which includes a physician, will evaluate this information. Sometimes, additional tests are required to support a claim.

The medical requirements for disability from lupus are very comprehensive, requiring not only a physician's diagnosis of lupus, but medical documentation of the existence of lupus-related symptoms as well as the impact lupus has had on you. In order to learn more about the requirements, as well as whether you are eligible, you may want to contact your local Social Security office; call the toll-free number, 1-800–772–1213; or go online. One website that has a lot of information is http://www.socialsecurity-disability .org/disabling-conditions/lupus-and-social-security-disability.

Be prepared to be denied. (No, I'm not being a pessimist! The majority of people applying for SSD are denied . . . the first time.) However, the good news is that when your disability application is eventually approved, you will start receiving benefits from the date you first applied, not the date that you're eventually approved.

SUPPLEMENTAL SECURITY INCOME

Once you apply for Social Security benefits, you also become eligible for Supplemental Security Income (SSI). Like the Social Security disability program, the Social Security Administration runs the Supplementary Security Income program. However, SSI comes from a general treasury fund, rather than from workers and their employers. SSI benefits are available to individuals 65 and over, the blind, and the disabled. The eligibility requirements for SSI include the same definitions of disability that are used for Social Security benefits. However, it is possible to get SSI coverage even if you did not work.

MEDICAID

Medicaid (the more commonly used term for medical assistance) offers benefits to individuals who are unable to pay for health care. This public assistance program is administered on the state or local level. Who qualifies for Medicaid? Virtually any low-income individual who demonstrates need can receive these public welfare benefits. Benefits are provided automatically for low-income individuals who qualify for Supplemental Security Income. Individuals who are sixty-five and over and who are receiving Social Security may qualify for Medicaid, and so may individuals who are under sixty-five and who have met the Social Security requirements for disability.

Medicaid will cover virtually any medical expense, as long as the health professional treating you is a participating provider. Your health care provider is then directly reimbursed by the state for the service provided to you. If you have any questions about qualifications or about the benefits themselves, check with your local Medicaid office for further information.

MEDICARE

Medicare, a federal health insurance program, provides coverage for Americans aged sixty-five and over, and for disabled people of any age. Anyone, any age, who qualifies for and receives Social Security Disability Insurance also qualifies for Medicare after having been approved for two years. The degree of coverage provided by Medicare varies widely, so it's vital for you to determine exactly what health services Medicare will cover in your case.

Medicare is divided into two parts. Part A provides for anyone who has reached age sixty-five or is disabled, and who is eligible for Social Security benefits. It covers hospitalization costs, as well as in-patient services in a skilled nursing facility. Part B covers doctor's charges, out-patient services, and specified medical items and services not covered under Part A. Part B insurance requires you to pay a monthly premium and a significant co-payment.

While Medicare does provide coverage for large costs, it will not cover everything. Especially in the case of a major illness, supplementary medical coverage is vital.

What Should You Do?

To determine whether any of these programs are applicable to you, contact your local Social Security office. In addition, consult your physician, your local support groups, or your local lupus organization. These sources can provide you with valuable information that will assist you in determining which programs can help you. But beware—these programs are strict. You can appeal if your application or claim is rejected, but this can be very aggravating. Want some advice? Talk to people who have been through it. The Lupus Foundation of America has put out a comprehensive guidebook to disability rights and programs. This book should be available from the national organization (see address in the Appendix) or from your local chapter. Fight for your rights—and for your dollars.

$umming Up

Financial concerns can be a big worry, but, despite high costs, it is possible to find ways to pay for appropriate treatment. The earlier you start planning and the more qualified professionals you consult, the greater the likelihood that medical costs will not become a major problem for you. You will then be able to concentrate on your most important goal: living successfully with lupus.

15.

TRAVELING

Ellen was a forty-two-year-old executive. One of the reasons she always enjoyed working hard at her job was that it provided her with an income sufficient to take her family on luxurious annual vacations. She and her family would spend many happy weeks in many different parts of the world. However, since she was diagnosed with lupus, Ellen had not taken any trips at all. Why? You see, Ellen was afraid that her disease would interfere with her sightseeing plans, so she didn't want to go at all. Need it be this way? Definitely not. Very few restrictions need to be placed on your travel plans. As a matter of fact, you can probably go just about anywhere!

If you think you might like to travel, discuss it with your physician first. Chances are that if you're able to get around your own neighborhood without assistance, you can probably handle traveling with confidence. If you do have difficulty getting around, you'll want to be more selective about where you go. (And obviously, if you're in the middle of a flare, this might not be the best time to travel. Want a tip? Always take out trip cancellation insurance, especially if you stand to lose a lot of money because of last-minute, nonrefundable cancellations.) If getting around is a problem, you may opt to use wheelchairs in order to reduce fatigue. Wheelchairs are a good idea for some people, others are afraid of being seen in a wheelchair, or are even more afraid that once they use them, they'll be stuck in them forever. Neither of these fears is valid, but both can interfere with happy travel plans. Work on your thinking to conquer these fears.

Do all individuals with lupus avoid traveling? No. Some don't travel simply because they feel it's too expensive. This may have nothing to do with lupus. But plenty of others do travel, whether their trips are short or long. Some travel simply to prove to themselves that they can. This doesn't mean that there are no fears attached. Many want to prove to themselves that they can do it—that traveling, one of life's pleasures, is possible for them, too. As with any other aspect of living with your lupus, planning ahead and taking the proper precautions can allow you to travel with a free mind (although not with free airfare!).

Let's explore some of the ways you can prepare for a comfortable—and safe—trip away from home.

Plan Ahead

You don't have to restrict your travel plans just because you have lupus. You'll want to acknowledge your physical strengths and weaknesses. Then you can plan a trip that takes both into consideration. With proper planning and preparation, you should be able to go virtually anywhere you want, by plane, train, automobile, or cruise ship. The following suggestions will help you better prepare yourself for your travels.

ESTABLISH CONTACTS

Ask you doctor if he knows of any doctors or facilities where you're planning to go. If your physician has no contacts, try to get some names on your own (try the local medical society or your local lupus organization), or plan your vacation at a place where adequate medical services are available. You might want to contact professionals at your destination in advance just to be reassured that they're there, that they know about lupus, and that they know you're coming. The International Association for Medical Assistance to Travelers (www.iamat.org, or call 716-754-4883) can provide contact details about doctors in different locations who speak your primary language, as well as a lot of additional valuable information.

GET A SIGNED LETTER FROM YOUR DOCTOR

Ask for a letter signed by your doctor stating that you have lupus. The letter should indicate the medications that you must take for lupus. To be safe, carry with you extra prescriptions for your medications with the generic name of the medications identified. Doctors and pharmacists in other countries may not recognize American brand names, so if you have the generic name on hand, you'll be ready if you need to buy medication during your trip. If you're going to a foreign country, you may want the prescription translated into the language of that country in case the pharmacist has difficulty with English.

RESEARCH YOUR DESTINATION

Research your destination to determine if it's best for your physical capabilities. For example, if you get tired easily, you may not want to go on a three-week walking tour of the Far East! Or if you're sun-sensitive, you know that this needs to be taken into consideration when you decide on your destination. (Of course, even if you can't sit in the sun, this doesn't mean you can't go to a sunny place! Just use proper protection, as we discussed in Chapter 7.)

Research your destination to find out how to get medical care. Try to get the names of doctors, hospitals, and local chapters of the Lupus Foundation of America in the area to which you will be traveling. This can be very comforting to have. Once again, the International Association for Medical Assistance to Travelers can be of great help if you're trying to learn more about medical care abroad.

PACK EXTRA MEDICATION AND SUPPLIES

Running out of medication or other supplies may be one of your biggest concerns about traveling. Bring more than enough of your prescription medication and supplies with you in case any unexpected situations arise, such as if your return home is delayed. Ideally, make sure any medications that you take with you are in their original containers (with prescriptions attached). This reduces the chances of questions. Make sure you take extra written prescriptions, as well. You may also want to ask your doctor if you can "keep him or her on call," so you can contact him or her in an emergency.

PACK OVER-THE-COUNTER MEDICATIONS

Nobody likes getting sick, especially on vacation. But if you're traveling far from home, there may be a greater chance that you'll experience diarrhea or nausea. You'll want to pack over-the-counter medications to treat gastrointestinal upset, as well as your typical cold symptoms, so that you can prevent any problems that may occur from becoming worse.

PREPARE FOR YOUR MODE OF TRANSPORTATION

If you're flying and have any physical restrictions, discuss these in advance, either with an airline representative or with your travel agent. Airlines frequently have special services for individuals with restricted mobility. For example, you may be able to board early, select your seat in advance, have wheelchair access to and from the gate, and have special meals, if necessary. If you have your own wheelchair and you plan on traveling with it, check with an airline representative to find out what regulations apply.

More and more cruise ships have special accommodations for people with physical restrictions. Some have rooms specifically designed for individuals with limited mobility. Ramps may have been built and doorways widened for greater accessibility on some ships. If you're planning on taking a cruise, make sure that you know what ports of call the ship will be stopping at. In certain Caribbean ports, for example, the ship does not dock at the pier. Rather, it drops anchor away from the pier, and small boats (called *tenders*) are used to get you ashore. This may be more difficult for you to handle if you have any physical restrictions. Again, if you're taking your own wheelchair, be sure to find out what regulations may apply.

Quite a variety of passenger trains exist throughout the country and abroad. Some trains are very accessible for individuals with disabilities. Others are not as accommodating. If you're thinking of traveling by train, speak with a railroad representative or your travel agent before making a final decision.

Bus travel is becoming easier for people with disabilities. Even if you need a wheelchair, it can probably be stowed, and somebody can help you to get on and off the bus.

KEEP MEDICATIONS AND SUPPLIES WITH YOU AT ALL TIMES

Carry your medication and supplies in a carry-on bag, rather than packing them in with the rest of your luggage. Why? Well, for one thing, if your bags end up in Birmingham when you're flying to Orlando, you'll be without some of the essential components of your treatment program. If you carry your supplies with you, you'll be sure that you have what you need when you need it, whether you're traveling by bus, train, or plane. (And, after all, it would be rather inconsiderate of you to ask the flight attendant to climb down into the baggage compartment to get it!) Although this may involve a little more carry-on luggage than you would like, the peace of mind you'll have knowing that you're prepared is well worth it.

Self-Care Away from Home

If you're smart about packing and you plan ahead, you'll have little to worry about—wherever you decide to travel. Remember, though, that if you're going to relax and have fun, you can't afford to take a break from your treatment program. The travel tips provided below will help you stay on track.

PACE YOURSELF

Pace yourself and don't overdo. Vacations can be very exciting. When you first get to your destination, you may want to do as much as you can. Calm down! Spread it out, and you're more likely to enjoy more of your vacation. If fatigue gets to you, don't beat yourself up for having to rest. Yes, you may miss certain things, but you want the overall experience to be positive.

IDENTIFY YOURSELF!

It's always a good idea to travel with complete identification, not just for your luggage but for yourself! This will make it easier for others to help you if, for some reason, you cannot help yourself. The Medic Alert bracelet is accepted worldwide as identification for people with medical conditions. In addition, make sure your wallet contains an identification card with complete details about your condition, a list of symptoms that require treatment, the medications you require, and the names of your physicians. The card should also list contact telephone numbers in case a friend or family member needs to be contacted.

If you're going to a foreign country, you may want to have the information on your card translated into the language of that country. You may need help with this if you're not fluent in that particular language. Try checking with a foreign-language teacher at a local school. Or you can contact a representative of an airline that travels to that country. Representatives who speak the language will probably be willing to translate for you. As a last resort, you may want to check with the foreign embassy of that particular country. This may take a little extra time, but your mind will be more at ease when you do travel.

If you're not traveling with family members or friends who know about lupus and what to do if a problem arises, make sure that you inform someone about your condition. For example, if you're going to be touring with a group, you might want to let the group leader know that you have lupus.

EAT, DRINK, AND BE MERRY . . . AND CAREFUL!

When traveling abroad, people need to be cautious about what they eat and drink. It's important to be on your guard and be aware of potential problems. Travelers are often warned not to drink tap water when they travel to certain countries. Unless you've been assured that it's okay, don't drink tap water or even water in thermoses provided by hotels. Avoid fruits and vegetables that may have been washed before being served. Avoid any other foods that include water in their preparation. Even something as simple as brushing your teeth can make you wish you were back home in bed. You've heard of

Montezuma's revenge? Well, Montezuma has traveled to many parts of the world! The best way to conquer the water problem is to use pure, sterilized, or distilled water. Some hotels will provide water purifiers so that you can take water from the tap, process it, and then be able to use it safely.

It is not always safe to drink even typical American soft drinks when abroad. The name of the soft drink may be American, and the packaging may look the same as it does in the United States, but that doesn't mean that it has been made in the United States. If the drink was manufactured or even bottled locally, you still run some risks.

In addition to being cautious of the liquids you drink, you should also be careful trying new and exotic foods. Any foods you do eat should be well cooked and properly prepared. Avoid foods that do not look or smell the way you'd expect them to. It's better to be safe and hungry than full and uncomfortable.

If you do want to eat fruits or veggies, peel them carefully, throw away the peels, and wash them with purified water. If any food has a broken skin or looks damaged, throw it away. You're usually better off not eating any foods that haven't been cooked. Canned baby foods that are available in large markets can be good dietary supplements (remember, you did like them once!). Here is a disappointing thought, however. Pastries, especially those made with cream, can be dangerous (and not just to your waistline)! If they're not prepared and stored properly, bacteria can grow in them. If you want to eat meat, be very careful about where you eat and what you choose to eat. American laws are very strict about the inspection of meats served to the public. Laws may not be as strict or may even be nonexistent in other countries. Therefore, you run the risk of eating improperly cooked meats, meats that have not been prepared appropriately, and so on. Use good judgment. You may ask, "Why can't I eat this when the people who live here eat it all the time?" Don't be jealous. You don't know if that's true. You don't know if they eat these foods or if they avoid them, too. Or maybe natives are used to these foods and their lead-lined stomachs can handle foods that your stomach can't. Perhaps hundreds of natives are home in bed with food poisoning! At any rate, be sure to protect yourself.

Are you beginning to think that because there is so much to be afraid of, you won't be able to enjoy your vacation? Don't feel that way. Just remember—you're not going on vacation merely to eat. (If you are, go someplace where you won't have to have such food worries!) Instead, try to emphasize the other, more enjoyable aspects of your trip. Adequate preparation and total awareness are easy to achieve and will certainly help to make your trip an enjoyable one.

BEWARE OF THE SUN!

If you are sun-sensitive, your vacation should be someplace that does not emphasize exposure to the sun. This does not mean you should avoid sunny cruises or trips to tropical destinations. You'll just want to make sure that there is plenty of opportunity to sit in the shade, and that there are plenty of things to do when other members of your traveling party may want to be out in the sun. (And don't forget the sunblock!)

All Aboard!

Remember, not everyone is like Ellen. Many individuals with lupus feel absolutely no reluctance to travel anywhere. If you haven't traveled recently, you may want to build up your confidence by taking short trips first. Taking a three-month trip around the world might be a bit much! Even an overnight trip might be traumatic. Start with a couple of day trips, then weekend trips, working your way up to short-distance, week-long excursions. Expanding your travel activities slowly is a good way to develop your confidence.

A lot of information has been provided here—mostly precautionary, but nevertheless realistic and sensible. You may need extra time to prepare for your vacation, but this extra preparation will enable you to enjoy a wonderful trip, just like any other globetrotter. Don't forget to send me a postcard!

16.

SEX AND LUPUS

This chapter is not rated R for Restricted. Rather, it is rated E for Essential. Why? If you are sexually active, you certainly don't want lupus to prevent you from having an enjoyable sex life. Sex can be very important for people with lupus. It's an activity of comfort, a way of connecting with someone special in the most intimate of ways. It's a way of having something pleasurable associated with your body, rather than the typical discomfort of lupus. It's even an excellent way of exercising, relaxing, and reducing pain.

Can lupus decrease your sexual appetite or ability? Certainly, some people with lupus experience a decreased interest in sex. As a matter of fact, decreased sexual interest is quite common with a number of chronic medical problems. This can have an important bearing on the closeness of the relationship with your partner.

Has lupus decreased your sexual appetite? What kind of sexual relationship did you have before you were diagnosed? If you had a good one, you may have an easier time getting over any obstacles that lupus may have thrown into your path. If your sexual relationship wasn't good, it is unlikely that having lupus will make it better! You may need some professional help to keep things from breaking down altogether. But hope is not lost. If you unite with your partner to work things out together, reassure each other, relearn how to please each other, and show a desire for each other—progress can certainly be made.

Sexual problems related to lupus can be physiological or psychological in origin, or they may be a combination of the two. Let's look at both types of causes and at possible means of coping with sexual problems.

Physical Problems

Can physical problems alter your interest in sex? You bet your hormones they can! Because lupus may affect the way your body feels, it may also affect the way your body is able to participate in sexual activities. The goal is to focus on what you can do, not on what you can't. Depending on the degree to which lupus and its treatment is affecting you and on your previous level of sexual interest and activity, a number of physical problems, including joint pain, mobility problems, fatigue, Raynaud's phenomenon, mouth or vaginal ulcers, or vaginal or other dryness may either alter sexual desire or make it more difficult to engage in sexual relations. Let's learn a little about these possibilities.

If you have pain in your joints, are you going to want to move around? Probably not. Sexual activity, offset by pain, is not too pleasant, causing the "ohhh, ouch" syndrome. Because painful movement or restriction of joints can make sex difficult, it's important to explore possible ways of changing this. Try procedures that can help relax your muscles or reduce pain, such as moist heat, warm baths, or compresses. Limbering-up exercises may pave the way to more pleasurable sexual encounters. (This gives new meaning to the phrase "warm-up," doesn't it?) If you're taking pain medication, take it early enough so that it is working in your body by the time you're planning on beginning your sexual experience. Try to plan sexual activities when pain is at its mildest.

You may want to try different positions. Some of them may put less of a strain on problem joints. If sexual activity is painful, you may be better off taking a less active role in your encounters. Discuss this with your partner. Together, you may be able to come up with a solution. On occasion, the use of simple devices such as pillows or kneepads can make sex a lot less painful. Or you can also use relaxation techniques to help enhance the pleasures of sexual activities and decrease the pain (see Chapter 9).

Is there any particular time of day when you experience less pain? For some people, it may be too uncomfortable to have sex late at night. Others may be too stiff in the morning (no comments, now!) or in the early part of the day. Working these problems out takes the cooperation of both partners. Schedule time for intimacy, when you are well rested. Don't wait for a time that you're not in pain. If you wait until you're in the mood, you may wait a long time. In many cases, once you begin an intimate encounter, the feelings (and hormones!) flow and it becomes more natural. Create an environment that is conducive to warm intimacy. Children, work, and other responsibilities may all interfere, but it's better to have sex at planned times than not at all. Frequently, sexual problems can be helped by using your imagination and experimenting with different varieties (in position, timing, and technique).

Finally, a satisfying sexual relationship can actually help relieve pain. Not only is it distracting, but sexual stimulation actually releases endorphins (those chemicals produced in the brain that block pain and produce pleasure).

Fatigue can be a factor. If you're tired, you're going to be less interested in sexual activity. This can be a real headache! (Sorry about that!) But if you're uncomfortable or fatigued, or in too much pain, hanky-panky will just have to be put on hold. Is this a poor choice of words? Actually, it may be an excellent idea. After all, just holding each other can be wonderful, too! So instead of shying away from sex because of the fatigue that so often is part of lupus, focus on the less active, less strenuous ways of enjoying intimacy.

The twenty-second kiss can revive the feelings that brought you together. The sixty-second hug is also a wonderful way to reconnect after a stressful day or when you are in pain. About halfway through a long hug, you will relax in each other's arms and feel a great release of tension. So explore other ways to enjoy intimacy with your partner. If returning to or increasing sexual activity seems uncomfortable or frightening, approach things slowly in order to get yourself back into a more normal routine. And be patient. Don't feel that you have to accomplish everything at once. By minimizing the pressure you place on yourself, you can maximize enjoyment and get back into the swing of things at your own pace. Feel free to experiment with various techniques and activities to determine the degree of arousal that is safe and comfortable.

Raynaud's phenomenon may reduce sexual interest as well. With Raynaud's, circulation of blood is restricted in the extremities. During sexual excitement, more blood concentrates in the genital area, further reducing the amount of blood that is available to the fingers and toes, potentially creating a lot of pain in these extremities. The use of medication, even aspirin, can help both joint pain and Raynaud's phenomenon. A warm bath can be very soothing, and a nice waker-upper to prepare you for a pleasurable sexual encounter. Raise the temperature in the bedroom. This can improve blood circulation in the hands and toes, adding to your comfort. Consider lying on a heated blanket. Or be aware of the times when your medication seems to be most effective, and try to plan your encounters during those times. Finally, how about wearing socks? It may not sound glamorous, but it does help!

Mouth or vaginal ulcers or sores may interfere with sex. Although painful, these ulcers need not prevent all kinds of sexual activity. Certain types of gentle physical contact can be enjoyed as long as both partners are willing. A warm, understanding relationship certainly makes this possible. And mouth or vaginal ulcers can be treated. Treatments include steroid applications, such as special mouth washes with added antibiotics for mouth ulcers, and steroid suppositories for treating vaginal ulcers.

Some women may experience tissue dryness. The dryness may be in your mouth, eyes, or vagina (this may be due to Sjögren's syndrome—see Chapter 7). This can be a problem. Vaginal dryness can make intercourse so painful that you'll want to avoid it. (It may also cause bleeding.) But don't think of vaginal dryness as a lack of excitation. Dryness is not an unusual complication of lupus. If dryness causes painful intercourse, what can you do? Keep in mind that a longer period of foreplay can increase vaginal lubrication. Be sure that irritants such as latex condoms, bubble baths, douches, contraceptive creams, laundry detergents, or spermicides are not the cause. And avoid products that may cause dryness, such as antihistamines, and others (such as douches, sprays, and colored or perfumed toilet paper and soaps) that can irritate delicate tissues. There are a number of commercial lubricants available that can enhance your comfort and pleasure during intercourse. Water-based lubricants, such as K-Y jelly, offer many advantages over other products because they are safe for use in the vagina and wash off easily after sex. Additionally, water-based lubricants are safe for use with latex contraceptives. On the other hand, oil-based lubricants, including those containing petroleum jelly and baby oil, should not be used inside the vagina because they may irritate the vaginal lining. Add moisture to your tissues by drinking eight 8-ounce glasses of water daily. Herbs such as dandelion leaf and oat straw, taken orally, may help restore vaginal lubrication.

What about drugs? Some drugs can have a direct effect on sexual desire. Sexual problems may be caused by such medication as painkillers, blood pressure medications, sedatives, and tranquilizers. It's true that small amounts of tranquilizers, for example, may make you feel more relaxed (increasing the possibility of sex), but too much can work against you, possibly suppressing sexual desire or your ability to achieve orgasm. Other types of "drugs," such as alcohol, are notorious in reducing sexual abilities because of their effect on the body.

Psychological Problems

Your body isn't the only thing that may affect your sexual interest. Your mind also comes into the picture.

What's the most important sexual organ? Think about this for a while. The correct response is . . . your brain! (Did I catch you?) So if a sexual problem has no physiological cause, then its cause must be psychological. In fact, the psychological variables that affect sexual activity are just as real as the physiological factors. Anxiety, depression, and fear can all form emotional blocks that significantly impair sexual enjoyment.

Many people with lupus experience a decreased interest in sex. This doesn't necessarily mean there's something wrong with you. As a matter of fact, decreased sexual interest is common in many chronic illnesses.

Let's learn about some of the psychological problems that may affect sexual relations and discuss how these obstacles can be overcome.

POOR SELF-IMAGE
Living with lupus can certainly affect your self-esteem. Do you feel like a different person now that you have lupus? Do you feel like "damaged goods"? Do you like yourself less because of your condition? If your answer

to any of these questions is yes, your self-image has suffered as a result of your lupus. Body image, an important component of self-esteem, plays a major role in one's sexuality. If you have a positive opinion of yourself, then your ability to respond to sex is positive. You are less likely to worry that your partner will reject or disapprove of your body. As a result, you may feel less need to limit your sexual activity simply to minimize this chance of rejection.

Why might you perceive yourself as being different as a result of your lupus? How has lupus affected your perception of your sexuality? You may feel that you are less masculine or less feminine (depending on your gender, of course!) now because of changes in your body. Or perhaps you have gained some weight, either before or since your diagnosis. You may even be afraid to get dressed or undressed in front of your partner. Alice, a forty-seven-year-old woman married for twenty years, was upset about her bloated appearance from long-term prednisone use. She feared that her husband would not want to touch her because of the way she looked. Do you fear that your partner may be less interested in sex because of the way you look? Actually, your partner may not feel this way. But you may try to avoid sex anyway, rather than risk rejection.

Dissatisfaction with your appearance can most certainly cause your self-esteem to drop. And you can't truly enjoy sexual intimacy if you don't feel good about yourself. So what's the answer? See what things you can change (consider getting advice about clothes, makeup, and other appearance enhancers). It makes sense to work on enhancing your looks in whatever ways are appropriate. If you are overweight, other than trying to lose weight, wear fashions that will trim down your appearance. If you're not happy with a rash on your face, apply makeup so as to make it appear more aesthetically pleasing. Whatever the problem, there is usually a way to correct or at least improve it.

Consider speaking to professionals about the changes that have affected you the most to learn about things you can do to eliminate or lessen any problems. And remember, although working on your physical appearance is an important part of looking good and feeling better, probably the most significant step you can take is to work on your attitude. Tell yourself that nobody's perfect—and nobody expects you to be perfect, either! Use some of the thought-changing procedures described in Part Three. Feel good about the things that are truly important in your life, and minimize the rest.

FEAR OF PREGNANCY

Research has shown that withdrawal from sexual activities is sometimes the result of a fear of pregnancy. This can even be a subconscious fear—one that you're not consciously aware of. Whether your reasoning is conscious or unconscious, the avoidance of sex may seem like the best way to avoid getting pregnant.

Why might you be afraid of getting pregnant? There are a number of reasons. You may be concerned that it will affect your condition. You may be concerned that your child will develop lupus! (Remember: Lupus is not considered to be a hereditary disease. Although small percentages of newborns may have lupus cells in their systems, these lupus cells tend to pass out of their systems within six to eight weeks following delivery. So fear of giving birth to a child with lupus need not be a reason to curtail sexual activity.) You may be concerned that you will be less effective as a parent because you have a chronic medical condition. And any or all of these fears can have an impact on your feelings about sex.

Let's say you just don't want to get pregnant. This creates a new problem: which contraceptive devices to use. Birth control pills should *not* be used because they can worsen a lupus condition or cause flares. Intrauterine devices (IUDs) should not be used because they also increase your chances of infection. You always want to minimize this. Many women with lupus prefer to use spermicidal jellies, foams, or creams. These preparations may not be as effective as birth control pills, but when used in combination with male contraceptive devices (such as condoms), they can minimize your chances of an unplanned pregnancy.

EMOTIONAL INTERFERENCE

Sexual activity—and sexual desire—may be impaired by a number of emotions. It is not unusual for people with lupus to have feelings of anxiety, fear, frustration, anger, resentment, hopelessness, depression, loneliness, guilt, isolation, and despair.

Depression may keep you from having any interest in sex. Anxiety concerning sex itself or the intimacy of your relationship can also hold you back. You may be concerned about possible rejection by present or future sex partners. Or you may fear that sexual arousal will increase pain. Certainly, negative emotions don't enhance the pleasure of sexual intimacy!

Your fear of pain may decrease your interest in sex. For example, if you've had vaginal ulcers, they usually go away with proper treatment. But what if you have a long memory of the pain you suffered from ulcers, and you worry that the friction of intercourse may bring about a recurrence of these ulcers? If so, the psychological effects of the ulcer may last longer than the physiological effects.

When negative thoughts and feelings affect sexual desire or performance, it's necessary to get at the root of the cause and to use coping strategies to eliminate troubling emotions. If anxiety or depression is affecting your sexual well-being, you'll want to improve your attitude. Use some of the thought-changing techniques described elsewhere in the book. They may be the key to your future happiness!

What else can you do to eliminate psychological obstacles to a fulfilling sex life? A very important part of sexual relationships is communication. All too often, sexual relations diminish because of physical or psychological concerns—on either side! This could be improved through constructive communication. If you and your partner can share thoughts and feelings, you'll be in much better shape to work out any problems that may occur as a result of your condition. Think about what's bothering you. Ask your partner what his or her concerns are. For example, you may need to discuss concerns about pain with certain positions. If necessary, work to alter the ways in which the two of you express your sexual desires. For instance, if there are times when you're in too much pain or just too tired for sexual activity, feel free to tell your partner how you feel. Talk about what feels good and what hurts during sex. Fully communicate your needs. And remember that problems get worse only when you chronically avoid the issues—not when you openly discuss them and work together to find solutions. If you feel unable to have these conversations on your own with your partner, enlist the assistance of somebody who has the compassion and expertise to guide you in a better direction.

Ruth, a thirty-eight-year-old housewife, had lupus. Her husband, Bill, felt incapable as her lover because he was unable to get Ruth aroused, and because she experienced pain whenever he attempted to make love to her. But Bill may be reassured to know that these problems could result from lupus rather than his inadequacy as a lover. Ruth and Bill should explore different methods of igniting sexual fires and should discuss these problems constructively. They want to avoid the prospect of unpleasant feelings developing between them.

Besides communicating your feelings and fears to your partner, you might also want to discuss any physical problems with your physician or with other health care professionals. For instance, perhaps you are concerned about the possibility of increased pain after sexual activity. That thought may be enough to kill a romantic mood! Discuss with your doctor different possible solutions to this problem. A qualified mental health professional or sex therapist who understands lupus might also be helpful for some couples. You can also take your partner with you to the doctor and talk about the problem openly and honestly.

So much of what's been said in this section assumes that your sexual interest or performance has been affected by psychological problems and that your partner is suffering as a result. But what if the opposite is true? What if you still have normal sexual desires and normal performance, but your partner is the one who's afraid? Maybe your partner fears hurting you or creating additional problems. Or maybe you're regarded as a fragile flower that is easily broken, and your partner is reluctant to be sexually spontaneous. Discuss this with your partner. Make sure that you communicate with each other, and be sure to set up ground rules so that you know which sexual activities are okay and which, if any, aren't. And if these one-on-one attempts at working things out don't help, don't hesitate to get some professional assistance. The results will be well worth the effort!

What If You're Single?

If you are single and dating, your concerns may be different from those of a person who is married or in another type of long-term relationship. For example, you may wonder when the best time is to tell the person you're dating about your condition. Should you mention it right from the start, or not until you're approaching a sexual encounter? In general, most experts believe that you need not say anything at the very beginning. After all, you want to get to know the person first, and you want the person to get to know you. Then, if the relationship seems to be proceeding in the right direction, you may want to consider a comfortable time to mention your condition. If you think that there is a future with someone you are dating, you definitely need to be honest and open. Your disease does not define who you are, but it is an important part of you that your partner will have to accept.

How should you share the news? There are as many different ways of saying something as there are people. The one most common piece of advice, though, is to show that you're handling your lupus well. Make it sound as if you're in control. The most frightening thing for a prospective partner is the feeling that you're so overwhelmed by your disease that it's definitely going to have an impact on the relationship. Test the waters first. You could say, "I have a disease that causes me pain in my joints," and then watch and see how much the person can handle. If your pain prevents you from going out on a date, you do need to let that person know that you have a medical condition. Proceed on a "need to know" basis. If the person is truly interested, provide additional bits of information, always making it clear that you're handling your condition. If the person shows some concerns, you'll know either that you need to wait before sharing additional information or that this relationship may not be for you.

Remember, sexual problems can be frustrating, especially if you don't have a partner. It may be uncomfortable for you to even think about finding someone new, knowing the problems you're having with lupus. Take things one step at a time. Be more social, look to make new friends, and try not to worry about the more intimate activities that might occur in the future.

And Now, the Climax

When dealing with any sexual problems that come along during your life with lupus, remember that much can be done to improve both your feelings regarding sex and your enjoyment of the activity. As a matter of fact, in many cases, people with lupus feel that expressing love and passion can be the most pleasurable experience they share with their partner while going through the ordeal of living with the disease. Psychological coping strategies can help you overcome many obstacles to interest and performance. But the most important one is to maintain open communication with your partner. Even if your sex life becomes less active, you can still have a warm relationship—but not if there are bitter feelings and misgivings. Honest discussions, marked by understanding, are a vital part of coping with sexual problems, just as they are a necessary part of coping with any other aspect of lupus.

Make sure that you do and be what is true for you, not to please someone else. A person who learns how to experience and direct sexual energy for the greatest possible pleasure will experience an improved sex life. Have a good attitude about being sexual. If you have a loving and sensual relationship with yourself, you will have one with your partner.

What if your interest in sex fails to increase after a period of time? Speak to your doctor, who may be able to make valuable suggestions. However, if this doesn't seem to be the solution to your problem, don't hesitate to seek help from a mental health professional or a sex therapist.

Remember: Having lupus doesn't mean that sexual activity must be reduced, curtailed, or totally eliminated! As a matter of fact, it can still be as pleasurable and as important as the partners want it to be.

17.

PREGNANCY

To have a baby, or not to have a baby: that is the conception. Whether it is nobler (or safer) to have children may be a big question mark. Why? Many people with lupus worry about pregnancy. You may be afraid that lupus will cause a difficult or unsafe pregnancy. You may be concerned that if lupus is genetically transmitted, your children may have a greater chance of developing it. Let's consider some of the important issues related to conception and pregnancy if you have lupus.

Before Trying to Conceive

If you are going to try to conceive, discuss your decision with your physician. You should discuss your desire to conceive with your gynecologist as well as your rheumatologist. This is especially important if your lupus is in a flare. Your doctor can best advise you whether this is the right time to consider conception. In fact, some experts believe that pregnancy should not be attempted until disease symptoms have been controlled or in remission for at least several months to one year.

IF THE TIME IS NOT RIGHT . . .

If pregnancy is not advised or for whatever reason you do not wish to become pregnant, the only way to make sure that you don't conceive is to use an effective form of birth control. Contraceptives available to women with lupus are the same as for other women . . . with one noticeable exception: Women with lupus should *not* use birth control pills, unless your doctor has specifically approved their use for you. Other acceptable birth control options include barrier methods, such as the diaphragm plus spermicide or condom. The risk of unplanned pregnancies with any of these birth control options is reduced as long as the techniques are used correctly. Talk with your doctor to find out which method will work best for you.

Certain immunosuppressive drugs should also be discontinued prior to conception. (This may apply to men with lupus also, if they are taking immunosuppressive drugs.) Discuss with your doctor any medications being used, to determine which may need to be stopped, and how long you need to wait before trying to conceive.

IF THE TIME *IS* RIGHT . . .

Will you have more difficulty conceiving because of lupus? Probably not, although some women have problems conceiving regardless of their medical condition. In some cases of lupus, menstruation may cease or periods may become irregular when they used to be regular. However, physicians have indicated that even if menstruation ceases, ovulation can still take place and conception can still occur. So if you are not menstruating, that does not mean you cannot become pregnant. Therefore, you should take normal precautions even if you're not menstruating.

When you and your partner decide to try to have children, check with your physician to make sure there are no other reasons to hold off. For example, it's probably not a good idea for women to attempt to conceive while in the middle of a lupus flare. (For men, this should not make a difference, depending on the drugs being used to control the flare. Speak to your doctor.) This doesn't mean that you can't try, however, or that something will go wrong if you conceive while in a flare. But you'll probably want your condition to be stable for a while so you'll be in the best possible shape for your pregnancy if it does happen. Should you try to conceive if you have elevated blood pressure or kidney involvement? Again, it's probably not the best idea, especially if your kidney trouble is more serious. But speak to your doctor.

Each case should be discussed individually. (In addition, you might not want to consider expanding your family if you're having difficulty fulfilling all of your current responsibilities.)

Are you concerned that there may be a possible genetic factor involved in lupus? You may be concerned about passing lupus on to your children. As we've discussed previously, although there is a genetic predisposition to lupus, and there are families in which several members do have lupus, it is less common for lupus to be transmitted genetically to your children.

Ensuring a Healthy Pregnancy

After you become pregnant, it is essential to remain in close contact with your doctor. This is especially important because you have lupus. This way, if any problems do develop, you'll be able to "nip them in the bud."

Although you may have had an obstetrician before you were diagnosed with lupus, be sure that he or she will take care of you now, considering your medical condition. Some may prefer not to take individuals with lupus and will suggest switching to a different obstetrician (a high-risk one, if possible). Is this unfair? You may not be happy about it, but you certainly want to know if a physician feels uncomfortable.

Does Lupus Affect Your Pregnancy?

Unfortunately, your pregnancy may not be without problems if you have lupus. Individuals with lupus have a statistically greater chance of premature births and neonatal complications. There is a greater chance of miscarriage (often due to the existence of antiphospholipid antibodies; see Chapter 7), and there might be a statistically greater chance of stillbirth. Pregnancy problems may also be due to hypertension (and preeclampsia—hypertension specifically related to pregnancy), gestational diabetes, and lupus activity. So what's the best thing to do? Discuss all these matters with your doctor.

Besides these problems, other things that can disrupt any normal pregnancy can still occur. Such pleasures as morning sickness, nausea, and fatigue are still possible. Thrilling, right?

Does Pregnancy Affect Your Lupus?

Pregnancy can cause a higher than normal level of stress, although it is impossible to predict what will happen during anyone's pregnancy. It's possible that you'll feel better than usual during your pregnancy. Or you may experience more marked symptoms and be in a flare for almost the whole time. As a matter of fact, some people first learn that they have lupus during or after their pregnancy. Why? Because symptoms develop that prompt them to go to the doctor and that's when they discover that they have lupus! In more than half of women with lupus, however, pregnancy has no bearing at all on the way lupus affects them. For the most part, be reassured that even if pregnancy does affect your lupus (either during or after the pregnancy), these problems are rarely so serious as to be life-threatening.

Elaine, a twenty-five-year-old mother of one, was one of the unfortunate ones. She had been diagnosed with lupus two years prior to her current pregnancy. She was feeling pretty good, though, so she decided to add to her family. However, within two weeks of conception, she went into a flare that made her want to crawl into a washing machine and spin dry! She then considered aborting the pregnancy, hoping this would end the flare. However, in most cases, physicians feel that having an abortion will not help a flare. If anything, it may even make it worse. Physicians prefer that you take steroids to try to control the flare.

Medication and Pregnancy

This physician preference leads us to another important point. If you can, it's usually a good idea to avoid most medication during pregnancy. But this is not always possible. Many women, for example, have used aspirin during their pregnancies without any damage to the fetus. Other medications, such as prednisone, have been used during pregnancy. Don't take decisions regarding medication and pregnancy lightly, however. And don't take decisions into your own hands. That's what you have a doctor for, right?

There are certain medications that shouldn't even be considered during pregnancy, such as immunosuppressive drugs. If you're on any of these, don't even attempt to conceive yet. Wait for your doctor's go-ahead after discontinuing their use for a period of time.

What if you discover that you're pregnant while you're on medication? Your doctor may want you to stop the medication as soon as possible. It's okay to stop certain medicines abruptly (your doctor will advise you). But remember that it is possible that you may go into a flare after discontinuing their use. And discontinuing the use of certain medications (such as prednisone) very suddenly can be dangerous indeed. Whether you should continue medication, stop it, or even consider pregnancy is a matter that you'll want to discuss with your family and your doctors (not just your rheumatologist, but your obstetrician and possibly a high-risk pregnancy expert).

Nutrition During Pregnancy

Nutritional planning is essential during pregnancy. You will need sufficient calories to support both your own strength and the growth of the baby. Doctors will determine specifically what your nutritional and weight goals are, depending on your size, pre-pregnancy weight, ideal weight, and other factors.

During pregnancy, you will probably need to increase your intake of protein as well as iron, folic acid, and calcium. You will also need additional vitamins and nutritional supplements to support the growing fetus. Discuss a nutritional plan with your doctor, nurse, or dietitian and follow their advice so you and your baby stay healthy.

As we discussed in the chapter on diet, controlling fat intake, eliminating additives, and eating a healthful diet will be even more important during your pregnancy.

Exercise During Pregnancy

Exercise is now just as important as, if not more important than, before you were pregnant. The same benefits that one normally gets from exercise, including relaxation, better fitness, better body image, increased sense of well-being, are necessary during pregnancy. So don't stop exercising, although you may want to lower the intensity of your workout. Being physically fit and staying that way will help you to better deal with labor and childbirth. It can also moderate or reduce the chances of excessive weight gain. Exercise will also increase your strength and stamina, and lower your anxiety level.

So how much should you exercise during your pregnancy? Ideally, moderate exercise done safely is the norm. The specifics vary, though, on a case-by-case basis. Because there may be risks, discuss your exercise program with your obstetrician, as well as your rheumatologist, in order to determine how much exercise is best for you.

After Delivery

To try to avoid flares resulting from delivery, steroids are usually increased just prior to delivery. You should also try hard to avoid any stressful circumstances (other than contractions!) because of your increased vulnerability at this time.

If you do go into a flare, it may occur in the short period of time (anywhere from two weeks to two months) following delivery (the postpartum period). Increased lupus problems often relate to kidney problems or emotional distress, although flares can occur for any reason. However, close cooperation with your physician can probably reduce the likelihood of such a postpartum flare or at least of such a flare becoming serious.

WHAT ABOUT THE BABY?

In general, the babies of mothers with lupus do not show any more evidence of lupus at birth than the babies delivered by women who don't have lupus.

Newborns of mothers who have lupus, however, may show a higher incidence of congenital heart block. This medical problem is usually associated with the presence in the mother of one of the antinuclear antibodies, called anti-Ro. Therefore, experts feel it would be reasonable to check all newborns of mothers with lupus for this problem, so that appropriate treatment can be started if necessary.

If your baby was tested for the presence of LE cells or given an ANA test when born, these tests might come back positive. But the results are most likely positive because the mother's blood has been circulating within the baby. The tests no longer usually show a positive result after the baby is a few months old.

WHAT ABOUT THE MOTHER?

The period of time following childbirth can be trying for any mother. Lupus adds more potential stress to the mix. Prepare for this. For example, prior to delivery, talk to other women with lupus who have had children. Here are some questions you may want to ask them:

- What has helped them to get used to their new addition?
- How did they deal with their lupus symptoms?
- How did they deal with the added physical and practical pressures around the house?
- How did they deal with any guilt they might feel if they couldn't do as much with the baby as they might like?
- How did they deal with the need to change certain responsibilities within the family?
- What would they do differently if they could?

In addition, you may want to ask if you can call them with additional concerns that may arise as you go through the first days and weeks following childbirth. After all, the best teacher is experience!

BREASTFEEDING

If you are planning to breastfeed your baby, you'll be happy to know that breastfeeding is perfectly safe for mothers with lupus. In fact, breastfeeding appears to offer some advantages over bottle feeding. For example, experts say that breastfeeding causes the uterus to return to its pre-pregnant state faster. Breast milk is an ideal food for your baby—it's packed with nutrients, and it also contains some of your own antibodies, which will help your baby fight off illness. (Please note: If you have more than just a mild case of lupus, or if you have been on moderate dosages of steroids for prolonged periods of time, you may want to consult with your doctor regarding breastfeeding, since the medication may get into the milk and may affect the baby.)

A Pregnancy Pacifier

Pregnancy is a joyous, exciting time for the mother-to-be and her family and friends. For women with lupus, however, there are plenty of questions to ask yourself before deciding whether you should become pregnant. You may have questions about your medication or feel selfish or guilty about your decision to have or not to have a baby. You may worry that you really won't be able to care for the baby if your lupus is so bad that you can't hold, diaper, or feed him or her.

If you and your partner are planning a pregnancy, bring all of the issues that concern you out into the open and discuss them with your family, as well as your obstetrician and rheumatologist. Everyone must get involved in the discussion. We're not dealing with simple questions such as, "Should I take two aspirin today or one?" We're talking about major considerations that have significant psychological overtones, too. Be open and honest in your discussion, and express any of your concerns about the potential risks of pregnancy. Make sure you fully understand all that's involved in ensuring a healthy pregnancy. Remember that in most cases, pregnancy should not be a problem at all, especially if you have only a mild case of lupus. What are the keys to a successful pregnancy? Awareness, supervision, and careful planning. Take all of these factors into consideration, and then—good luck!

18.

MEN WITH LUPUS

It's hard enough to live with lupus. But if you're a man, it may be even harder. Why? You've read the statistics. You've heard that far more women have lupus than men. Some people have even called lupus a woman's disease. So now, not only are you living with lupus, a disease that may already make you feel different, but now, as a man, you may feel even *more* different, even from other people with lupus!

Have people been surprised to find out that you have lupus? Have you been reluctant to even share that news? This may bother you, too. What should you say about all of that? *So what!* Yes, you're a man. But men *do* get lupus. Yes, you have lupus. But focus on dealing with the physical manifestations, coping with it, and living the best life you can with lupus, rather than wasting energy feeling different, feeling sorry for yourself . . . or like less of a man.

Just the Facts, Please

Actual numbers vary, but it is estimated that approximately 150,000 men in America have lupus. Men of any age can get lupus. Statistically, it is estimated that:

- One in four children with lupus below the age of puberty will be male.
- During teenage years and in adulthood, nine to ten females will be diagnosed with lupus for every male diagnosed with lupus.

• After age fifty, approximately eight women will be diagnosed with lupus for every man diagnosed with lupus.

Experts still are not sure about the exact explanation for these numbers, although because of how the statistics vary according to age, hormonal theories continue to be suspected . . . and investigated.

MEN VERSUS WOMEN: SIMILARITIES

Men are diagnosed with lupus in exactly the same ways that women are diagnosed. There are no specific differences in diagnostic methods. The same diagnostic guidelines, using a minimum of four out of eleven criteria, are used.

Lupus symptoms that may affect you are basically the same, regardless of gender. The most common symptoms for both men and women include pain, fatigue, and skin manifestations. The course of the disease is basically the same for both genders, and treatment is generally the same as well.

Some men fear that, because of the idea that it is a "woman's disease," a diagnosis of lupus implies that they are less masculine than men who don't have lupus. Nonsense. One thing has nothing to do with another. Sex hormones, sex drive, sexual functioning, reproductive abilities, and even sexual preferences are virtually the same in men with lupus as in men who do not have lupus. (Of course, if a man is experiencing a significant flare, sexual performance or even desire may decrease, but both men and women may experience this.)

MEN VERSUS WOMEN: DIFFERENCES

Studies have suggested that men with lupus have an increased frequency of seizures, blood clots, and other cardiac-related problems. (This may explain why more men than women suffer from drug-induced lupus, since some of the medications used for heart abnormalities and high blood pressure, such as antiarrhythmic drugs and antihypertensive drugs, are on the list of possible catalysts for drug-induced lupus.) Pleurisy, renal disease, discoid lupus, and hemolytic anemia may also be more common in men with lupus than in women.

What Can You Do?

In general, the emotional reactions of men and women with lupus are basically the same. Men can be depressed, anxious, or angry—the same as women. But the reasons for these reactions may be different. The way you show these emotions may be different. Your thinking may be different. And because the way you think leads to your emotional reactions, it's important to pinpoint the ways in which your thoughts about lupus are affecting you emotionally. Let's talk about some of the things that may affect you, and how you can change your thinking:

- *Are you less able to be physically active than you would like to be?* Many men are affected by activity-related changes. This can apply to work, sports, recreational activities, or sex. Yes, you'll need to deal with any lupus-imposed limitations. For example, make sure you pace yourself, get enough rest, and don't overtax your body. Trying to do too much can wear you down. Do-it-yourself projects may not be as practical, and you may not be able to be a "weekend warrior," for example, attempting to paint your whole house! Don't let it bother you if you paint only one room (or even only one wall!) in a weekend. There's always next weekend to continue the project. Don't feel guilty about doing less, or resting more. Remind yourself that you're doing what you must to take care of yourself. And, of course, focus on what you *can* do; don't dwell on what you can't.
- *Are you concerned about intimacy issues?* Be reassured that *anyone* with a medical problem may have intimacy concerns, male or female, and not just you. Talking about this with your partner is very important, and can be very helpful. If necessary, bring the issue up with your doctor, or discuss it with a mental health professional. In the meanwhile, go give your partner a big hug! (There is more about this in Chapter 16.)
- *Has lupus affected your family life?* If so, pinpoint the ways in which this is a problem. Family responsibilities may need to change. Other family members may be concerned about the impact of your lupus on

them, as well as being scared about the future. But this can all be handled, primarily through good communication. Have family pow-wows to share feelings, make plans, and reorganize responsibilities. It will bring everyone closer, and you'll certainly feel (and deal) better.

- *Are you having problems being able to work?* If this is an issue, or you are concerned about being able to provide financially for your family, discuss this with experts. Look into what other options you may have, both for working and for obtaining financial support. And, as always, focus on doing the best you can; work on your thinking so you can better deal with and accept that which you cannot change.

- *Are you affected by physical symptoms or changes?* Are you bothered by changes such as hair loss, bloating, weakness, or rashes? Learn what you can do to better deal with these symptoms. Get advice about what you can do to help your appearance. Work on the positive ways to look at yourself, instead of dwelling on any changes that may have occurred.

- *Are you having difficulty dealing with other people because of your lupus?* First, be honest with yourself. Are these difficulties because of the ways others are treating you, or because of your own sensitivities? Once you recognize the answer to that, you can start working on improving things, either by communicating more effectively with others, or by working to feel better about yourself. Part Four of this book has a lot more about relationships and the many strategies that can be helpful to you.

- *Are you simply having a hard time coping?* Pete, a thirty-seven-year-old father of three, felt as though he was falling apart. Everything was building up inside of him, and he found (perish the thought!) that he was crying every day. Not only was he having difficulty dealing with lupus, but he was having a hard time with his reactions! The emotions of living with lupus can be overwhelming, for men as well as women. But there's a lot you can do about it. Pinpoint the specific ways in which lupus is bothering you the most. Work on your thinking, and use coping strategies that can help you deal with any of the issues affecting you. Reach out to your support network—your family members and friends you know are there for you. And don't hesitate to speak to a

qualified mental health professional who can give you the support you
need when you need it the most.

WHAT ELSE CAN YOU DO?

I've said it before, but it bears repeating: There are *always* things that you
can do to help yourself. This book contains plenty of information and strategies about lupus and coping more effectively with it, for *everyone* with lupus,
including you! So start using the coping strategies that are most appropriate
to address your concerns. You especially may benefit from learning more
about working on your thinking to control your emotions (see Part Three),
pacing yourself (see Chapter 8), and handling your activities and any limitations better (see Chapter 13).

Would you like to be able to talk to other men with lupus? You may find
it helpful to take advantage of support services, such as counseling or support groups. But here's an interesting reality: if they reach out at all, more
men end up choosing one-on-one counseling, and are less likely to take
advantage of support groups offered by organizations (because they tend to
be more heavily populated by females).

Organizations have become aware of this, and there have been efforts
made to establish men-only support groups. The focus and content of these
groups is often very different than for traditional groups. Men getting together
are less likely to discuss symptoms, impact, and body image, for example,
and more likely just to share stories about their lives, work, sports, and other
topics of common interest. Check with your local lupus organization about
the existence of such a group. If none exists in your area, request that one be
formed. You might even express a willingness to "run the point" on setting
one up. At the very least, mention that you'd like to speak with other men
with lupus, if the organization can connect you. (Read more about support
groups in Chapter 33.)

You might also consider taking advantage of online support or social networking, a way in which you can maintain your anonymity. There are *many*
men with lupus who have confided that they spend a lot of time learning
about lupus in this way. For more information about online support groups
and social networking, see Chapter 34.

A Manly Conclusion

So, sir, hold your head up high. You are not alone. Many other men have lupus; you just may not know who or where they are. Focus instead on feeling good about who you are. Yes, you're a man with lupus, but remember which word came first: "man" . . . that's what you are. And lupus does *not* change that!

19.

CHILDREN WITH LUPUS

How did you react when your child was diagnosed with lupus? Did you feel angry? Did you feel numb? Did you break down and cry?

It's common for parents to have trouble coping with a child's illness. Raising a healthy child is challenging enough, after all! As a parent, you are responsible for your child's physical and emotional well-being. So a diagnosis of lupus can be devastating for your family. You may fear that you'll never be able to deal with the medical reality of the condition. You may wonder if your family can possibly adapt to the lifestyle changes a disease such as lupus requires. And, like so many parents of children with lupus, you may worry that your child will never lead a "normal" life.

This chapter addresses the important issues of your child's life with lupus. The information here applies to any child, regardless of age. However, adolescents can have (and cause!) additional issues, and that's why the next chapter is devoted just to them!

How can you begin to help your child cope with lupus? Parents (as well as others who are close to the child) should learn as much as possible about lupus. The more knowledge you have, the more understanding you can be. You can then be more supportive of your child.

Accept the fact that lupus won't just "go away," but remember that lupus management must not take over your family's life. Love, guide, and discipline your child as if lupus were not a factor. And tell yourself that a diagnosis of lupus is not totally negative—people grow and change not only when things are going well, but also during times of adversity.

This chapter will first look at what you can do to help yourself cope with the problems involved in caring for a child with lupus. Remember, there will be times when you'll have to reach out and get help for yourself so that you can be as strong as you possibly can for your family. Then, we'll look at how you can give your child the tools and self-confidence it takes to manage his or her own care.

Coping with Your Emotions

When your child was first diagnosed with lupus, you may not have been able to react at all; you may have felt "separated" from your emotions. Or you may have felt intense anger, sadness, fear, guilt, or despair. Maybe you even felt relieved to find out the cause of your child's illness. Chances are, you experienced each of these emotions at some point after the initial diagnosis.

Of all the feelings you might have experienced after the diagnosis, guilt and fear are probably the most destructive emotions. Why? These two emotions can interfere with your acceptance of lupus and its treatment as a part of *your* life. And your ability to care for your child ultimately depends on your acceptance of his or her condition.

It is important to try not to let your child see your pain or unhappiness. Imagine how the child will feel seeing unhappiness in loved ones. You can be sure the child will feel guilty. This will only make things worse. So let's take a moment to discuss guilt and fear, and the steps you can take to overcome these emotions.

GUILT

Because of the "genetic predisposition" to lupus, many parents are afraid that they did something to contribute to the onset of their child's illness. They feel guilty for bringing the child into the world, only to develop lupus. Additionally, some parents believe that if they had taken better care of their child (and themselves!), the condition would never have developed. These are the kinds of negative thoughts that contribute to feelings of guilt.

Your feelings of guilt will not positively affect your ability to care for your child. Rather, guilt can lower your self-image and exhaust your emotional resources, leaving you with less of the emotional energy you need to help your child cope. So if you catch yourself feeling guilty because your child has lupus, work on restructuring your thinking. Instead of telling yourself that you're a "bad" parent because your child developed lupus, remind yourself of how much you love your child. Ask yourself if you've ever done anything that a "good" parent might do. (You're sure to come up with more than one example, right?)

In learning to overcome your feelings of guilt, it's important to remember not to dwell on what might have been had your child not developed lupus. Instead, focus on the present and the future. Concentrate on learning how to help your child cope with lupus. The idea is to turn your mind's negative thoughts into reasonable, constructive, positive ones.

As you learn to cope with lupus in your family, never underestimate the benefits that support groups have to offer. Groups provide a forum for the exchange of feelings and ideas. You'll hear how others are dealing with feelings of guilt, and you'll gain valuable information and strategies to help you conquer this destructive emotion. Most important, support groups remind you that you're not alone—and it's much easier to live with a difficult problem when you know that you're not alone. (Read more about coping with guilt in Chapter 26.)

FEAR

When you first learned about your child's condition, were you overwhelmed by feelings of fear? It's certainly natural to feel afraid when someone you love is diagnosed with a serious illness. And when that illness requires the care and lifestyle changes that lupus does, you may be fearful that you won't be able to provide the kind of care your child needs to grow up healthy and well-adjusted. "How will I ever make sure that she takes her medication properly?" "What if he never tells me that he's in pain?" "How can I teach her to take care of herself?" "What will school be like for him?" "What if her condition gets worse?"

Education is the key to overcoming your fears about your child's well-being. Learn as much as you can about lupus—what it is, how it affects your child, and how it's treated. Knowing the facts will help you feel more confident in your approach to treatment and will enable you to communicate more effectively with your child's doctor. Perhaps most important, you'll be well equipped to teach your child about the importance of good lupus management.

When you first set out to gather information on lupus, keep in mind that you don't need to learn everything all at once—otherwise you can easily become overwhelmed. Some parents get so caught up in learning about lupus that the disease seems to take over their lives! Don't allow this to happen. Your goal is to adapt to lupus as a normal part of your life, not to make lupus treatment the focus of your life. (There is more about coping with fear in Chapter 24).

Finally, take care of yourself. It is important for you to maintain your own emotional health in order to be strong for your child. Maintaining a positive attitude not only is essential to help you get through difficult times, but also serves as a valuable role model for your children. If you find that you're getting too negative, take definitive steps to work on this and to improve your attitude and feelings. Recognize, however, that negative emotions are understandable and normal. Be prepared, therefore, to deal with them, rather than be overwhelmed by them. This is essential if you really want to take good care of your child. Make sure you take the time to reenergize yourself, and do things for yourself. You can't feel as though you are "on call" all the time.

Understand Your Child Better

It's not a surprise to know that children living with lupus (or any other chronic illness, for that matter) may have difficulty adjusting and adapting to their new lives. They may find that the emotional consequences of the disease are just as painful to them as physical manifestations.

Learning to adjust to a diagnosis of lupus takes time, for children as well as for adults. Don't feel the need to push your child to accept the disease more quickly, simply because it would make it easier for all concerned if it's accepted. Recognize that it takes time to work through the varied emotions that typify the acceptance of the diagnosis of lupus.

Children with lupus will feel differently from those children who don't have the disease. There can be a stigma attached to being sick, having to go to the doctor, being hospitalized, taking medications, or any of the other very real problems that may exist for a child with lupus. Then there are also the additional psychological concerns, such as when children fear that being labeled as sick makes them different enough to be excluded or ostracized. Any of these issues may contribute to children having difficulty dealing with their peers.

There are many similarities between adults with lupus and children with lupus. There are certain symptoms that children are more likely to complain about: arthritic symptoms (such as swelling and joint pain), fatigue, fever, weight loss, and the butterfly rash. The most common serious problem for children is kidney involvement that may not be symptomatic until serious. This may make it more difficult to get children to comply with treatment programs.

An important factor in determining how well a child will adjust to lupus and its treatment is how well the child handled stress before the onset of the condition. (Does this sound familiar? Of course. This also helps determine how adults will adjust to lupus!) But having lupus is very difficult for a child, especially if physical restrictions interfere with normal activities. You'll want to do everything you can to help the child deal with this. Other problems that may occur for adults, such as feelings of isolation, pain, unhappiness with their bodies, and the side effects of medication, can also plague children. So how do children react to their condition? Some withdraw, sleeping as much as they can, staying away from friends (and even family), and keeping their bodies covered at all times. Others are very open about their condition. They almost flaunt it, trying to get extra attention. But most children with lupus fall somewhere between these two extremes.

Let's briefly mention some of the difficulties experienced by children with lupus:

* Most children want to be like everyone else. They may have difficulty feeling different, or being seen as being different. (Of course, adults with lupus feel different from other adults, too!)

- Children with lupus may experience a variety of emotional reactions, including denial, fear, frustration, anger, and depression.
- They may not be able to do what other children can do. Their pain and/or fatigue may not be understood by their peers. They may experience, or fear experiencing, rejection.
- Symptoms may affect them, making them look or feel different. They may require medication, and experience side effects.
- They may have to go to the doctor more often and possibly be hospitalized more often than other children.
- They may feel uncomfortable getting extra attention from teachers, or other individuals in a position of authority. (This may cause resentment among peers, similar to the reactions of siblings that may occur if parents spend too much time doting on their child with lupus.)

HOW DO CHILDREN COPE?

The way children cope with lupus is based on a number of factors, including:

- *Their personality, emotional state, and their attitude.* For example, some children seem to be able to take virtually everything in stride. They may handle lupus in much the same way that other children would handle any obstacles they encounter. And, of course, having lupus can certainly be an obstacle!
- *Their family environment.* What are the parenting values and philosophies in place? How solid is the "family dynamic"? Does each child have the opportunity to be in the "spotlight"?
- *The specific manifestations of their lupus.* Children (like adults) deal with different symptoms in different ways.
- *Their intellectual abilities.* Related to this is how much children understand about lupus, and to what degree they can participate in self-care.

How Old Is Your Child?

For adults as well as children, coping with lupus depends on the physical symptoms being experienced, and the personality of the individual with lupus. It may be less common for lupus to be diagnosed in children, especially in very young children, but for them, coping often depends on the age of the child, since one's ability to understand and deal with the disease increases as the child gets older. Other factors, including your child's intelligence, emotional makeup, and maturity, all play a role in determining how your child copes with lupus. Let's talk about the unique ways that lupus affects children at different ages. Remember: These are generalizations!

- *Children up to age three:* Very young children (infants, toddlers, and preschool children) tend to understand very little about what's affecting them when they're sick. They do react, however, when they don't feel well. Pain will affect them, and it's even harder when they don't understand why they're in pain or what they can do about it. Due to the strange, uncomfortable experiences that may possibly occur, such as hospitalizations, blood tests, and the like, the presence, support, and comfort of parents is most critical at this age.
- *Children from three to five:* Children of preschool years may have more of a sense of what getting sick is all about, but that doesn't mean they understand why they're getting sick or what the implications are. Children, for example, may not understand whether their symptoms are caused by the disease, side effects of medication, or their activities. Although young, children at this age may begin testing the limits, pushing to see how much they can get away with. They may become resistant to taking medication. Children at this age are not too young to have meaningful conversations with their parents to discuss involvement in their own self-care. Parents may find it helpful to give children "forced choices" to help them learn how to choose how they are going to take care of themselves (for example, "Do you want to take your medication now, or after this television program?").
- *Children from five to twelve:* School-aged children become more aware of what their disease is all about, even if they're still not sure what caused it. They're also more aware of what they need to do to take care of themselves, even if they don't always want to do it. Communication is essential in order to encourage children to be more independent and, at the same time, be appropriately involved in their own self-care.

These children are better able to accept the need for doctor visits or hospitalizations. This is difficult for children of any age, but it becomes less difficult as the child gets older and better understands the reasons for treatment.

Eventually they will be better able to express their thoughts about what's going on with them. They may talk about how lupus is affecting them, but their thinking may not always be accurate. Parents should try to correct misconceptions that may be upsetting, counterproductive, or just flat-out wrong, and provide information in a constructive way in order to help them help themselves. Parents should also be helping children to be more actively involved in their own self-care. The more children learn to help themselves, the more empowered they will be to live successfully with lupus.

- *Children from thirteen up:* Adolescence is difficult for many children, due to increased responsibility, peer pressure, and concerns about approaching adulthood, among many other factors. Having lupus makes all of these factors more difficult. Normally, adolescents are encouraged to be more independent, in socially and morally responsible ways. Parents need to continue to encourage this independence, but balance that with the need to make sure that adolescents continue to take care of their lupus appropriately. (Adolescents with lupus are discussed in the next chapter.)

CHILDREN DENY, TOO!

Both children and adults may attempt to deny that they have lupus or that their life has changed. (You, as a parent, may want to deny that your child has lupus as well!) How do children deny? They may fight fatigue, for example, trying to do everything they used to. Or they may "forget" to take their pills. But denying or ignoring their illness won't make it go away. Children, especially adolescents, are more likely than any other age group to say, "I'm fine!" and try to do everything they normally would, rather than admitting or giving in to lupus. Often, this expression of being "fine" is more important as an attempt to convince themselves than it is to convince parents or doctors. Denial can make it more difficult for parents (and physicians!) to try to keep lupus symptoms in check.

You want to protect, and take care of, your child. But you also want your child to do what's best. Keep in mind that there may be times when children may be able to do more than you think. In many cases, children are less sensitive to pain and other negative aspects of the illness than adults. You may often be more concerned than your child about the lupus. Try not to be overprotective. However, you should still guide your child in the right direction. Even when your child pushes too hard, there are times that it may be better to let the child learn for himself or herself what can and cannot be done. In order to mature while having lupus, your child must be aware of the limitations that exist.

LASHING OUT

Rebellion against authority is a normal part of a child's development. When it happens, be sure that you are prepared to deal with it. At the same time, be assured that a child with lupus will probably not seriously hurt himself or herself with tantrum behavior. So deal with rebellion the same way you would if your child didn't have lupus. Ignore it, wait until the child has calmed down, and then talk to your child. However, if your child throws things around or hurts himself or herself, do try to minimize the physical effects of these outbursts. Try to keep the home environment emotionally calm, stable, supportive, and loving.

How to Help Your Child

If your child has lupus, you'll be much more careful in every aspect of your child-raising than if he or she did not have this disease. You'll want to be certain that your child follows all of the components of the prescribed treatment program. Remember, however, that your child's health care team is there to support you and help make this a smooth process.

Now, let's take a look at some of the ways you can ensure the success of your child's coping with lupus.

HELP YOUR CHILD CONSTRUCTIVELY

Managing your child's lupus should be done matter-of-factly. Make it a regular part of life. It's usually not a good idea to reward your child just for routinely following the lupus treatment. You want your child to learn proper self-care habits—not to expect a reward. Set a good example—teach your child that compliance and consistency are essential to lupus management, and emphasize the idea that the reward of his or her hard work is good health. This way, when your child is ready to take on the challenge of self-care, he or she will already possess some good habits.

PREPARE YOUR CHILD FOR LIFE WITH LUPUS

Prepare your child as much as possible for things he or she may experience. This can include symptoms, treatments, side effects, hospitalizations, and difficulties dealing with other people. For example, by preparing your child for fatigue, it may not affect him or her quite as much as if he or she felt weak and had no idea why this was happening. Consult the doctor with any questions. In addition to providing information realistically, at a level appropriate for the child, and on a need-to-know basis, communication must be honest. For example, telling the child preparing to undergo a procedure that "this won't hurt a bit" will damage the relationship and affect credibility of future communication if it turns out that it hurts a lot!

Teach your child as many different coping strategies as possible for any specific encountered situations. Strategies should involve things that the child should do, as well as improved ways for the child to think. Be willing to reach out to others, health care professionals or other experts, when the coping strategies that seem to be needed are beyond your expertise or awareness.

ENCOURAGE COMMUNICATION

As you help your child learn to cope with lupus, it's essential to keep the lines of communication open. Encourage your child to communicate with you. Why is this so important? Good open lines of communication are essential to help your child deal with every facet of the disease. Only through communication will you learn how your son or daughter feels, physically and emotionally. And only by knowing how your child feels will you be able to help. Encourage your child to share feelings, fears, and practical concerns. For example, don't accept, "I feel fine" as a statement of fact if you see changes in your child's physical appearance and ability. Make sure your child knows that talking about the way he or she feels is not only beneficial, but it's essential. And if your child is depressed, you want to know that, too. Children who get depressed need their parents. You're helping by being there for your child, and by making him or her aware that you care.

How can you encourage communication? Try setting aside some special time when you can chat with your child. Make it a routine—a regular time for good conversation. And you don't have to talk just about lupus. Take an interest in what's going on in your child's life apart from lupus. But let you child know that you'll be ready to talk about any issues related to lupus when he or she feels comfortable discussing these topics.

Listen to your child. Be as aware as possible of everything that your child is experiencing. Work together to identify and come up with solutions to the problems caused by lupus. Children need to be given the opportunity to ask any questions that they may have. You may be surprised at what is most important to your child!

What if your child is reluctant to talk or ask questions? Don't try to force your child to open up if he or she isn't ready. Reassure your son or daughter that you'll be available to talk—or listen—whenever he or she would like. If you remind your child of this often enough, you can be sure you will be sought out when the time is right.

As your child grows older—particularly as he or she enters into the teen-age years—communication may become a bit more strained. Remember, this can happen in any parent–child relationship, whether or not the child has lupus. We'll discuss the special problems that parents and adolescents face in the next chapter.

RESPONDING TO THINGS YOUR CHILD
MAY SAY, ASK, OR BE THINKING

Certain things that your child brings up to you may be easy to handle. But there may be other issues that are more difficult . . . for your child, and/or for you. Honesty and appropriateness are the keys. For example, you can't guarantee that a child will not experience pain. What you can focus on, instead, is the reality that people with lupus can live a long time, and pain comes and goes. Tough questions may be asked, questions that you may not be sure how to answer. Don't hesitate to defer answers until you've had the opportunity to speak to somebody about them, or to bring somebody else into the conversation.

When you try to provide answers to your child, make sure that you consider the unique personality characteristics of your child as well as what your child needs from you. Let's discuss some examples:

- *"It's my fault that I got sick."* It's hard enough for a child to deal with having lupus; it's harder if the child believes that he or she is to blame for the diagnosis. For example, your child may worry about things he or she did in the past that might have led to getting sick. You want to do everything in your power to eliminate self-blame.
- *"It's not fair that I got sick."* If your child verbalizes this, you can honestly agree. This may not change the reality of the situation, but you want to encourage your child to be able to share these feelings. It's an unfortunate lesson for children that some things in life may very well be unfair. But that doesn't change the need to cope with them, and everything else, as well as possible.
- *"I hate being in pain."* You can honestly say that you hate it, too; you hate seeing your child hurting. But remind your child that pain comes and goes. Even though pain is an unfortunate, unpleasant part of living with lupus, there are things that can be done to help. (See the discussions about pain in Chapter 9.)
- *"I'm so afraid of all this."* If you sense that your child is upset, or living in fear, it's important to be able to try to help the child identify the fears as specifically as possible. Hopefully, this will help you respond to them in a way that will help the child feel better. You don't want to patronize the child, and you don't want to say that there's nothing to be afraid of, but you do want to help your child develop a more positive attitude.
- *"Will you still love me?"* You want to reassure your child that he or she will always be loved. Having lupus does not mean your child is any

less deserving of your love than always. (And reassure healthy siblings that the same holds true for them.)

- *"Am I going to die?"* Although you'd love to reassure your child that this will not happen, there are never any guarantees. It is realistic to say that everyone is going to die eventually, but there is no reason to believe that your child won't live for a long time. Doctor visits, going to the hospital, being on medication—none of these mean death is imminent. Rather, they're all part of the process of feeling better.

UNITE THE FAMILY

An important goal is to unite your family. The way to best achieve this is for parents to be united whenever possible. Any disagreements concerning your child or your child's health should be aired privately. It can be very damaging for any child to learn that he or she is the source of parental disagreement or dissension between a parent and another sibling. Family routines should continue as before. It may be a challenge, but each family member must learn to live with any restrictions that lupus may impose.

ESTABLISH A GOOD DOCTOR–PATIENT–PARENT RELATIONSHIP

Your child's primary care physician is the "hub" of the wheel as far as lupus treatment is concerned. He or she takes responsibility for your child's overall health, coordinates the efforts of any other health care professionals that are necessary, and provides guidelines for any lifestyle changes that may be beneficial or necessary.

Of course you want the very best for your child, so you must choose a doctor in whom you have confidence medically. (As your child gets older, he or she should be part of the decision-making process as well.) This is only part of the equation, however. Just as important, you'll want to find someone with whom you and your child are comfortable personally. Naturally, you should feel confident that the doctor can address your questions and concerns. But you should also be assured that the physician you choose has the consideration and patience to address your child's concerns. Make sure that your child feels comfortable asking questions. Children, especially very young ones, will be less able than adults to understand the facts about lupus. Your child may ask: "Why do I have to go through all this?" "Why do I have to take all these pills?" "Why do I always hurt so much?" "Why can't we go to the beach anymore or go out in the sun?" "Why do I always have to put that stuff on when we're going outside?" "Why can't I do a lot of what I used to?" "Why do I have to rest so much?" Other questions may also occur.

BE AWARE OF YOUR CHILD'S EMOTIONS

Children may experience many of the same emotions as adults in dealing with lupus. The causes for these emotions, however—the thoughts behind them—may be different, and the ways of dealing with them may be different as well. Let's discuss three of the most common emotions, and what causes them. Then we'll talk about what can be done about them.

Fear

Both children and adults may initially be afraid when diagnosed with lupus. Children may fear how it's going to affect them—if it's going to hurt, if they're going to be sick all the time, how it will affect their school experiences, and if it will affect their friendships. Children may be afraid of frequent doctor visits and of the need for hospitalization. They may also be afraid of an increased need for needles, blood tests, scans, and other components required for treatment.

Anger

Both children and adults may be angry that this is happening to them. Children may be angry that they are, or appear to be, different from other children, both in terms of physical appearance and with regard to the responsibilities and obligations of having an illness. Children may be angry that their activities are limited: they can't play as long or as hard, they need more rest periods, and other children may not understand and may tease them. Children may be angry about the ups and downs of lupus. For example, they may get frustrated that plans that have been made need to be canceled at the last minute because of lupus symptoms. Children may be angry at the unpredictability of lupus. They may feel helpless, knowing that they don't know what to do to make it go away.

Depression

Both children and adults may be depressed because of lupus. Children may be depressed because of the helplessness of living with both the symptoms of lupus and the disease itself. They may be depressed because of the impact lupus has, not only on themselves but on other members of their family, too. They may be depressed because of limitations in their activities, or the impact on their schoolwork. They may be depressed because they need others to help take care of them. This depression may go hand-in-hand with a lower self-esteem. They may be depressed because of pain, fatigue, weight changes, or other physical manifestations. They may be depressed because they feel different from their peers (either because of appearance issues, or by simply having an illness such as lupus), and even more depressed if their peers are unkind in dealing with these differences. This may be even more significant for adolescents. They may be depressed as a result of the medication they take for their lupus. For example, some symptoms require corticosteroids, which can cause mood swings. They may be depressed because of lifestyle changes necessitated by lupus, or its treatment.

How do you know if your child is depressed? There are certain symptoms that you can watch for, including irritability, grumpiness, sadness, demonstrations of feelings of worthlessness, suggestions of hopelessness, decreased interest in normal activities, changes in appetite, changes in school behavior as indicated by teachers, lower grades, emotional outbursts, weight changes, decreases in energy, reduced interest in day-to-day activities, or sleep problems or changes. In general, you know your child. If you see changes in your child that have no specific, tangible explanation, monitor them, and don't hesitate to contact your child's pediatrician. There are times that some of these changes may be a reflection of lupus, rather than depression. This makes it important to consult with your doctors to figure out how to proceed. Stay on top of this.

WHAT TO DO ABOUT YOUR CHILD'S EMOTIONS?

Watch out for warning signs of emotional difficulties. These can include significant changes in normal routine, changes in personality, or school reports about inappropriate or unacceptable behavior. And remember the most important thing: Your child is learning how to adjust to living with lupus as well as possible. If you see signs that your child is having a difficult time with this, don't hesitate to reach out for some professional support. Why make your child suffer any longer than necessary, when professional help can ease the transition into acceptance?

Both children and adults dealing with the emotional consequences of living with lupus need to work on their thinking (more about this in Part Three). Negative emotions come about as a result of negative thinking. Children need to learn to identify when their thinking is negative, so they can work on changing their thoughts in a more constructive way.

Communication between parents and children is critical, regardless of whether the problem is denial, depression, fear, anger, or any other emotion. It is so important for parents and children to be able to talk about how the child is feeling. Parents need to know that lines of communication are open, and children need to know that parents understand the way they feel. In an ideal world, this communication will always be successful and focused. But because of the potential for children to tune out their parents, or even rebel if they don't like what they're hearing, open lines of communication are essential, and need to be gentle, calm, constructive, and sensitive to the needs of the child. For example, if you sense your child is not listening, rather than hammering away and insisting on continuing the conversation, know when to terminate a talk and suggest revisiting the issue at another time. Gently remind your child of the reason for these conversations: not to be annoying, but to be helpful, positive, and realistic.

If you're having difficulty communicating with your child, and you believe that your child is depressed or having other emotional difficulties dealing with lupus, it is important that you inform your child's physician. Together, your child's treatment team can determine how to proceed. In some cases, your child may benefit from supportive services, such as counseling or a support group. In more extreme cases, medication may be warranted. Your child's doctor will be able to guide you and your child in the right direction, and make suggestions for referrals if necessary.

HELP YOUR CHILD TALK WITH OTHERS ABOUT LUPUS

Children who are able to talk about their lupus tend to deal with it better. Conversely, children who have more trouble talking about it, or who are reluctant to share details, tend to have more adjustment problems. Children usually have a sense about whom they're able to talk to about lupus. They know which friends can handle this information and deal with it in a supportive way, and which may not. Decide which things your child is willing to talk about, and how he or she will do it, and identify those things that may be more difficult to discuss. You can even help your child by rehearsing explanations to make him or her feel more comfortable.

HANDLING THE REACTIONS OF OTHERS

You also want to help your child deal with different types of reactions he or she may receive. For example, what if peers want to know more? What if they tease your child? What if they're afraid of lupus being contagious? These and many other issues can be discussed and prepared for in ways that will help your child be more confident dealing with peers.

Teasing is a big problem for many children. It's hard enough when children are teased about nonsense. But if they're teased about lupus, they may feel more defensive and ostracized, and may be more likely to withdraw.

Discuss what is being said and done and what possible things your child can say or do in response. There may be times that situations should be ignored. There may be other times that they can't be ignored. It may be important for your child to learn how to be more assertive. You may want to have practice sessions, "rehearsing" potentially helpful responses. Approaching the teasing peer one-on-one is often more effective than responding to a group. Parents may sometimes need to speak to parents of the teasing children, and teachers or other school officials may need to be informed. As upsetting as this may be, if children know that there are always things that can be done to handle these situations better, they may feel less out of control and overwhelmed.

How observable are your child's lupus symptoms? This is important as part of a discussion about how to get a child to talk about lupus. Some lupus symptoms are unobservable. Pain and fatigue, for example, are hard to see. Children may not want to talk about them, figuring others won't get it anyway. On the other hand, a child's malar rash may lead to curiosity, or even teasing. Peers may also have contagion concerns, which can make the situation even more strained.

In responding to teasers, some children may feel the need to withhold information, or they may "stretch" the truth because they're afraid of any negative reactions. (For example, if someone teases a child about a butterfly rash, they might attribute it to a sunburn so as not to invite any further comments.) Discuss the pros and cons of doing this with your child, and, if necessary, help your child prepare for these interactions.

EMPHASIZE "NORMALCY"

Above all else, you must make sure your child feels normal and accepted. Although at times it may seem very difficult, you want to treat your child with lupus as normally as you would treat any other child. The realities of the condition may warrant certain differences, but whenever possible, raise your child with the same family rules and values that you would under any other circumstance. For example, you do not want to overindulge your child, or let your child get away with behaviors that you would not normally accept. Make sure that normal routines are followed.

Emphasize the child rather than the illness. It is better to still think of or talk about your child as a child who just happens to have lupus. This way, your child will grow up with an identity that is separate from the illness.

Make sure your child continues to be as active a participant as possible in household responsibilities. The goal is to encourage normal development as much as possible, despite the existence of lupus.

Encourage your child to continue to be involved in school and social activities. There may need to be changes in specific activities depending on your child's physical abilities. But help him or her feel good about doing as much as possible, rather than dwelling on what has changed. Try to maintain as normal a life as possible for the child or adolescent. Focus on the need to continue to have good peer interactions.

Continue enjoyable family activities. Although it is important for the family to sit down and discuss lupus and how it's affecting each member of the family, it's also important for the family to do things together and spend time talking about things that have nothing to do with lupus. The best way for the family to work together and move forward is not to focus on how things have changed. Rather, the reality is that someone in the family has an illness. The goal for each person in the family should be to make the best of this, and still enjoy being a family.

Some children can be encouraged to learn other enjoyable activities. Swimming is a great sport and may be good for your child's body. If your doctor approves of this activity, why not encourage it? Other nonphysical activities, such as chess or arts and crafts, can be good outlets. And, of course, doing well academically and developing good reading skills can be a great boost psychologically.

In addition, try to maintain a calm, emotionally stable home. This is crucial to keeping the family together. It is harder to change the behavior of more distant family members. How can you communicate to friends and relatives that you don't want them to bring gifts or to shower extra attention on your child? You want your child to be treated like any other child, despite the condition.

Continue to encourage independence in your child. Keep him or her focused on strengths and abilities, and keep reminding your child, as often as necessary, that having lupus is simply one component of his or her life. Parents need to remind children that each and every person has difficult things to deal with in life. The successfully growing child is the one who learns how to most effectively deal with these difficult things, not the one who avoids (or is protected from) having difficult things to deal with.

Be careful about what your child hears. Anticipate how your child might react if he or she hears something upsetting and try to be as protective as realistically possible. This does not mean hiding the truth, just using discretion about what you share, how you share it, and when.

It is important for parents and children to recognize that the goal is for life to be as normal as it possibly can be. Obviously, this is easier when symptoms are controlled. But when symptoms are active, or your child is in a flare, changes have to be made, and these need to be approached constructively, intelligently, and maturely.

KEEP CAREFUL RECORDS

Establish a health care looseleaf binder that you will use specifically for your child's lupus. By keeping a written or computerized record of all aspects of your child's life with lupus, you will be reassured that all information will be in one place, and nothing will be forgotten.

You'll want to keep records about all doctors involved in your child's care, specifics about treatment, such as dates of implementation, medications (including dosage and times of administration, as well as side effects experienced), appointments, unusual or important experiences relative to the lupus, and a running list of questions to ask health care professionals at subsequent appointments. (Does this sound familiar? Yes, it's the same kind of record-keeping that can help adults with lupus.)

You may want to use a day planner, with sheets covering a day at a time, week at a time, or, if there isn't as much information being recorded, a month at a time.

An excellent website for information, forms, and even an entire notebook that you can download and use for this purpose is the Center for Children with Special Needs, www.cshcn.org.

Have your child be directly involved with record-keeping as soon as it is realistic and possible. Even if your child is just putting smiling or sad faces next to each day, it enables more involvement on your child's part. But there will be times when your child will write more information about what's going on, some of which may even surprise you because you weren't aware of it!

As with everything in life, balance is key. You want to teach your child the importance of good self-care skills, but stress the fact that lupus management should not be all-consuming. And you need to be ready to relinquish control as your child begins to demonstrate the maturity to take over his or her own care.

Does this seem like a tall order? It doesn't have to be, as long as you avoid the following pitfalls:

- **Overindulgence.** Some parents believe that the rigors of self-care are too intense for their child to handle, so they offer special treats while providing little discipline. As a result, the child learns poor self-care skills and may feel incapable of handling self-care when the time comes.
- **Overprotection.** In this case, the parents are so worried about their child's health that they continue to handle most of the details of lupus management, even when their child is old enough to assume responsibility for treatment. A child raised in this type of environment tends to be over-dependent, lacking the self-confidence necessary to be fully responsible for self-care.
- **Indifference.** Indifferent parents are the opposite extreme—they don't fuss *enough* over their child's care and don't provide the discipline and support necessary for the child to learn good self-care skills. The danger here is that the child may "rebel" and seek attention through negative behaviors, such as overdoing, skipping medications, or staying out in the sun. Obviously, these behaviors can have some very harmful physical effects.

No, you're not perfect. (Who is?) You won't always make the "right" decisions when it comes to parenting. Even parents of healthy children struggle with issues such as discipline versus indulgence, and overprotection versus indifference. Just don't lose sight of the bigger picture. Overall, your goal is to raise your child to be a responsible, well-adjusted adult. And when all's said and done, isn't that what every parent wants?

WORK TO IMPROVE YOUR CHILD'S SELF-ESTEEM

Self-esteem is an important issue for children of all ages, and parents should do everything they can to foster a positive view of self. Lupus, and its impact, can adversely affect self-esteem. It is important for everyone involved—the child, the parents, even the physicians—to work together to minimize any adverse impact on self-esteem.

How can that be done? It's important to help the child feel good about who he or she is and to recognize all of his or her various strengths. Keep looking to build on these strengths and look to work on improving weaknesses to offset any lupus-related negatives. It's important to keep reminding your child that "lupus is not who you are, lupus is what you have." (More about self-esteem strategies can be found in Chapter 22.)

GET SCHOOL PERSONNEL INVOLVED

Obviously, you can't be with your child every minute of every day. When school starts, you'll have to entrust your child's care to teachers and other school personnel. Open communication with school personnel will help ensure that your child has a comfortable, safe, and happy school experience.

It is very important for you to discuss your child's lupus with his or her teachers. There are certain aspects of this disease that are essential for a teacher to understand. It's important for teachers to know about the physiological impact of the disease and possible treatment-related tips. It's also important to make sure that teachers are sensitive to the emotional needs of your child, so they can monitor the situation in the classroom (and even outside the classroom) with peers.

It may be helpful to provide informational materials such as brochures or videos. This is helpful both for the teacher's peace of mind and to allow your child to attend school without being concerned about an insensitive teacher. It can also be helpful for teachers to be aware of any potential problems from other classmates, such as those who don't understand or who tease the child with lupus.

A child who has lupus should be able to participate in many normal school-related activities, with exceptions based on pain, sun sensitivity, or other symptoms as they occur. When you talk with your child's teacher, emphasize the idea that your child should not receive special treatment. Most school children just want to feel "normal"—they don't want their peers to see them as being different. Although special considerations may be needed from time to time, this should be balanced with your desire for your child not to be singled out in a way that will cause problems within the school setting. Let teachers know what they should watch for and, if all is going well, that you want your child treated as a normal member of the class. Your child will be expected to complete his or her own work and should be rewarded or disciplined like his or her classmates—as if lupus were not a factor. The teacher should not allow your child to get away with behavior for which other students would be disciplined. Not only would this do a disservice to your child, but it might also foster peer conflicts. By the way, your child should be encouraged to communicate with teachers as well. It can be very comforting for your child to know, firsthand, that teachers understand and are supportive.

EXPLORE PROFESSIONAL COUNSELING

Making the adjustment to living with lupus can be very difficult for a child, especially if any restrictions imposed by the condition interfere with normal activities. Some children may react by denying that the condition exists. They may believe that if they ignore lupus, it will just go away. So they may continue to do the wrong things. Other children may become angry and lash out—temper tantrums are not uncommon among children who are learning to live with lupus. Depression may also be more likely to occur in children with lupus. Naturally, you want to do everything you can to help your child. But sometimes, even a parent's support and understanding are not enough.

If your child is having a great deal of difficulty coping with lupus—if learning to live with the disease is just too painful—then professional counseling may help. Your child may feel that he or she can be totally honest with a counselor and can express feelings that may otherwise remain hidden. At the same time, the child can get feedback that can help him or her better deal with these feelings. If you don't know an appropriate professional, you can get a referral from your child's physician, from your local lupus organization, or from a local hospital or professional organization.

A support group can also help your child overcome negative feelings about lupus. There your child will meet kids his or her own age who are learning to cope with the same challenges and issues. Support groups can provide a great feeling of fellowship and inspiration. Your child can share his or her feelings more openly in this kind of nurturing, supportive environment. (There is more about support groups in Chapter 33.)

Look into special services that can help your child. For example, consider camps with special approaches, such as Camp Sunshine (www.campsunshine .com), a camp that was established for children with illnesses (including lupus) and their families. You may want to check out the kidshealth.org or teenshealth.org websites, which have a lot of valuable information about illness-related topics, with some pages written specifically for children or adolescents. You may even want to spend some time on these sites together with your child, and they may want to use the sites themselves.

HANDLING SIBLING RIVALRY

Lupus in a child can affect the whole family. (Of course, lupus in any family member can affect everyone else, but there are additional issues to deal with when it's your child who has lupus.)

One of the most significant ways in which lupus in a child affects the family is in sibling relationships. Sibling rivalry is normal in any family, whether or not one child has a chronic illness. When one of your children has lupus, the other children in your family will definitely be affected. They may resent the extra attention that they feel is being lavished on the child with lupus, and begin to believe that their needs are secondary. This problem is certainly compounded if friends and relatives fuss over the child with lupus. Brothers and sisters may think that the whole illness is being blown out of proportion—that the child with lupus is making a big deal out of nothing, just to get some attention.

Remember that siblings play many roles in the family: friend, enemy, teacher, student, partner, competitor, role model, leader, follower, confidant, and advisor, among others. These roles tend to evolve over time between siblings, in many cases without parents even being aware of this. It's up to you to help to maximize the positive sibling roles, and minimize the negative ones. Provide information, love, and support. Don't ignore, reject, or be unaware of the changes that have taken place and the needs of each member of the family.

There are more reasons that siblings may have difficulty with lupus in a brother or sister. For example, they may be afraid they're going to develop the same disease. Siblings need to be reassured that just because their brother or sister has lupus, it does not mean it's going to happen to them. You want to make sure that they don't become obsessed with any symptoms they may experience, worrying that they're going to be "coming down with lupus."

Siblings may feel guilty that they, in some way, caused their brother or sister to get lupus. Reassure healthy siblings that they did not say or do anything that led to the diagnosis of lupus in their brother or sister. This is especially true if there has been any sibling rivalry prior to the diagnosis. For example, maybe one sibling said to the other, "I wish you would get sick," or, "I wish you would die." If something like this did happen, the sibling who said it might not dare bring it up to you or anyone else. But if it's harbored inside, it can be devastating.

How can you keep sibling rivalry from breeding bad feelings among your children? Good communication is definitely a key. Siblings need to understand more about what's going on, the role they can play in helping the situation, their right to be able to express the way they feel, and that they are going to get plenty of attention, too. Let siblings know that you understand why they might feel left out, and that you certainly do not intend to push them aside. Remind them that they're every bit as important as the child with lupus, and that you love all of your children equally. And make sure they know that you'll be available to listen if they feel their needs aren't being met.

Have regular family powwows. Use this to keep the lines of communication open. Confront any problems head-on, in a positive, constructive way, so that your children can learn better ways of interacting with their peers and respond more effectively to any negatives that they may encounter.

Make sure you spend quality time with each sibling. (Make sure you stick to this. Empty words here can really backfire.) Although it is realistic that ill children may occasionally require more time, it should always be possible to have time devoted specifically to healthy siblings. Even as little as ten or fifteen minutes a day of quality time can be enough to make each child in the family feel loved and accepted. Include this in your schedule! In this way, you'll know in advance when you're going to spend time with each child and, of course, you want them to look forward to this time as well. Quality time may be in different forms, and at different times in certain circumstances, all determined by what's realistic given everyone's situation. But quality time for a sibling *must* be set aside.

Just as it's important to share information about lupus with your child's teacher, it is important to speak to the teachers of your other children. You want to let them know that their students have a sibling that has lupus. Request that they watch your healthy children and let you know if there are any signs of changes of behavior or emotional difficulties.

It can be very helpful for healthy siblings to be included in some of the medical activities necessitated by lupus. For example, having them go with you and your child to the doctor can be a bonding time. And hospital visits can be stressful for all family members; sibling support can be very important for your sick child. Talk often to each child about this, and make sure everyone's on the same page.

If you sense that healthy siblings are continuing to have difficulty dealing with lupus in the family, make sure you address this. Talk to them about it, and encourage them to air their feelings.

If sibling problems continue to exist despite your best efforts, it may be helpful (if not essential) to reach out to knowledgeable professionals for additional support, understanding, and strategies to help siblings get through this difficult change. Don't hesitate to reach out to health care professionals for advice and support strategies whenever necessary.

Farewell to Childhood

Because your child has lupus, you will have to deal with special challenges that parents of healthy children will never face. Initially, you'll have to take full responsibility for every aspect of your child's treatment. But as your child grows older, you must relinquish some of this control—and that may not be easy.

Childhood is typically considered to be a time for fun and innocence. The responsibilities of lupus may result in an earlier end to innocence and greater responsibility. But if handled correctly, it doesn't have to reduce the fun of childhood—either for your child, or for you!

20.

ADOLESCENTS WITH LUPUS

A h, the joys of adolescence! Adolescence can be one of the most difficult periods in one's life. It's a time of insecurity, sensitivity, rapid physical and emotional growth, and friendships made and broken. It's a time when teenagers struggle to forge a new identity, while attempting to fit in with their peers. Adolescents are swingers, not because they have such active social lives (although they may), but because their behavior and moods may swing so extremely, from the childish dependence of years gone by to the mature independence of adult years approaching.

Adolescents are children, after all. As such, a lot of the information presented in the previous chapter is relevant for all ages of children. Lupus is the same disease, whether you're an adult or an adolescent. But due to the unique changes occurring during adolescence, the ways of dealing with it may be very different. So let's discuss the special characteristics and needs of adolescents.

The adolescent years tend to be sensitive ones. Adolescents are frequently insecure and unstable. Self-esteem becomes even more of an issue, because of increasing participation in social activities and the potential consequences of peer pressure. Although teens can be resentful and rebellious, adult understanding often goes a long way to diffuse emotions and bring a family closer together.

For young children, the restrictions of both lupus and its treatment may be unpleasant but tolerable. However, for adolescents living their "glory days," the changes that accompany lupus may be much more upsetting.

Having to experience ongoing pain and to restrict activities, in addition to feeling lethargic and unattractive, may be very depressing for the adolescent. Adolescents, especially, may be noncompliant regarding their medications or other treatment requirements. Once they find out the ways in which steroids, for example, affect both their mood and their appearance, they simply choose not to "participate."

Then again, many adolescents with lupus cope better than their parents do. Parents may feel guilty. They may feel that they could have done something to prevent their child from having lupus. Parents frequently feel that it is their responsibility to protect their child from harm, disease, or injury. Remember: Adolescents can handle pain more effectively than other age groups and also deal well with fatigue by resting or pushing themselves in spite of it. The adolescent who feels only some occasional pain and fatigue can usually maintain a fairly normal, active life, despite lupus.

Let's learn a little bit about the trials and tribulations of adolescence, and how lupus can compound these problems.

The Need for Acceptance

Many adolescents are embarrassed that they have lupus. As we discussed earlier, children with lupus don't want to be different—they want to be a part of the crowd. Peer acceptance becomes even more important in the adolescent years. Remember, social relationships are very important at this stage of life—friendships eclipse all the other facets of daily life. So a teenager with lupus may try very hard to hide his or her condition from classmates and friends. Or the teenager may be more reluctant to develop social relationships because of concerns about feeling different.

If you sense that your child is feeling lonely or excluded, talk about it. Remind your teen that *everyone* is different. It's our differences that make us unique individuals. Ask your child to think of other teens they know who have to deal with their own differences. Your teen will come to realize that his or her schoolmates aren't as similar as they appear, even though they may look and act alike.

Your child may have a hard time deciding whether to tell friends about lupus. He or she may be concerned that this information will hurt friendships, that friends may be afraid or upset—even hostile—when they hear the news. Some friends may even be scared that they'll "catch" lupus. Your child may feel pressured to hide the truth from friends, and this can certainly take its toll on his or her emotional well-being. So how can you help your son or daughter in this situation? Remind your child that he or she may feel more relaxed if one or two close friends knew about the problem. Reassure your child that true friends will take the announcement in stride, and won't let lupus stand in the way of a good friendship.

Perhaps your teen wants to let friends know about the situation, but can't find the right words. If this is the case, then you'll need to do some brainstorming. Sit down with your son or daughter and think of ways to talk about lupus. Once your teen has settled on a comfortable way to approach the topic, spend some time rehearsing what he or she will say. If your child is uncomfortable participating in this kind of discussion with you, you might want to ask your child's physician or another health care professional for assistance in how to educate others about the disease.

In some cases, your child's lupus may, in fact, be the cause of broken friendships. This can be a problem for anyone, but especially for the adolescent. Making friends is probably one of the most important activities during the adolescent years. Restrictions because of lupus reduce available activities. The adolescent may not be able to spend as much time as desired with friends. It may not be possible to go out as often or keep late hours. It may be necessary to cancel plans at the last minute due to illness. Your child's friends may become annoyed or irritated by these restrictions and may decide not to bother to maintain the friendship.

If your child loses a friend because of factors related to lupus, ask your child why he or she thinks this happened. For example, did your child inadvertently push the friend away? Could the friendship have been saved if the friend knew a little more about lupus? Or was the friend simply uninterested in learning about the condition? It's important to examine these possibilities, so that your child can learn from the situation (although it's certainly a painful lesson).

The Need for Independence

Adolescents want to be more independent. They are approaching adulthood and feel that they should be treated as adults, with all of the freedoms that come with the territory. Adolescents usually work hard at this and like to assert their independence in front of parents. At the same time, they don't want to be too different. This is one reason why adolescents may have great difficulty accepting lupus. Naturally, it's difficult for parents to begin to let go as their children grow older. When teenagers demand more freedoms than their parents are ready or willing to concede, the result is rarely a healthy compromise. Instead, the parents usually find themselves with a rebellious teen on their hands.

Rebellion is just a part of growing up. It's the result of a child's attempts to define a new identity as an adult. Again, this stage of adolescence may be more painful and volatile for children with lupus. Why? Because the natural tendency of any parent is to become overprotective when a child is sick. Your teen with lupus may resent what he or she perceives as interference on your part. Clearly, closer supervision is the *last* thing a teenager wants at a time when independence is of utmost importance!

How can you resolve these conflicts? Realize that your teenager expects support and understanding during these trying times. Let your child be more responsible for self-care. Try to keep an eye on his or her progress, but don't send the message that you don't trust your child. Even when your child pushes too hard, try not to interfere. Some way or another, your child must learn what he or she can or cannot do. If your child is forgetful or careless in his or her approach to self-care, engage him or her in constructive discussions. You'll find that gentle reminders are much more effective than put-downs or confrontations.

Some parents try to protect their adolescents by withholding information about their lupus. This is not a good idea. If you expect your child to be responsible for lupus management, then he or she needs to know all the facts—even if the truth is a little scary. By attempting to protect your child too much, you will actually be hindering his or her adjustment to living with lupus. This can breed anger and bitterness, which can have serious long-term effects on your relationship.

Rebellion may occasionally lead to more serious physical problems for your adolescent. Why? A rebellious teenager may be less diligent with lupus self-care. On occasion, the adolescent may even deliberately try to make the condition worse, by sitting out in the sun or by not getting enough sleep.

There are many reasons why your teen might engage in these negative behaviors. Some teens neglect their health when they want more attention. Others might do it just for spite. Still others neglect to follow their treatment programs as a way of avoiding the situation altogether. Before you can deal with this behavior, you need to understand your child's motives for acting out. Then you can take steps to improve communication. Try to make your child understand that these negative behaviors are extremely dangerous and that there are healthier ways to express feelings. If you are unable to get through to your child, try talking to your child's physician.

It can be very helpful for your adolescent to participate in a teen support group. Of course, if your adolescent is rebelling, just your suggesting it can virtually guarantee the rejection of this idea! But often these groups are *only* for teens (parents aren't invited), and the prospect of meeting other adolescents who are going through the same things can be enticing. Check with your local lupus organization to see if such a group is available in your area. If not, discuss with your child the potential for online support groups, using appropriate discretion (see chapters 33 and 34).

Who's My Doctor?

It is usually preferable for lupus to be treated by a board-certified rheumatologist. This is true for adolescents as well as adults. It would be even more desirable for a pediatric rheumatologist to be the primary physician treating your adolescent, because of his or her expertise in dealing with this age group.

One of the anxiety-laden concerns for adolescents is the transition from pediatrician to adult physician. This can be especially true if your child has become comfortable with his or her pediatrician, and may create a significant conflict. The pediatrician may be a warm, comforting type, typical of this specialty. But your adolescent, wanting to be an adult, may feel that going to a pediatrician is "childish," and may be torn about what to do. Of course, the need to work with a rheumatologist may eliminate any questions about how to proceed. And it may be more comfortable for all concerned if the pediatrician is the one who recommends a particular rheumatologist. Communication is important here, with your adolescent and with all doctors involved, in facilitating this inevitable transition.

Questions About the Future

As your child gets older, he or she may become troubled by questions about the future. Your child might ask: "Will I be able to finish my education?" "Will I be able to get married?" "Will I be able to have children?" "Will I be able to perform my job well enough to keep it?" "Will I be able to make and keep my friends?" "Will I be able to lead a normal life?" These questions bother almost all adolescents. Having lupus just makes them more worrisome. What are the answers? As long as the new condition is taken into consideration and the necessary lifestyle changes are made, the adolescent with lupus should be just as able to answer these questions as any other healthy teenager. These and other questions should be discussed with health care professionals, to provide as much reassurance as possible. These questions can also be discussed in support groups, where a teen may learn how other adolescents with lupus handle these issues.

From Adolescent to Adult

The goal is for your adolescent to have the best possible life, despite lupus. Although there are many issues that need to be addressed, by being aware of and sensitive to your adolescent's needs, by maintaining open lines of communication, and by doing everything you can to smooth the path to effective coping, you're doing the best you can to pave the way from adolescence to adulthood.

21.

COMPLEMENTARY AND ALTERNATIVE MEDICINE

A growing number of people are interested in learning more about complementary and alternative medicine (CAM). Why? Some people with lupus, in looking toward the best possible ways of living with this disease, may want to use these therapies as a means of strengthening their bodies and controlling side effects while undergoing conventional treatment. Or they may prefer the more holistic and noninvasive approach of complementary and alternative therapies—hopefully with fewer side effects. In short, most people with lupus want to do everything possible to help themselves. Many look to complementary and alternative medicine as another area to consider for inclusion in their comprehensive treatment plan.

Because of the growing interest in complementary and alternative medicine, a division of the National Institutes of Health (NIH) was established, called the National Center for Complementary and Alternative Medicine (NCCAM). NCCAM defines CAM as "a group of diverse medical and health care systems, practices, and products that are not presently considered to be part of conventional medicine." This agency attempts to evaluate as many complementary and alternative therapies as possible, determining whether they are safe and effective. However, the agency warns the public that, for the most part, there is no way of knowing for sure how safe these methods are in general, and specifically if they work for lupus. Regardless, the interest in CAM will inevitably continue to grow.

What's the difference between complementary and alternative medicine?

Complementary medicine strategies are designed to *accompany* traditional treatment protocols. Alternative medicine strategies are used *instead* of traditional medicine. Because of the significant risk attached to discontinuing prescribed conventional medicine, in this book we will focus primarily on complementary therapies, ones that can be used in conjunction with approved treatment methodologies.

Let's learn more about these types of treatment—how they aim to help lupus, about the many different alternative therapies available, and how you may choose one or more of these as part of your program.

Similarities of Complementary and Alternative Treatments

Despite the fact that there are a number of different types of complementary and alternative treatments, they do have common "themes." Many of the complementary and alternative therapies, for example, are based on the belief that a truly healthy body is much less vulnerable to the ravages of a disease such as lupus. All of these methods are designed to create (or re-create) the healthiest body possible by reducing or eliminating the vulnerability that allowed the disease to develop in the first place. The hope is that a healthier body state will enhance the body's healing process, to eliminate or reduce the lupus.

Complementary and alternative treatments normally use a holistic approach. That is, their goal is to treat the whole body, rather than just the lupus symptoms being experienced. Many complementary and alternative treatments also work at a number of different levels, including physical, mental, spiritual, and emotional.

Categories of CAM Treatments

There are many appropriate complementary and alternative treatments that may be beneficial for people with lupus. According to NCCAM, the five main categories of complementary and alternative medicine are: whole medical systems, mind-body therapies, biologically based practices, manipulative and body-based practices, and energy therapies (also called energy medicine). Let's briefly discuss each of these.

WHOLE MEDICAL SYSTEMS

This category does not focus on any one strategy or technique. Rather, it combines a number of practices into a treatment philosophy. An example of a whole medical system is traditional Chinese medicine, or TCM. This system, developed centuries ago, views disease as an imbalance of yin and yang, the female and male life forces that flow throughout the entire body. It also considers disease to be a condition of stagnant energy (chi) and blood.

Traditional Chinese medicine and Western medicine may work well together. TCM encompasses the treatment methods of acupuncture, Chinese herbs, dietary change, and massage techniques in different combinations. Traditional Chinese herbs come in their raw form, such as sliced root or bark and are boiled for a period of time. They may be consumed as tea or are available in pill, capsule, or powdered forms. They should be prescribed by and obtained from a licensed practitioner.

Other examples of whole medical systems include homeopathy (which uses small doses of a substance to stimulate the natural, self-healing responses of the body) and naturopathy (which uses noninvasive strategies to "motivate" your body to heal itself, and includes specific focused practices such as massage, acupuncture, and exercise).

ACUPUNCTURE/ACUPRESSURE

Acupuncture and acupressure are examples of traditional Chinese medicine. Acupuncture is administered using very fine needles inserted into specific body points. Acupressure is a form of massage that applies finger pressure on acupuncture points. Practitioners often use a combination of these methods. Both are used to stimulate or sedate the body's flow of vital energy along channels or meridians. This helps disperse and dissolve any kinds of blockages that may be in those meridians. With lupus, the belief is that anything that can improve immune system functioning and increase the flow of vital energy in the body is likely to help.

MIND-BODY THERAPIES

The concept of mind-body is also called the biopsychosocial model or approach to health care. This may be one of the more potentially beneficial areas for individuals with lupus to consider. Mind-body strategies focus on understanding how the psychosocial aspects of your life can impact your physiological functioning, and they generally work to increase the ability of your mind to have an influence on your physical symptoms and health. The strategies attempt to enhance the communication between mind and body, hopefully resulting in improvement in both. Examples of mind-body therapies include relaxation techniques, guided visualization strategies, meditation, biofeedback, tai chi, and gentle yoga. Many of these strategies have a large enough body of research supporting their effectiveness that they are less likely to be considered alternative or even complementary strategies. In fact, many strategies, including relaxation techniques and biofeedback, for example, are far more commonly used as part of a comprehensive treatment program. (More information about relaxation techniques, biofeedback, and imagery can be found in Chapter 9.) Physicians tend to be more supportive of this type of therapy than some of the other types of CAM.

BIOLOGICALLY BASED PRACTICES

This category primarily includes dietary supplements and herbal remedies, virtually all of which use ingredients that are naturally occurring. These substances are available in a number of forms, including tablets, capsules, powders, compresses, extracts, salves, syrups, oils, and teas.

The medicinal benefits of herbs have been known for centuries. Working with herbs, making herbal preparations, and using them for health and healing can be very therapeutic. Herbs are effective when used over an extended period of time to strengthen the immune system. Herbs are also powerful *adaptogens*, meaning that they help the body to adapt to the ever-changing environment and the stresses of life. They provide support for the body while the body is experiencing symptoms or undergoing treatment that may sap its energy.

There are numerous herbs, vitamins, minerals, and other supplements that may be helpful for some people with lupus, including black currant oil, ginger, feverfew, and turmeric. They are best used in combination with conventional medical treatment and should be considered only after consulting with your health care professionals. (You can read more about herbs in Chapter 11, "Diet and Nutrition.")

A number of additional supplements and herbs are being investigated because of the promise that they may have in helping the inflammation of lupus. (Discuss any of these with your physician before using them.) They include:

Fish oil supplements containing omega-3 polyunsaturated fatty acids. These have been found to have anti-inflammatory capabilities. Some research has suggested that they may lower the inflammation of lupus and improve other symptoms, all of which may decrease the need for other anti-inflammatory medication. However, it seems that the dosage must be high for relatively little benefit. There also can be side effects with fish oil supplements, including nausea, experiencing a fishy taste in your mouth, and flatulence.

Flaxseed. This contains another type of fatty acid that can be beneficial for decreasing inflammation. Some research has suggested that there may be improvement in kidney function for patients on flaxseed. However, much more research is necessary. Side effects of flaxseed may include abdominal pain and bloating. Flaxseed may also be incompatible with certain medications, so make sure you speak to your doctor before trying this.

Yucca. This is an herb that has been found to be helpful in treating some symptoms of arthritis. It may be helpful for people with lupus as well, because of its ability to reduce inflammation and pain.

Other supplements are said to have immunosuppressive capabilities. Examples of these so-called immunomodulators include cloud mushroom, thundergod vine, and lotus.

DHEA (Dehydroepiandrosterone). Some clinical trials suggest that a hormone supplement, DHEA, synthetically derived from wild yam, has helped some patients with lupus. Anecdotal reports suggest patients have experienced an improvement in the quality of their life, and some may even have been able to decrease their dose of prednisone. Unfortunately, research at this point has been inconclusive. Even though some people have been helped by DHEA, there is still not enough evidence to indicate that this should be a complementary treatment.

CAUTIONS ABOUT SUPPLEMENTS AND HERBAL REMEDIES

These supplements may be labeled and promoted as being "natural," but they are still scientifically unproven. As such, be very careful. Another problem is that you can't be sure of the exact dosage necessary to achieve the desired results, and you also have to be concerned about toxicity and side effects. In addition, you can't always go by manufacturers' claims (really?). Make sure these products are safe . . . and that your doctor approves.

Many supplements contain a number of ingredients, and only certain active ingredients are actually targeting your symptoms. Different products may have different percentages of active ingredients. So, as you can see, there are many questions and fewer answers.You may feel a little more comfortable if you're working with a credentialed professional who is knowledgeable about these supplements. But even so, given how many uncertainties continue to exist, make sure there is communication between this professional and your physician. Many holistic practitioners also sell the products they recommend. Is that something to be careful about? Hmmmm, yes!!!!

Certain herbs should be avoided. For example, echinacea and astralagus are frowned upon because it is believed they can stimulate the immune system (not what you want!). This is the same reasoning behind the recommendation that alfalfa sprouts be avoided by people with lupus, because they contain an amino acid that can stimulate the immune system and increase inflammation.

MANIPULATIVE AND BODY-BASED PRACTICES

These techniques attempt to help physical manifestations of lupus by manipulating or moving one or more parts of the body. They include massage therapy, chiropractic, tai chi, yoga, and osteopathic treatments. Because of more widespread use, these treatments are more accepted than they were in the past. Although there is still a paucity of research that proves the effectiveness of these strategies for the treatment of lupus in general, many of them have proven to be helpful for specific symptoms, such as fibromyalgia or chronic pain (which may occur in lupus or a number of other medical conditions).

MASSAGE THERAPY

Massage may be the most ancient and natural (and pleasant!) pain reliever of them all. Massage offers many physical benefits for people with lupus, such as decreasing muscle tension and stiffness, lowering blood pressure, stimulating circulation, and relieving pain. Therapeutic massage is deep and relaxing and gives our bodies a chance to rest and sleep (a time for repair and healing). Some people believe that healing energy is locked in the muscles and that a massage will release energy blockages and help eliminate chronic pain. (See Chapter 9 for more information about massage.)

ENERGY THERAPIES

These strategies focus on the belief that there is a specific invisible energy that flows through your body. This energy has different names, including chi, and life force. Healthy bodies have healthy flowing energy. Unhealthy bodies have energy that is blocked or unbalanced. Energy therapies work to unblock or rebalance the energy flowing through your body. Examples of energy therapies are qi gong (pronounced "CHEE gong"), reiki, magnet therapy, and therapeutic touch.

Is a Treatment Right for You?

Regardless of how exciting some of the "discoveries" are, much care must be used in trying any of these techniques or substances. And remember, your physician should be consulted before you take or do anything. You want to make sure that any complementary substances you take do not interact negatively with your current treatment. By all means, don't give up your prescribed medication, or change your currently prescribed treatment protocol, without your physician's approval and guidance. You know by now that a number of the medications prescribed for lupus should not be stopped abruptly. Be more than wary if any holistic practitioner suggests this. Don't do it. Discuss this with your physician.

In choosing a complementary treatment that's right for you, your first step should be to fully understand your prescribed conventional treatment. Why? It's important to understand why your doctor recommends it, and what the benefits and the side effects may be. Even if you're considering a complementary strategy, you owe it to yourself to understand all your options. What you choose to include as part of your lupus treatment program depends on your preferences, as well as your physician's advice. Some may view complementary therapies as the way to go. Others may think that conventional treatments alone make sense and that supplements or mind/body techniques, for example, won't make a difference. Each person has many choices—both conventional and complementary.

In learning about conventional treatments, you'll probably find your doctor or other health care professional to be a valuable resource. While speaking to them, though, don't hesitate to ask about complementary treatments as well. They may have had patients who tried complementary therapies or may know of other professionals who have had some experience with less conventional treatments. Try to get information from other people with lupus. Some organizations and websites, in addition to having a lot of information, may even connect you with people who use their programs. Don't hesitate to contact these people and see what helped them. Take everything you learn, however, with a grain of (low-sodium) salt.

If the doctors you contact aren't able to help you evaluate the complementary therapies that have interest, you can learn about complementary and alternative therapies from a number of sources. Contact educational organizations, patient-referral services, or legitimate Internet websites that provide information on these treatments. By visiting libraries and bookstores, contacting health organizations, and exploring online websites that focus on lupus (remembering, of course, that not all information available on the

Internet is accurate—be careful!), you should be able to obtain up-to-date information both about your lupus and about all available treatments.

As you would do with any health care professional, it is important to find a credentialed practitioner who specializes in CAM and with whom you feel safe and comfortable. Ideally, these professionals should be willing to consult with your regular physicians in order to eliminate treatment incompatibilities or conflicts, and optimize your treatment protocol. When screening alternative practitioners and clinics, ask about their success in treating lupus. Ask, for example, how many cases of lupus they see every year. Keep in mind that an effective therapy for one person's disease won't necessarily be effective for yours. Ask to see supportive studies, documented cases, and patients' testimonials.

What is the biggest problem with complementary medicine? Not enough research. Rarely have complementary medicines been investigated extensively in clinical trials. As a result, there's often no hard evidence validating the effectiveness of these treatments for lupus. In addition, risks from these treatments are not known, either. View all information with a healthy dose of skepticism, and pin the practitioners down as much as possible as to whether you can expect long-term improvement, short-term improvement, or reduced pain. Also make sure that the therapy is being used in addition to conventional treatment, rather than instead of it.

A Complementary Conclusion

There are a lot of things you may want to add to your treatment program. Consider carefully whether a complementary therapy fits in with your own individual lifestyle, personality, and belief system. Some therapies, for instance, may require a degree of practical, emotional, or financial commitment that you are not willing or able to make. Some may require more time than you have, especially if you work full-time. Others may require too much travel. Some may simply be too expensive. Remember: It is not being suggested that you avoid complementary strategies. Just consider any such strategies in a careful, knowledgeable, and intelligent way. Widely respected healthcare practitioners are increasingly combining the best aspects of conventional medicine with supportive complementary treatments. You want your choice to be the best possible complement to treatment that can truly help your life with lupus. (Check the Appendix at the end of this book for examples of websites that may be able to provide you with current or updated information about mind/body therapies, supplements, physical or body manipulative strategies, TCM, and other CAM methods.)

PART THREE

Lupus and Your Emotions

22.

LUPUS AND YOUR EMOTIONS: AN INTRODUCTION

How do you feel about having lupus? It can have a tremendous emotional impact on you, your family, your friends, and everyone around you.

Each person's emotional responses to lupus are different. Even your own reactions to the condition will vary from time to time. The more severe your reactions are, the more they will interfere with your ability to cope. In fact, studies have suggested that a vast majority of individuals with lupus experience anxiety and depression that affect their physical and emotional well-being.

Your emotions ride the roller coaster just like lupus does. As a matter of fact, emotional ups and downs are very common. It is estimated that far more than half of all people with lupus experience emotional problems because of their illness. But one of the most important aspects of being able to cope with lupus is the ability to control your emotions.

The Factors Shaping Your Emotional Reactions

A number of factors may play a role in determining how you react to lupus. Keep in mind, though, that because there are so many factors, no one can predict just how a person will react at any given time. How did you handle problems before your condition was diagnosed? What was your general coping style? Were you calm or nervous? Were you persistent or did you give up easily? The way you've handled life's problems in general will suggest how well you will cope with lupus and its treatment.

Your age will also have a bearing on how you respond emotionally. Your general physical health prior to the onset of lupus, too, will play a role in determining your coping ability. What about your relationships? In many cases, your emotional reactions may reflect the responses of significant others in your life. For example, if family members or friends are anxious about your medical condition, this may have an impact on the way you feel. And if there is any central nervous system involvement, there may be organic, physiological causes for emotional disturbances.

Emotional Problems

Have you ever felt intense anger because you have to go through all this? Are you angry that your life will change because of lupus? Are you afraid of the medication you may need? Do you become depressed when you compare your present life to the way things used to be? Are you afraid that you won't be able to cope? Do you fear facing a bleak, if not hopeless, future? So many people who are diagnosed with lupus become angry, anxious, and depressed. Feeling this way doesn't mean that you are weak. Rather, it means you are normal! Because of the importance of coping with these and other emotions, a separate chapter has been devoted to each. But other than these specific emotional responses, what else might you be experiencing?

Do you like yourself less since your diagnosis? Previous feelings of confidence can be quickly shattered. Loss of self-esteem can have a very unpleasant effect on you. You may not feel or behave the way you used to. You may feel disoriented. Do you sometimes feel that things around you are unreal? One of the most frightening feelings is that you're not yourself, especially if you don't know why you're feeling this way. It can be reassuring to understand that these episodes do occur from time to time, both because of lupus activity and because of the medication, such as steroids, that you may be taking. It is helpful to be aware of these effects and to know that by just riding them out, or by changing medication dosages, these episodes will go away.

How about mood swings? Do you ever experience these? Everyone experiences mood swings from time to time. It's not uncommon to have some problems adjusting emotionally during times of major life changes, such as adolescence, going to college, starting a first job, getting married, or going through a pregnancy. You may be concerned that your mood swings are caused by the illness. For example, it is possible that medication, especially high dosages of steroids, can increase the range of these mood swings. But let your physician know what's going on so changes can be made.

Have you found yourself "bargaining"? This often occurs without your even being aware of what you're doing or why. You start thinking about or making "deals" as to what you can do to make this go away. You start thinking, "If only I find out I don't have lupus, I'll take much better care of my health, I'll be a better person, I'll be a better parent, spouse, friend, colleague," you name it. It almost sounds like an act of desperation, and in some ways it is. But as common a reaction as this may be, it can interfere with your efforts to be more in control of your emotions. So recognize it when it occurs, and remind yourself of what your true goals are: to be in as much control of your life as you can be.

Managing Emotional Reactions

Because your emotions play such an important role in your life with lupus, you'll certainly want to do the best possible job you can of controlling them. How? Let's discuss some of the more important ways in which you can manage your emotions.

GET THE BEST MEDICAL CARE POSSIBLE

If you haven't already done so, you'll want to establish a good working relationship with your physician, someone who not only has expertise in treating lupus and is informed of the most up-to-date research, but also is understanding, available, and sympathetic to your emotional needs. You'll want to be sure that your physician watches your condition carefully, so any problems that may arise can be caught as early as possible. Your physician must also monitor your dosages of medication carefully, so that they are used most effectively and so that any side effects are minimized. (See Chapter 32 for tips on creating a good relationship with your physician.)

JOIN A SUPPORT GROUP

Self-help or support groups can be incredibly helpful and are some of the best sources of support for people with lupus. Groups provide a forum for the exchange of feelings and ideas. Perhaps most important, these groups will show you that you're not alone—and it's much easier to live with a difficult problem when you know that you're not alone. It's helpful to meet new people who know what you're going through because they've gone through it themselves. (More information about support groups can be found in Chapter 33.)

LEARN ABOUT MEDICATIONS THAT CAN HELP YOU COPE

There may be times when your emotions may get too intense. In some of these cases, you may want to consider medications that can help you cope. A number of medications can be effective in dealing with depression, anxiety, anger, and many other emotional reactions to lupus. Antianxiety medications can be helpful, as can mood elevators and antidepressants. If you feel that you might benefit from treatment of this type, be sure to discuss the possibility with your doctor.

EXPLORE PROFESSIONAL COUNSELING

Professional counseling can help whenever some aspect of your life becomes overwhelming, your emotional problems become severe, or you want to prevent problems from getting worse. Certainly, any period of change can be made easier with the help of a support professional such as a psychiatrist, psychologist, social worker, psychiatric nurse, pastoral counselor, or other professional with the necessary credentials, compassion, and expertise.

Having somebody to talk to can be a big help, especially with an up-

and-down illness such as lupus. When you're speaking to your counselor, it may be one of the few times when you can be totally honest in releasing your feelings and at the same time get feedback that can help you better deal with your emotions. Yes, it can be helpful to talk to family and friends and to other people in your situation. But none of these people can provide you with the kind of frank intervention you can get from a therapist who is familiar with the feelings that exist because lupus is in your life.

If you don't know of an appropriate professional, you can get a referral from any of the physicians who are treating you, from your local lupus organization, or from a local hospital or professional mental health organization.

USE EFFECTIVE COPING STRATEGIES

There are a number of coping strategies you can use to better manage the emotions that may be troubling you as you deal with lupus. Any of these strategies can help you feel more in control.

Make a conscious, constructive agreement with yourself. Tell yourself that you're going to set aside a little time each day to work on strengthening your emotional self and preparing yourself for the next day. During this special time, include activities such as relaxation, imagery, goal setting, or positive thinking to improve your attitude. By consciously devoting time to this, you will improve your overall emotional state and increase your feelings of control because you're doing something to help yourself.

Let's discuss some of the best techniques you can use to improve the way you feel.

DEVELOP A POSITIVE MENTAL ATTITUDE

It is *so* important to have a positive mental attitude. People with good mental attitudes are much better able to control their emotions. A negative mental attitude may exacerbate any emotional problems that may occur because of, or in addition to, lupus. Your primary goal should be to do all you can to improve your attitude so that you can improve every other aspect of your life.

Concentrate on the good. Why waste valuable time and energy focusing on the bad? Many books offer suggestions that can help you generate a more positive attitude. Look into some of these. (Some good ones are included in the Appendix.) If you get just one good idea out of a 300-page book, the effort will be worthwhile.

Focus on wellness, not illness. Yes, you have an illness. But everything else in your life can focus on wellness. Take control of your attitude and work on your efforts to enhance your mind, body, and every facet of your life. Work on what you are going to do moving forward, rather than just dwelling on the way your life has changed.

Improving your attitude is a very important part of getting the most out of your life. If you think positive thoughts, you'll feel better, regardless of what's going on around you. The more positive you are, the more everything else falls into place. Isn't that worth the effort? Walk tall, hold your head high, and feel good about who you are. (And read more about thinking more positively, later in this chapter!)

LAUGH A LITTLE

Laughter truly is the best medicine—and is one of the most effective coping strategies there is. Laughter can help improve your health as well as reduce your stress. Having a good sense of humor may not cure your lupus, but it certainly can help make everything appear to be better. There are more and more positive things that humor can do. Research has shown that chemicals called endorphins—our body's own natural painkillers—are released by the brain whenever we laugh. These endorphins can block pain and give us a feeling of well-being. Haven't you felt better and experienced a greater sense of well-being after having a good laugh? You can enhance the process of getting and staying better by developing your sense of humor and making laughter an important part of your treatment program.

Humor can actually bring about many physical changes. Your heart will beat stronger and you'll breathe better, enabling a better blood flow and the delivery of more rich oxygen to the cells and tissues of your body. It will stimulate the efficiency of your muscles. It can offset the negative physical effects of stress. It can have a positive impact on your immune system. It can reduce pain, strengthen your body, and facilitate and stimulate healing. It can increase protection against viruses and bacteria.

Humor can be an amusingly pleasurable and effective way to deal with emotions. There are many psychological benefits of humor. Laughter is one of the best ways known to release tension and reduce anxiety. It can lift depression and diffuse anger. It can dispel worry and distract you from those feelings or thoughts that are bothering you. It can momentarily "break the chain" of any stressful or upsetting event, action, or thought, enabling you to deal with it better. When you're involved in something humorous, you often feel a lot better. Think back, for example, to a time when you were depressed or uncomfortable, and somebody asked if you had heard a certain joke. Initially, you may have been reluctant to hear it. But before long, you were probably totally absorbed in the joke, wondering what the punch line would be!

Humor can help you to come up with new possibilities in difficult situations, and can help you see things from a different perspective. So you may be able to look at something more objectively, which can help you handle it more effectively. It can provide a catharsis, the ability for you to release negative emotions. It can make you feel more optimistic. It can increase your ability to be creative and make your thinking more flexible. It can improve your ability to be tolerant—of others as well as yourself. It can inhibit, interfere with, or offset crying or unpleasant emotions. It can improve your ability to deal with physical—and psychological—pain. It can help your self-esteem. It can improve your social interactions and your ability to communicate. (You know the saying, "Misery loves company"? Well, laughter loves company as well!)

Whether you're listening to someone else's joke, laughing at yourself, or telling your own joke, humor can be a big help in troublesome situations. Although there may not be anything funny about having lupus, it helps to look on the bright side and lighten up a bit.

Finally, the ability to laugh at yourself is a helpful coping strategy. Find more humorous ways to look at your own situation. Learn to laugh at yourself by exaggerating your situation. Make fun of yourself in a way that is positive and constructive, not demeaning. Work to detach yourself from your problems, and take serious situations less seriously. The degree to which this works, however, depends on what you're going through. It's just about impossible to laugh at yourself while you're going through a crisis. However, as you adjust to your condition, you will be better able to use humor as a coping strategy.

Of course, be aware of the things that are *not* funny. For example, it's okay to make fun of yourself or look for the humorous aspects of your situation. But it's not appropriate to do that to others. (You wouldn't want them to do that to you, would you?) Make sure that you use good judgment in determining what's funny and what's not.

So make laughter-filled experiences a part of your everyday life. Develop a more playful frame of mind. Become more flexible in your perceptions, thoughts, and attitudes. Determine the type(s) of humor that you prefer. Know your *own* sense of humor and ability to laugh. Watch funny shows on television. Borrow humorous videotapes or DVDs. Read amusing books or magazines. Listen to comedy albums. There's nothing like a great CD to make you healthy. Read the comics. Accumulate some jokes and funny stories (either through books or from others) that you can use in social situations.

Any of these things will help you have fun and feel better. Not only can they give you a quick boost by helping you distance yourself from what may be troubling you, but they can also improve your overall mood and physical well-being.

So what should you do right this second? Smile! Force yourself! Even if you don't feel like it . . . smile . . . right now! Bigger. Bigger! See? It works! Try to do this much more often. And try to include some fun and laughter in your life . . . *every day!*

Set Goals for Yourself

Goal-setting can be a very good way of coping with your emotions. What types of goals might you set? A good short-term one might be the purchase of a new book by one of your favorite authors. A long-term goal could involve the planning of a family vacation or activity, or, perhaps, a reunion with out-of-town friends. By setting realistic and positive goals and working to achieve them, you'll be giving yourself pleasurable events to look forward to and a reason for getting through every day.

Be Nice to Yourself

Because you've been diagnosed with lupus, you may feel that you've given up some control. You may even feel—incorrectly—that you're being punished. It can be very helpful to offset these feelings by emphasizing the fact that nice things can still happen to you. Often, because you have lupus, it may be important for you to be just a little bit more "selfish"—that is, to initiate the kinds of activities or changes that will make you feel better. Of course, this should not be done in a way that is offensive to others. Instead, it should be done in a way that conveys the message to yourself, "I am a worthwhile person, and I deserve to have nice things in my life."

Some people find it very difficult to be nice to themselves. Others may take it to the opposite extreme. They may be so nice to themselves that they have to temper their enthusiasm so as not to appear totally self-centered!

What are some of the ways in which you can be nice to yourself? Why not buy yourself little goodies, give yourself some special time to relax, involve yourself in favorite activities, spend more time with the people you enjoy, or take a break and sit in the . . . shade? You may want to make a list of those things that would be most interesting and pleasurable—just for you. More about being nice to yourself shortly, in the section on building your self-esteem.

BE NICE TO OTHERS

Sometimes one of the best ways to boost your own self-esteem is to be nice to other people. The feeling of pleasure you get from helping others can be very gratifying and can improve the way you feel about yourself.

What are some of the things you can do to be nice to others? You can help virtually any person in practically any aspect of his or her life, whether at home, work, or play. Visiting people in places such as hospitals, nursing homes, or assisted living facilities is one way to spread sunshine. Performing voluntary services in such organizations as churches, schools, and civic organizations is another possibility.

Helping others will make you feel better about yourself not only because you're performing a kind deed, but also because you're doing something tangible to cope better with your disease. Helping others with lupus can make a big difference in your life. You'll feel more productive. You'll feel like you belong and are an important member of society. And, perhaps just as helpful, you'll find new ways of reducing boredom and channeling any excess energy or tension.

BUILD YOUR SELF-ESTEEM

Our self-esteem, the way we think about ourselves, is one of the most important components in a strong, emotional foundation for growth, progress, and health. Negative self-esteem, on the other hand, can make everything harder. Having low self-esteem can have an impact on virtually every facet of one's life.

Many people think, incorrectly, that there's nothing they can do about their self-esteem. There are always things that you can do, even if your self-esteem has been low for a long period of time. If that's the case, it may take longer, but it still can be done.

The key to improving self-esteem is to improve your thinking. So what can you do about this? Start by identifying your negative thoughts, those that contribute to low self-esteem. These may be self-critical thoughts, thoughts about your inability or difficulty in dealing with a situation, or thoughts about bad things that have happened or are happening to you. Remember: It is *not* the bad things that are happening to you that cause low self-esteem. It's the way you *think* about these bad things, and the way you believe you're dealing with them.

Become more aware of why you're thinking these negative thoughts. Think about what contributes to your negative thinking. Maybe your values are not the way you want them to be. Maybe your interpretation of a situation is inaccurate, or even irrational. Maybe you just feel so down on yourself that you always seem to think negatively. Use this as a starting point to change the negative thoughts to positive.

Note how you react to the negative thoughts that affect your self-esteem. You may react physically, behaviorally, or emotionally. By being aware of these "signals," you're in a better position to recognize them right away and turn them around before they have more of an impact on you.

Look for more positive responses to your negative, self-esteem-hurting thoughts. Start with the premise that the way you have been looking at something is not the only way. In fact, there may be many other more positive ways of looking at things that you have previously been unable to figure out. Your goal is to discover these more positive ways of thinking, in order to counteract the ingrained negative thoughts.

Make a list of the positive characteristics or attributes that you see in yourself. (Don't be discouraged if this list initially is short. The longer your self-esteem has been low, the more likely it is that this list will be short.) Your goal is to add items to this list, in an ongoing process, through better awareness of the good things about you, or by working on improving what you do and how you think. Then make a list of the negative characteristics or attributes that you see in yourself. Rather than considering these to be permanent and carved in stone, look at these as characteristics and attributes that you want to work on and improve. You will get great satisfaction from crossing items off this list and moving the improvements onto the positive list.

Replace negative values and beliefs with more positive values and beliefs. This may take time and requires effort, but the more you work on it the easier it gets. In addition, instead of dwelling on the negative components of your life, reframe them and look for the more positive aspects of your life. *Always* try to focus on the positive.

Replace hopelessness with hopefulness. Be warm and encouraging to yourself instead of allowing discouragement to shape your thoughts and behaviors. Acknowledge and condone your mistakes. Nobody is perfect. Sure, you make mistakes. Everyone does. But by perpetually blaming yourself for mistakes, you are also perpetuating your low self-esteem. Instead, focus on how and what you can learn from them. Give yourself permission to do so, and you will feel better as you do.

Use positive affirmations. Keep telling yourself positive things. Examples include: "I deserve to be happier and feel better." "I am a good person." "I can still like myself even if I occasionally make mistakes." "I can still like myself even if I have lupus!" Be realistic in your affirmations, but make sure they lean in a positive direction. The more you say them to yourself, the more you will absorb them, and they will improve your self-esteem.

DERIVE COMFORT FROM SPIRITUALITY AND FAITH

Being spiritual enables you to learn more about your inner self, the essence of your being. This may help you to better deal with your outer self, including your life with lupus. It can help you improve your attitude. It can be a very effective stress reducer and help you cope more effectively. This section is not designed to teach you how to be spiritual or even to encourage you to be spiritual. Rather, it's just information about how spirituality can be very comforting . . . and strengthening!

Being more spiritual makes you feel less in need of controlling every facet in your life. It can help you to better "go with the flow." It can also help you be more accepting of things that are beyond your control. People who are more spiritual tend to be healthier and better able to cope with life's adversities.

In order to enhance your own spirituality, concentrate on learning more about yourself and your values. What are the things that are important to you? Be more comfortable with them. Be more accepting of yourself and others. This self-introspection is very important, and can be facilitated through relaxation strategies, meditation, or prayer.

Being spiritual is not the same as being religious (involved in a specific religion). Rather, it suggests being more connected with who you are, feeling more comfortable within yourself, focusing more on your core values, and the place you see yourself in life. It can help you to determine your priorities. It tends to accentuate your positive personal values, and can, at the same time, "deprioritize" issues that are less important.

There can be an overlap between spirituality and religious faith. Yes, for some, spirituality simply goes hand in hand with one's religious beliefs, behaviors, and activities. But for others, spirituality can be embodied in music, nature, or calm introspection.

People with strong religious faith often derive a tremendous amount of solace from prayer. The religious beliefs of family and friends can also be a source of comfort to both you and them. However, the degree to which you exercise your religious beliefs is up to you. Don't feel that you have to turn to religion if this doesn't seem natural to you. Yet if others have religious beliefs, let them derive the comfort and support this provides for them, even if you don't share their intensity.

What steps can you take to derive spiritual or religious comfort? Work on being more accepting of yourself and of others. Look for the good in people, as well as in yourself. Read inspirational stories of others. (These may or may not include religious overtones.) Speak to others about their spirituality, how they have benefited from it, and how they have accomplished it. If you choose to move along a more religious path, have conversations with members of the clergy.

MAKE USE OF RELAXATION TECHNIQUES

Relaxation is the opposite of tension. Therefore, if you learn to relax, you'll be much less tense! But relaxation techniques by themselves will not totally control your emotions. So why use them? Because if you're feeling more relaxed, you'll be better able to identify those problems that are affecting you, and you'll be better able to figure out how to deal with them. So relaxation procedures can be an essential step in coping with your emotions. (Refer to Chapter 9 for specific relaxation techniques.) There's also a procedure called imagery, in which you view pictures in your mind to help you relax. (More information about imagery can also be found in Chapter 9.) Books on any of these procedures are available in your local library and can really help you to start feeling better.

Remember that if you have difficulty learning to relax on your own, there's nothing wrong with working with a professional who can help you learn these skills.

PINPOINT WHAT'S BOTHERING YOU

As you learn to relax, you're ready to proceed to the next crucial step. In order to deal with anything that's upsetting you, you have to determine exactly what it is that's bothering you! Make a list of these things. Then go over what you've written. In reviewing your list, you'll see that just about every item can be placed in one of two categories. The first category contains the "modifiables"—the problems or emotions that you can do something about. The second category includes the "nonmodifiables"—the things you can't do anything about. Why separate them? Because different strategies should be used to deal with each of these two categories of problems.

For the first category, you'll want to figure out what techniques you can use to improve the situation. As for the second category, you'll still be planning strategies, but of a different kind! Where do your emotions exist? In your mind, right? Therefore, your plan for this category is to work on the way you're thinking.

WORK ON YOUR THINKING

We talked before about the importance of having a positive mental attitude. It goes without saying that positive thinking is a key to successful living. It is a vital component of having that positive mental attitude. You've heard the old saying, "The glass is better half full than half empty." But what if you too often look at your life as half empty? And what if you don't know how to change that and make it half full?

The power of positive thinking focuses on your glass's being half full rather than half empty. Research has shown convincingly that the more you follow this type of thinking, the better off you will be. Given the fact that one of the problems of living with lupus is the feeling that lupus does control too much of your life, everything you can do to improve your thinking will help you in your life with lupus.

We all think about a lot of things all day long. This is called our self-talk. Some people are more likely to engage in positive self-talk than others. They invariably are the people who are happier and healthier. People who have negative self-talk often believe "that's the way it is and I can't do anything about it." Nothing could be further from the truth. Negative thinking is a habit. You're used to it, just as you're used to other things in your life that you do all the time. But that doesn't mean you can't change it. It takes effort. Anytime you want to break a habit, it takes effort. In fact, thinking more positively can improve virtually every facet of your life. For example, you can reduce your stress, improve your physical health and reduce the impact of physical symptoms, improve relationships, and improve your emotional health. You'll be less likely to experience depression or anxiety. You'll be more effectively able to use positive coping strategies. You'll be better able to deal with adversity, if and when it occurs.

How can you change the way that you think so that something will bother you less? The technique you choose should depend on the specific emotional reaction that's bothering you. For example, if you're afraid of something and you want to conquer this fear, a procedure called *systematic desensitization* may be helpful. (We'll go into this later, in Chapter 24.) Then again, if you're feeling guilty or angry about something, or if something is depressing you, it can be very helpful to learn how to change or "restructure" the way you're thinking. (You'll learn about more techniques for this in chapters 23, 25, and 26.)

How do you deal with uncertainty? One of the first things to do is to focus on living as a person who happens to have lupus, rather than seeing yourself as a victim of lupus. Try to live life and enjoy as much as possible. Concentrate on what you have, not on what you don't. Concentrate on what you can still do, not what you can no longer do. Those who are successful are the ones who live life one day at a time, making the most of each day.

What other things can you do to change your negative thinking to positive? Actually, any of the techniques discussed can be used to cope with just about any problem. It's simply a question of deciding what works best for you. In general, be as aware as possible of your negative thoughts. Catch them when they occur. If you're feeling any negative emotions, recognize that these are because of negative thoughts. Ask yourself, right then and there, what you're thinking. Then write down the negative thoughts, and follow that by writing down more reasonable, realistic positive thoughts in response. Think about other people you know who generally are more positive thinkers. Ask yourself what they would say in response to your negatives. Use humor as a way to respond to negative thoughts. This can lighten your mood and enable you to come up with alternatives that are more positive. Spend time with positive people. Watch them and try to identify what they might think in different situations. And finally, practice, practice, practice. Remember that learning positive self-talk is a skill. Any skill requires repetition in order to make it part of your normal behavior.

A Final Emote

If you are currently experiencing intense emotional reactions, have faith that these feelings will diminish, either due to the passage of time or because you're doing something to help yourself. You can expect to experience more emotional reactions during those times when your symptoms are more pronounced, so you'll probably experience a range of emotional reactions from time to time. But even when these feelings do occur, you should be able to point to so many positive things in your life that it may be easier to deal with these feelings. In this way, you'll be able to develop the positive mental attitude that you want to become an integral part of your life.

The purpose of the following six chapters is to help you understand the different emotions you may be experiencing. You'll discover where these emotions come from and come to recognize that many other people have gone through exactly what you're going through now. In addition, a number of strategies will be presented to help you cope with these emotions more effectively. Remember that "practice makes better." (There's no such thing as perfect!) Just reading about a method to control an emotion doesn't guarantee success. You have to keep on practicing. So don't be afraid, depressed, angry, or guilty. Instead, read on!

23.

DEPRESSION

Jackie was depressed. A thirty-three-year-old mother of two, married for six years and living in a comfortable home in a good neighborhood, she apparently had everything she could ask for. But she certainly hadn't asked for lupus! She found herself feeling increasingly upset with the changes that had to be made in her life. She felt that she could never make plans to do something and that she could never see her friends. She couldn't spend time with her children. She felt both helpless and hopeless. Jackie was suffering from depression.

Depression is a serious problem. The very mention of the word can sometimes knock the smile right off your face. Although actual numbers vary, it is estimated that up to ten million Americans or more need professional care for depression. Because it is so widespread, depression has been nicknamed the "common cold" of emotional problems.

Just what is depression? The noun *depression* is not the same as the adjective *depressed*. Anyone can feel depressed. You might be depressed because you missed the first ten minutes of a movie, or because the Yankees lost their latest game (although many of you might be depressed because the Yankees *won* their latest game!). Day-to-day things might make you feel a little depressed, but they usually have little impact on your life in general.

However, the topic of this chapter is what we call *clinical depression*, an extremely unpleasant feeling of unhappiness and despair. It can range from a mild problem—feeling discouraged and downhearted—to a severe disorder—feeling utterly hopeless, worthless, and unwilling to go on living. You may believe that there is no reason to remain a part of the world. You may be afraid of being a burden to your family, and you may think that everybody would be better off without you. Or you may just feel useless. And the feeling goes on and on, often for weeks or more.

Depression can be painful. Imagine how it must hurt to feel (or say), "I wish I were never born. What good am I? I'm not helping anybody around me, and I'm not helping myself." You may feel as if the whole world is against you. Life may seem unfair—a constant struggle in which you can never win. And that hurts.

What Are the Symptoms of Depression?

There are a number of possible symptoms of depression. If you notice that you're feeling excessive amounts of sadness, despair, discouragement, or melancholy; if you're unable to eat, and this problem has nothing to do with the lupus or its treatment; if you're sleeping either too much or too little; if you feel totally withdrawn from social activities; if you find yourself crying often, and that's not typical behavior for you; if you're brooding about the past and feeling hopeless—any of these feelings may indicate depression. And there are other symptoms, as well. If you're experiencing excessive amounts of irritability or anger; if your fears seem to be extreme; if you feel inadequate and worthless; if you are unable to concentrate on virtually anything in your life, whether it be work, family, or other interests; if you seem to have little or no interest in activities that previously gave you pleasure; if you have reduced amounts of energy that don't seem to be related to the disease or treatment; if you have little or no interest in sex or intimacy; and if your cognitive style (the way you speak, think, and act) seems to be generally slowing down—these, too, can be symptomatic of depression. Depressing, right? The more of these symptoms you experience, the more likely it is that you are depressed and should take some action to help yourself.

How Does Depression Affect You?

Now that you are familiar with some of the many possible symptoms of depression, you should also be aware that its effects are not isolated problems. Depression can affect your physical well-being, take control of your moods, and make it difficult to enjoy—or even carry out—the simplest activities. Let's take a look at some of the ways in which depression can affect you in your day-to-day life.

HOW DEPRESSION AFFECTS YOUR BODY

Some of the more noticeable symptoms of depression are physical in nature. Nervous activity or agitation, such as wringing of the hands, may occur. You may be restless or have difficulty remaining in one place. On the other hand, you may become much less active and remain motionless for abnormally long periods of time, appearing to be almost in a trance, with no desire or energy to do anything. Jim became very concerned when his twenty-eight-year-old wife, Jane, remained seated in a chair in the living room for hours at a time. When he asked her a question, she would respond in monosyllables. When friends called on the phone, she never wanted to talk to them. Jane's depression was causing her to lose interest in just about everything.

If you're depressed, most of your physical activities will also slow down—and not just because of physical limitations. You're probably feeling exhausted. This may be surprising, since you're not doing much of anything. But constantly telling yourself that you're no good can be tiring in itself! You really don't want to believe this, but you feel as if you have no choice. And in attempting to escape from these feelings, you may become even more depressed—as well as more physically drained and exhausted.

Depression may also cause you to feel physically sick or to experience a change in appetite. Of course, it's wise to remember that any of these symptoms might be related to lupus, or another physical disorder, or even the medication you're taking. So even if the symptoms go away once your depression improves, don't just assume that they're related to the depression.

A medical examination may still be a good idea. This way, you'll be sure that there is no organic cause for your depression.

HOW DEPRESSION AFFECTS YOUR MOODS AND OUTLOOK

If you're depressed, you may experience frequent mood swings. For example, you might feel worse in the morning and better in the evening. This may be because of joint stiffness and pain, as well as depression. The nightly improvement may occur because each evening you realize that it's almost time to go to sleep—the "great escape." But depression may also make sleep difficult, even if you weren't doing much of anything during the day.

If you're mildly depressed, you may have difficulty concentrating, and your attention span may be much shorter. When you speak, and you'll probably do less of that, too, your conversation may suggest, or even express, feelings of worthlessness and despair.

When you're depressed, it feels as if your mood keeps getting lower. You like yourself very little, if at all. Your thinking is very negative and very different from the way it was when you were feeling good. In fact, it is this negative thinking—not just a particular triggering event—that leads to depression in the first place. (But more on this later in the chapter.)

Naturally, your day-to-day activities may suffer as a result of these negative feelings. You may, for instance, spend the day in your bathrobe, simply because you don't feel like dressing. Or you may "go through the motions" of your everyday activities, even though your heart isn't in them. Many people, in fact, simply withdraw from their usual activities during bouts of depression.

HOW DEPRESSION AFFECTS YOUR RELATIONSHIPS WITH OTHERS

If you're depressed, you may feel that people around you have no need for you. You may feel the same way Jackie did. She used to complain, "Why should my friends want to see me or make plans with me? They know that I'm probably going to have to change my plans. Even if I don't cancel my plans, they probably think I'll be so tired that I won't be much fun to be with anyway, so why should they even want me as a friend?" It doesn't matter how they behave toward you; you're convinced they are doing so out of obligation or necessity.

Do you now feel less at ease talking to others? Does it seem as if others are having a hard time talking to you, even if they have been close to you for a long time? As already discussed, due to your depression, you may be less interested in conversation and you may feel less confident. You may project your negative feelings about yourself onto others and believe that they really don't want to talk to you. And the more depressed you become, the better you may get at convincing those around you that you're no good. You may feel that others have no need for you. You may think that they consider you to be an uninteresting, boring person.

What Causes Depression?

There are many possible causes of depression. Each person is different, so it's impossible to predict how it will begin in any given individual.

A bout of depression frequently seems to start with one specific thing, an event or occurrence that makes you unhappy. Gloria had been planning a big dinner party for over two months. Although she had been more tired recently, she still was able to go with a friend to buy a beautiful cocktail dress. In the weeks prior to the party, she tried to get as much rest as possible. The big day finally came. Gloria felt so physically weak that she had to talk herself into getting through it. She tried to think about seeing her friends and relatives, the money she had spent on her dress, and the feeling that she did not want to give in to her lupus. But what happened? She had no choice but to sit the entire evening, because she was too weak to get up. When the party was over, she was so depressed and weak that she remained in bed, crying and miserable, for over a week. That one evening seemed to open the floodgates, and triggered a long depression. She felt as if even the most important things to her were ruined because of lupus.

What happens after that first depressing event occurs? A kind of chain reaction follows. This one occurrence creates feelings that spread like wildfire.

It's almost as if the bottom has dropped out of your world. You may feel less able to control your thinking (although this is not true, as we will see later). But keep in mind: The deeper you go into depression, the harder it is to climb back out again. Therefore, you certainly want to catch these feelings of depression as early as possible, to try to keep yourself from spiraling further downward.

What we also know is that depression doesn't always result from one precipitating event. It often results from an ongoing, draining accumulation of upsetting and hopeless feelings. So, in other words, the chain reaction may have already started, but the triggering event brought it all to the surface. Why does this happen? Where does depression come from, and why does it affect some people more than others? Sometimes we can figure this out, and sometimes we can't. But before we give up, let's discuss some of the possible causes.

HOW ABOUT THE NORMAL "DOWNS"?

A certain amount of depression is normal in anyone's life. We all experience ups and downs. If we never experienced some of the downs, how could we ever fully appreciate the ups!? However, when depression becomes more than just the normal "downs," it must be attended to. Stopping it quickly can keep it from becoming much worse.

Of course, certain events—traumatic experiences such as losing a loved one, being diagnosed with a chronic medical problem, requiring major surgery, or being fired from a job—can lead anyone to depression. However, this doesn't mean that you should ignore the problem or wait until it goes away. It's necessary to learn how to deal with depression, as this is an essential part of coping.

HOW ABOUT ANGER YOU CAN'T EXPRESS?

What if you get so angry that you feel like you're going to burst? But you don't—or can't—do anything about it, so you decide to "swallow" your anger. It seems strange that a powerful feeling like anger can turn into a withdrawn, helpless feeling like depression. But it can. If you become increasingly angry about something and feel unable to do anything about it, you may turn the anger inward. You may feel so much frustration or hopelessness that you "shut down" in an attempt to keep yourself from experiencing these terrible feelings. This leads to withdrawal, which is one symptom of depression. (For more information on anger, see Chapter 25.)

COULD IT BE A CHEMICAL IMBALANCE?

In some cases, depression may be caused by biochemical deficiencies—chemical imbalances in our bodies. Treatment for biochemical deficiencies may involve the administration of drugs in an effort to rebalance body chemistry. But this usually isn't the whole answer. Regardless of whether your depression is caused by this or, more typically, by your reaction to the people and events around you, there are still things you can do. For example, you should still try to modify your thinking. Many experts believe that even if the cause of depression is biochemical, by working on the way you handle your day-to-day living, you can have a positive effect on your emotions.

LUPUS AS A CAUSE

Can lupus cause depression? Absolutely. Some research has suggested that depression is more common for people with lupus than it is for people in the general population. It also seems to recur more frequently and may last longer. The pain and other symptoms of this disease can certainly either create, or magnify already existing, depression. In fact, the most common lupus-related causes of depression are any changes in physical appearance encountered, as well as physical symptoms and changes. So it would not be surprising to experience some depression if you are living with lupus.

The depression you felt after being diagnosed with lupus is understandable. But it can get better as you begin to adjust to your new life situation. There's a problem, though. Because life with lupus has its ups and downs (physically), your feelings may bounce up and down as well. This can be a problem, considering what depression can do to you. Unfortunately, it may take quite a while to adjust to having lupus. So, if your depression lingers, don't wait until you've fully accepted having lupus before you start learning how to cope with depression.

The way your body feels or looks may depress you. You may want to throw out any mirrors in your entire house. Experiencing a lot of pain, especially for prolonged periods of time, can be depressing. Joint and muscle pain, along with intense fatigue that just doesn't seem to lift, can be depressing. In many cases, it's less the physical symptoms that depress you. It's more the limitations they impose. And when the way you feel or look doesn't get better, whew! Depression!

You might get depressed because you have to take medications, regardless of whether you're concerned about their side effects, the damage to your body, or the way they change your appearance. Most people do not like having to take medication. You may feel depressed because of being torn between taking medications, which you don't want to do, and feeling worse, which you certainly don't want.

Flares can be depressing. Because the "downs" of flares often follow the "ups" of feeling better, your thoughts probably are: "Here we go again." And, of course, worrying when (or even if) you'll get out of the flare, with no predictable answer to that question, can be depressing.

Problems involving other people may depress you. You may feel helpless at not being able to share what you're experiencing or the way you feel. You may get depressed if others don't understand what you're going through (not that you want to be pitied, though!). People may expect more from you than you're able, or want, to provide. They may lose confidence in you, feeling you're less reliable because of the effects of lupus. You may be depressed over the possibility of damaged relationships, lost friendships, or family friction. If you're single, you may become depressed because you think you'll never meet anyone or be able to develop a meaningful relationship because of the changes in your life necessitated by lupus.

What else about lupus might depress you? You might become depressed thinking about the future, not knowing what your prognosis is or how it will affect your life. Knowing that you'll probably need medication to keep your condition from getting worse can be depressing. You might get depressed if you read misleading information in books or magazines, hear things from others ("Gee, that's a bad illness, isn't it?"), or realize how little is known about the illness. Changes in habits necessitated by your condition and its treatment may also be depressing.

Depression can result from changes in lifestyle. You might not be able to participate in activities you used to enjoy. You might have to change your work routine as well as your family routine. Money problems, with no immediate solution imminent, can certainly be depressing. Just having lupus, with its intangible effects on your day-to-day living, can get to you.

You may be saying to yourself, "If I'm depressed over my lupus, how can I expect to get over my depression unless I get rid of this disease?" That kind of thinking will get you nowhere. Even if you go into remission, you still can't ignore the fact that lupus is a chronic condition—and you don't want your emotional state to depend on your physical state. This and other triggers can even cause anxiety, which can affect lupus symptoms, which can make you even more depressed. So if your depression lingers, don't wait. Work on it, and learn how to cope. We'll talk more later about how you can improve your thinking.

What Maintains Depression?

If you're depressed, you may be blaming yourself—or your lupus—for everything that is wrong. You may tend to become more and more withdrawn, and pull away from the world around you. Why? Well, if you believe that your condition is causing all these horrible things, isn't it better to "escape" and not think about it? Realistically, escaping won't solve anything. But you may feel that withdrawal is the sole way to stop feeling terrible. Unfortunately, this will only keep you depressed. (In fact, it may make you even more depressed.)

Although you may even seem sullen and withdrawn to others, you're probably in deep emotional pain. Part of what is making you, and keeping you, depressed is your failure to protect yourself from this emotional pain. When your mind does allow any thoughts to enter, you tend to feel overwhelmed by feelings of doom and destruction. You feel that nothing good can possibly happen—that only bad things can happen. So what do you do? You try to block everything out of your mind!

So why do you stay depressed? Why doesn't it just go away? It may be because you don't feel like talking to anybody or won't even consider counseling. Therefore, the thoughts and feelings that lead to your depression are kept hidden. You may ask, "Is my unwillingness to talk the only reason I'm still depressed? If I start talking more, will that get me out of my depression?" Not necessarily. But it can be helpful to talk out your feelings. It would probably be beneficial if a close friend or family member took the initiative and coaxed you into some kind of conversation—therapeutic or otherwise—or, at least, encouraged you to do something constructive. But then again, you might feel too depressed to respond!

How Can You Cope with Depression?

Can anything be done to alleviate depression? Of course! One of the most important strategies in your effort to get out of depression is increasing your control. Depression often embodies a horrible, total, out-of-control feeling. So every little bit that you can do to retake control of your life will help.

One of the first things you can do is make sure that, in your efforts to help yourself feel better emotionally, you also concentrate on taking care of yourself physically. Your next step will be to tell yourself that the main reason you're depressed is that you haven't taken the proper steps toward emotional wellness. Start doing this now. These steps can begin the process of pulling you out of your rut and reacquainting you with the more positive, pleasant aspects of living—the aspects that you'd like to experience.

You want to learn to accept any limitations in your life. Admit that you can't control or become involved in *everything*. This doesn't mean that you are powerless, but it does mean that you may have to alter your views about what you can and can't do. Once you accept your limitations, you'll be able to focus your energy in appropriate, constructive directions instead of lamenting what has changed. How can you accept your limitations? Well, let's say that you were previously able to do twenty-five things in your life, and now, because of lupus, you're unable to do ten of them. Instead of wasting your energy thinking about the things you can no longer do, focus your energy on feeling good about the ones you can do! Remember the Serenity

Prayer, "Grant me the serenity to accept the things I cannot change, the courage to change the things I can, and the wisdom to know the difference." Keep repeating it . . . and believing in it.

Another strategy you can use to alleviate depression is to exercise choice. Demonstrating that you have the ability to choose certain things in your life will help increase your feeling of control. Sure, there may be certain events that are beyond your influence. But you can still focus your energy on all those things that you can do.

Regardless of what you have to do and what mountains seem to stand in your way, the most you can ask of yourself—the most that anybody can ask—is to take one step at a time. Just keep taking one more step. This will be helpful, especially if you're feeling overwhelmed because there are so many things to do.

Alleviating depression is not easy. Unfortunately, once you've fallen into depression, it takes hard work and a certain amount of persistence to pull yourself back out. The result, however, is surely worth the fight. And, of course, the fight will be easier if you know of specific techniques and activities that will help. Don't be afraid of depression. Rather, expect it and prepare yourself for it. This will help you better deal with depression when it does occur.

The strategies and techniques that are most effective in dealing with depression can also be effective in preventing you from becoming depressed. Unfortunately, this doesn't mean that you'll never again feel depressed. It may happen. Anticipate it, so that if it does recur, you won't completely fall apart. And if this feeling does come back, won't it be good to know that you *can* do something to help yourself?

Now that you're ready to fight your depression, consider two major ways of dealing with it: being more physical (in other words, doing something) and working on your thinking.

It can be very helpful to make a list of all the things that are depressing you. You may feel there'll be at least fifty items! But in actuality, you'll probably start running out of ideas after six or seven. Next, divide this list into two more lists: first, those things that you can do something about, and, second, those things you can't do anything about. So get physical and do something about those items on the first list, and get thoughtful—work on your thinking—regarding those items in the second list.

LET'S GET PHYSICAL

There are two ways of getting physical in order to deal with depression: actively working to accomplish goals and increasing physical activity. Hopefully, as suggested above, you've listed all the things that are depressing you and have made a separate list of those items that can be changed. Now think about ways in which you can modify or eliminate the items on this list. Be realistic but aggressive in planning ways to reach your goals—even if it can't be done all at once.

Where does the physical activity come in? Unknowingly, you may be using a lot of energy to keep yourself depressed. You may be working hard to keep that anger inside, even if it appears to others that you're simply withdrawing. If your depression is anger turned inward, we can logically assume that by releasing your anger, you'll be able to reduce your feelings of depression. But what should you do with those feelings? You must find an object toward which your anger can be expressed. This may be difficult. However, it's important to release the trapped anger so that it doesn't build up further and deepen your depression.

Think about the following scenario. You're sitting there, depressed and withdrawn. Somebody makes an innocent remark, and you practically bite that person's head off! What's happening? Whatever was said triggered the release of the internalized anger that was contributing to your depression. Look out, world!

What kinds of activities can help you release your anger? Many physical activities can be effective. Exercise helps by lowering your blood sugar level, and it also causes the release of neurotransmitters called *endorphins*. Endorphins make people feel good and can give them a more positive attitude about life.

Before you begin any exercise program, you should schedule a complete physical to make sure that exercising is safe for you. Your physician or exercise specialist will help you develop an appropriate exercise regimen. Your program has to take into consideration any symptoms you're experiencing; you need to make sure that physical activity will not contribute to further harm. It's very important that you're clear on which activities are safe for you, so you must work closely with your physician or other health care professionals to plan a program that will provide maximum benefits with little or no risk. (Refer to Chapter 12 for a complete discussion on setting up—and sticking with—an exercise program.)

Make sure you get enough sleep. This may seem to contradict earlier comments about sleeping too much because you're depressed. But you need the wonderful, restorative power of sleep to help you emotionally. Yes, too much sleep may be indicative of a problem. Yet if your physical symptoms are depressing you, sleep can help your body heal. And that can help your depression. (You may want to review Chapter 8, on fatigue, to learn more about the role of fatigue, and rest, in lupus.)

Finally, because physical symptoms can be an integral part of the cause of depression, you want to make sure these symptoms are addressed in treatment. Be assertive with your doctor. Explain that not only are the symptoms affecting you, they're depressing you. You want to work together with your doctor to do everything you realistically can to feel better, physically and emotionally.

LET'S GET THOUGHTFUL

Although getting physical may help lift your depression—and can also provide a great distraction, which may help you to look more objectively at what's going on—physical activity will not teach you ways of fighting inappropriate thinking. Besides, lupus may not even allow you to participate in intense physical activity! Remember: It's your *thoughts* that have made you depressed. Clearly, changing and improving your thinking is a key element in alleviating depression and dealing with any negative emotions.

If you can think yourself into depression, then you can think yourself out of it. How? Your thoughts are the way in which you talk to yourself. In fact, when it comes to talking to yourself, you're probably the biggest chatterbox you know! But if you're depressed, you're just talking yourself *down.* All your comments—or at least most of them—are probably put-downs: harsh statements that can make you feel even worse. You want your inner voice to help you, not hurt you. Let's see how you can do that.

DISTINGUISH FACT FROM FICTION

When you're depressed, you tend to distort reality. Clinical research with depressed patients has proven this. Recognize, therefore, that your thoughts are not necessarily based on what is really happening, but may, instead, be based on your own distorted views. This is called *cognitive distortion.*

Is this bad? You bet your happiness it is! *Cognitive* refers to your thinking. *Distortion* means you're twisting things around and, in general, losing sight of what's real. We all tend to do this from time to time. But when you're depressed, you do it a lot of the time—if not all of the time—and it keeps you depressed. So how do you stop? First, you must become reacquainted with what is really happening. But how can you do that if you keep distorting reality? Right now, you're better off accepting somebody else's perceptions of the situation, because that person is probably a lot more objective and accurate. Since so many feelings of worthlessness are based on distorted facts, depression can be reduced, if not eliminated, once these facts are straightened out.

Angela kept moaning because none of her friends were calling her. "They don't call as much as they used to. I guess they just don't care." Her sister, Stephanie, asked her to estimate how often her friends used to call. When Angela compared this number to the current number of calls she was receiving, she realized that the numbers were almost the same. She then realized that she was probably just more sensitive because of all the changes going on in her life! Although she did not feel a hundred percent better, Angela did feel a good deal better, because she could now see that she wasn't being abandoned.

So make sure you know what's true and what's not. Provide your own assessment of the situation, and be as objective as possible. Then, if necessary, ask other people—people whose opinions you trust—for their evaluation. Work to become more comfortable with any differences in perception and to adjust your thinking so that it more closely resembles the actual circumstances.

MAKE MOLEHILLS OUT OF MOUNTAINS

Does this imply that if you're depressed you have no real problem? Is it "all in your head"? No. Everyone has problems. If you feel good, you can handle them, but if you're depressed, you may feel overwhelmed. Each and every obstacle and task, regardless of how trivial or slight it may be, will tend to depress you. Do your best to view each problem objectively—to avoid blowing it out of proportion. Eventually, as your depression lifts, you will be able to deal with all of life's problems, both big and small.

AVOID SELF-FULFILLING PROPHECIES

We've discussed several different thoughts that are characteristic of depression—thoughts that you may be having right now. Are all these thoughts and feelings irrational and untrue? No. But, ironically, although some of them may start off being far from the truth, the longer you feel that way, the greater the chance of them becoming self-fulfilling prophecies. In other words, you'll begin convincing yourself that nonsense makes sense. The more you allow yourself to think negatively, the greater the likelihood that your fears will turn into realities. For example, if you begin telling yourself that friends and relatives don't care, this may become a reality because your negative attitudes may alienate the people close to you. And if you feel less able or less willing to do the things you used to do, your inactivity is likely to magnify and confirm your feelings of worthlessness, leading to even greater depression and helplessness. Not a pretty picture.

Once you begin feeling depressed, your negative thoughts will soon lead to negative actions. These negative actions will lead to more negative thoughts, which will in turn lead to more negative actions, and so on. It is an ongoing, vicious cycle that will spiral you further downward into deeper depression. Eventually, you'll feel trapped in this vicious cycle and believe there's no way to escape.

Are you getting depressed just reading this? In all probability, if you've ever been depressed, you've said to yourself at least once already, "Wow, that sounds just like me!" So if you find that you're starting to believe in your negative thoughts, stop yourself. As we've said before, depression both results from and causes a lot of negative thinking. Negative thoughts automatically pop into your mind and you cannot stop that from happening. It's like trying to keep your eyes open when you sneeze! You just can't do it. But once you become aware of these thoughts, you *can* do something about them. People who remain depressed feel incapable of doing anything about their negative thinking and allow these thoughts to pull them into that vicious cycle mentioned earlier. Try to think of more positive thoughts, so that if one of your thoughts does turn into a reality, it will at least be a positive one.

Ann, a thirty-four-year-old housewife, was resting when the telephone rang. "I'm sure that's Katherine, calling to cancel our lunch plans," she thought to herself. Within the thirty seconds it took her to get to the phone, she had become so depressed that she considered not even answering the call. Imagine how she felt when she reluctantly answered the phone and discovered that it was a wrong number! Ann had allowed her negative thoughts to run wild—she became more and more negative until she was about ready to give up. And for what? There was no clear-cut reason for thinking the way she did.

Once she realized that she was thinking this way, what could she have done? She could have countered her thoughts. She could have told herself, "It may not even be Katherine on the phone. Or if it is, maybe she's just calling to confirm. I won't let it bother me now. After all, I don't even know who it is." This is the beginning of positive thinking.

DWELL ON BRIGHTER TOMORROWS

Marie was depressed because she constantly compared her present condition to the way she used to be. She couldn't swim anymore, stay out late with the girls, spend hours in museums, or participate in many of her other favorite activities. She allowed these thoughts to overwhelm her, and, as a result, certainly did not give herself a chance to enjoy her life.

If you find yourself unhappily comparing your present life to life before lupus, try to modify your thinking. Start planning fun things for the present and future. Anyone can come up with some enjoyable activities, regardless of physical restrictions. But it takes effort. Don't wallow in self-pity, because that will only allow your depression to strangle you. Work on your thinking, develop some positive plans, and translate them into pleasure. Then wave good-bye to your depression!

Of course, if you clearly reflect on your past, you may find that it wasn't much better than the present! In the past, you may have had other physical problems. You may have made some mistakes. Naturally, this may make you even more depressed about the future. However, you can't change the past.

What's done is done. Keep telling yourself that. Don't punish yourself for the past. Tell yourself that you're going to work on making the future better. Set up some specific goals, starting with the easy-to-reach ones. You'll be helping yourself just by *thinking* about all the positive things you can do!

REDISCOVER WHAT'S MISSING FROM YOUR LIFE

You may have laughed when you read the heading to this section. "Good health," you might respond. "Mobility without pain!" Sure. But why discuss this? Because depressed people frequently lament the fact that something is missing from their lives. But another important element that might very well be missing—an element that can be regained!—is the feeling of satisfaction, accomplishment, and pride that normally comes from others' praise. You may be missing the attention and interest of other people, and this can cause you to feel worthless. What can you do about this? Think about your positive qualities. (Yes, you do have some!) Think about how you can interact more with people, spark their interest, and obtain more of the satisfaction that makes you feel worthwhile.

SHOOT FOR THE EARTH, NOT THE MOON

We all have goals for ourselves. It's normal to become depressed when we don't reach a particular one, especially if we've tried very hard to get there. But sometimes our goals are not realistic. Try to judge if the goals you've been setting for yourself are realistic. If not, reset them, keeping your abilities and limitations in mind. Once your goals are more realistic, you'll have a much better chance of achieving them and less chance of falling short.

Jenny had not returned to work since a major flare had required a six-week stay in the hospital. Finally, after a long period of rest and medication, she was feeling better and was looking forward to getting back to work so she could catch up on everything. When her doctor finally gave the go-ahead, she practically flew to her office . . . and after two hours of phone calls, typing, dictation, and meetings, she was exhausted, and her spirits plummeted. She became worried that she wouldn't be able to handle all the pressure and that she was in danger of losing her job. Wrong! Jenny had simply set her sights too high. Expecting to return to her old schedule as if she didn't have lupus was just not realistic. Try to return to your old activities slowly. Build up your stamina. Isn't the end result more important than the initial gains? And if your goals are more realistically set, you'll have a much better chance of achieving them, and less of a chance of falling short.

TALK ABOUT IT!

Now you know how to cope with depression both through physical activity and by changing your way of thinking. But there's one more thing you can do—something we've mentioned before. You can talk about your problems and concerns with others. Often, the very act of talking will help lift your depression. If there are family members or friends to whom you feel close and whose opinions you trust, talk to them. Air your feelings, and listen to their feedback. They may be more objective and better able to come up with constructive solutions.

If your depression is so intense or prolonged that friends and family are unable to help, then by all means consider speaking to a professional. Counseling is a very effective way to treat depression. So don't deny yourself this invaluable assistance. Why not do everything you can to help yourself feel better?

When Are Antidepressants Appropriate?

In a small percentage of cases, depression may be caused by biochemical deficiencies—chemical imbalances in our bodies. If depression is persistent, and nonmedical coping strategies are not effective, then antidepressant medications may prove helpful. Examples of new-generation antidepressants include selective serotonin reuptake inhibitors (SSRIs) such as Lexapro (escitalopram), Zoloft (sertraline hydrochloride), Prozac (fluoxetine hydrochloride), and Effexor (venlafaxine); and drugs such as Wellbutrin (bupropion) or Cymbalta (duloxetine). These medications work in different ways and may have different possible side effects.

There is always the chance that certain medications may not be appropriate in your lupus treatment program. So *always* check with your doctor!

Question, learn, and help yourself. If you need to take many different pills, it's important to avoid self-adjusting your dosage, changing the times you take them, or moving around the number of pills you take at a particular time. Follow your doctor's prescriptions as carefully as possible. In addition, be careful about bad mixes. Some mixes can make your symptoms worse, interfere with the action of the prescribed medication, or cause additional problems. Don't hesitate to ask questions.

Because medication causes chemical changes within the body, side effects may occur whenever a drug is taken. And, unfortunately, the more powerful the drug, the more potent its side effects may be. If the side effects you experience are slight, you will probably want to ignore them—especially if the medication you're taking is having the desired effect. If side effects are having a harsh impact on you, let your physician know, so together you can weigh the disadvantages of the medication against the advantages. In fact, any side effects should be reported to your doctor so that he or she can determine if the drug therapy should be continued, changed, or ended.

Regardless of whether your depression is caused by a biochemical deficiency or by your reaction to the people and events around you, you should still try to modify your thinking. Many experts believe that even if the cause of depression is biochemical, by working on the way you handle your day-to-day living, you can have a positive effect on your emotions.

An Antidepressing Antidote

The best way to work on negative thoughts is to prevent them from continuing. Try to be realistically positive. Deal with reality the way it actually exists. Deal with thoughts from a more factual point of view. Handle them the way they might be handled by somebody else—somebody who is not depressed and who can be more objective. Try to make your perceptions more accurate, your awareness more realistic, and your thoughts more constructive. Remember: Your thoughts lead to your emotions. If your thoughts are negative and critical, your emotions will also be in bad shape. But if you can turn your thoughts around to a more positive, constructive point of view, you'll see that your emotional reactions will most certainly improve as well.

24.

FEARS AND ANXIETIES

Don't be *afraid* to read this chapter! It may help you to discover what you're *anxious* about!

The two sentences above may help you to distinguish between anxiety and fear. What's the difference? Anxiety is a general sense of uneasiness—a vague feeling of discomfort. It is an agitated, uncertain state in which you just don't feel at peace or in control. There is a premonition that something bad may happen, something you have to protect yourself against. You feel very vulnerable. However, you're not exactly sure what the source of your anxiety is.

Fear, on the other hand, is usually more specific. It's often directed toward something that can be recognized, whether a person, an object, a situation, or an event. We experience fear when we become aware of something dangerous, or when we feel threatened. When we are afraid—much like when we're anxious—we feel out of control and less confident. So the feelings of anxiety and fear are basically the same, the main difference being whether the source of the feeling can be identified. For this reason, from this point on I'll be using the two terms interchangeably.

Fear is so common that many words are used to describe it: scared, concerned, alarmed, worried, uptight, nervous, edgy, and shaky. Then there's wary, frightened, and helpless. Is that it? Nope! How about suspicious, hesitant, apprehensive, tense, panicky, disturbed, and agitated? Of course, there are more, but if I went on, this book would have to be renamed *The Fear*

Synonym Book. The important point is that all these words mean the same thing: "I'm afraid." The source of this fear may be either real or imaginary.

Fear and Lupus

Unfortunately, people with lupus all too commonly experience anxiety and fear. They may be afraid that the pain will never stop. They may worry that lupus will affect their social and vocational activities. They may be scared of the treatment or of symptoms worsening. Many are fearful of the powerful drug treatments and their potential side effects.

Becky, aged twenty-nine, was afraid to go to sleep at night. She was worried that she'd wake up in the morning with painful lupus symptoms. Since she felt fine at night, she didn't want to go to sleep. If Becky was stronger (emotionally), she might still be concerned about new symptoms, but would not let them disturb her sleep. Becky, however, wasn't strong; she was frightened. Her fear kept her awake, she got less sleep, and she became more vulnerable to the very symptoms she wanted to avoid!

Often, the emotions experienced by people living with lupus parallel the course of the disease. Feelings are usually the most negative during flares or more painful periods. During periods of time when you genuinely feel good, emotions may be much more positive. But even during periods of remission, anxiety is often common. (For example, you may be afraid of symptoms returning.) And because anxiety can interfere with your ability to deal effectively with any medical problem, it's vital that you learn to cope with this emotion.

The best way to start dealing with your fears is to obtain as much information as you possibly can. By gaining knowledge and understanding, you will equip yourself to fight and conquer your fears. Just as important, both you and your family can implement successful psychological strategies that will help you deal more effectively with your fears, enabling you to better adjust and cope.

What Are the Symptoms of Anxiety and Fear?

What happens when you become extremely anxious? Your body may react physiologically. You may become short of breath, your heart may beat rapidly, you may feel shaky, and you may think, "I've got to get out of here!" You may try to relax but be unable to do so. You may try to breathe deeply but find that the breath keeps catching in your throat. You may try to "shake the feeling" but find that you can't. This inability to calm down can be frightening and may increase your anxiety even more. A vicious cycle can quickly develop. Before long, you may be completely out of control.

Which came first, the anxiety or the symptoms? That's not really important. What's more important is doing whatever is possible to reduce both. And it *is* possible to conquer your fear—to regain control of your emotions and improve your day-to-day life.

Is Fear Good or Bad?

Believe it or not, fear is usually good! Now you're probably wondering, "If I'm shaking with fear, how can it be good?" Fear mobilizes you. It tells you that something is frightening you and you need to prepare to attack the source of your fear. You react in a way that leads to action. In this regard, fear is similar to stress. It serves a necessary and critical purpose. In a way, it protects you.

Anxiety is bad only when the source of your fear becomes overlooked, ignored, or denied, or when the feeling is so excessive that it paralyzes you. In such cases, the threat or danger is allowed to continue and nothing—or, at least, not enough—is done to control it.

What Determines the Intensity of Our Reactions?

Fear ranges in intensity from mild to severe. It is impossible to measure just how much fear there is in anyone's life. This varies from person to person and from time to time.

What determines how fearful you get? Usually the intensity or closeness of the feared object, person, or event is important. (Wouldn't you be more afraid of getting an injection within the next thirty seconds than if you were getting it in thirty days?) How vulnerable are you? (Do you truly hate injections, or are you just tired of feeling like a pincushion?) Finally, how successful are you at defending yourself? (Can you calmly accept the needle, or do you scream a lot?) These are some of the factors determining how you handle fear. Your own strength and the success of your defense mechanisms also play a role.

What Is Panic?

Although this chapter focuses on anxiety and fear, we really can't discuss these emotions without also considering panic. Panic is the most intense form of anxiety—it's what you feel when your anxiety increases beyond the "typical" level. In fact, with panic, the degree of anxiety is so profound that you feel as if you've lost total control. Panic is anxiety "running amok." Research suggests that approximately 5 percent of the general population suffers from panic disorders.

Panic may strike suddenly and without warning. Occasionally, there may not even appear to be a specific trigger. Or the trigger may be perfectly clear, but you may find yourself unable to prevent the panic attack.

Although there are times when anxiety can be beneficial, panic is usually so intense that there are few, if any, benefits to the experience. So let's talk more about panic attacks and learn what can be done about them.

WHAT ARE THE SYMPTOMS OF PANIC ATTACKS?

The most common symptoms of panic attacks are palpitations, increased heart rate and blood flow, pounding heart, chest pain, sweating, dizziness, shortness of breath, imbalance, disorientation, a feeling of suffocation, rubbery legs, flushing, tingling in different parts of the body, faintness, numbness, nausea, shaking, trembling, a lump in the throat, and lightheadedness. This even *sounds* frightening! But the list doesn't end here. There are also psychological symptoms, including the feeling of going crazy, fear of dying, fear of losing control, a feeling of impending doom, and an urgent desire to escape.

CAN I STOP A PANIC ATTACK?

When you are experiencing a panic attack, it may be very difficult to rationally view the situation and realize that there is nothing to be afraid of—or, at least, that your fears may be out of proportion with reality. Rather, you may be unable to think objectively at all, and your emotions may take over. The fear then becomes more intense.

The more you feel unable to control panic attacks, the more often they may occur. This happens in part because you're already out of control, so that it takes less stress to trigger an attack.

There are times when panic attacks are of very short duration. They may last for only a few minutes, and then pass. At other times, though, they may last for up to an hour or more. This can be devastating!

The desire to avoid panic attacks may lead to the onset of phobias. Why? Phobias—irrational fears of a situation or object—actually begin as avoidance behavior. You may start associating the discomfort of panic attacks with whatever situations you were in at the time the attacks began. You'll then try to avoid these situations more and more, becoming phobic in your intense need to avoid the seeming triggers of these attacks.

Fortunately, many of the techniques that are helpful in dealing with anxieties and fears will prevent your emotions from escalating into panic, and help you deal with panic when it occurs. These strategies include pinpointing possible reasons for your fear and panic, using relaxation techniques to prevent or overcome your panic, and restructuring your thinking. If your feelings of panic continue, though, medication or counseling may be necessary. There are also many successful programs designed to help people cope with panic attacks.

How Can You Cope with Anxieties and Fears?

Obviously, the more fears you have, the more difficulty you'll experience in making a successful adjustment to your new situation. Recognizing your fears and learning how to deal with them will help you live more happily and comfortably. How? I was afraid you'd never ask! Let's look at some of the ways in which you can help yourself better cope with your fears.

PINPOINT THE SOURCE OF YOUR FEARS

The first step in coping with your fears is to use the "pinpointing" technique discussed in Chapter 22. Identify and list exactly what you're afraid of and exactly why you are afraid. Then think about what you can do to alleviate your fears.

For Claudia, this was not hard. She knew she was afraid of how people would react when they saw the rash on her face. She quickly realized that what she feared was rejection. She was concerned that they wouldn't want to be with her because of their own fears ("Is it contagious?" "Will it affect me?" "I don't want to be seen with her," and so on). She planned a course of action (no, not a one-way ticket to Brazil!). She decided she'd simply do the best she could, expecting her friends to accept her the way she was. If they didn't, that was *their* loss. She was less afraid almost instantly. As you begin planning your strategies and gradually putting your plan into operation, you'll feel better and better.

RELAX!

Because relaxation is the opposite of tension, the use of relaxation techniques can be very helpful in coping with anxieties and fears. As mentioned earlier in the book, there are many types of relaxation techniques: progressive relaxation, meditation, autogenics, deep breathing, and more. Regardless of what is provoking your fear, learning to relax is an important part of improving emotional well-being. (Detailed information about relaxation techniques can be found in Chapter 9.)

DESENSITIZE YOURSELF

One great technique for conquering fear is called *systematic desensitization.* Using this technique, you gradually desensitize yourself—that is, make yourself less vulnerable—to the source of your fear.

Here's how it can work for you. Sit in a comfortable chair and relax. Then create a movie in your mind by imagining whatever it is that makes you afraid. If you get tense, stop imagining it and relax. When you've calmed down, try imagining it again. The more you try to imagine your fear, and alternate this "movie" with relaxation techniques, the less it will bother you. Try it! It will give you a great feeling of relaxation and control. There are many books that provide much more information on systematic desensitization. Check them out.

LEARN TO COPE WITH ANXIOUS THOUGHTS

It was stated earlier that anxiety is a vague, uneasy feeling with an unknown source. So how can you cope with anxiety by following the steps listed above? Surely, if you can't pinpoint the source of your fear, you can't follow these specific steps. So what can you do? Well, a number of things may work. Try the relaxation techniques discussed earlier in this book. Work on changing your thinking to make it more positive and productive. Find somebody to whom you can express your fears—somebody who will listen to you, talk to you, and try to help you deal with your fears. Even if you can't pinpoint a specific fear, these techniques will greatly help you cope with general anxiety.

LEARN MORE ABOUT LUPUS

Things that are unknown are often feared. And unfortunately, there are still a lot of unknowns regarding lupus. However, the more people you speak to, the more questions you ask, and the more information you obtain, the fewer "unknowns" there will be. Knowledge is power! The more you know about lupus, including the different symptoms and treatment options, the easier it will be to eliminate many of your fears, or at least reduce them to the point of being manageable.

Let's Talk About Specifics

When you were first diagnosed, many fearful questions probably came to mind. "What will the future be like? What will become of me?" These are all typical, legitimate questions of people who are diagnosed with any chronic medical problem—not just lupus.

As time has gone by, in all probability, some of these questions have been answered and you have started to adjust to living with lupus. But once your initial fears are reduced, new fears may arise.

In the previous pages, we looked at some general coping strategies. But you're probably more interested in seeing how these and other strategies can help you better deal with the specific fears that you're struggling with right now. Let's discuss some of these fears and see what methods of coping may help.

FEAR OF A FLARE

One of the most common fears experienced by people with lupus is going into a flare. Wow, can this be upsetting! Hopefully, you're doing everything you can to help yourself remain healthy and minimize the chances of a flare. But sometimes, even if you're doing everything perfectly, you'll still go into a flare.

Can you defeat this fear? Yes. Try to plan what you're going to do if and when a flare occurs. For example, if you're afraid that a flare will affect your work, plan in advance how you're going to handle your job, your employer, and your responsibilities if and when it does happen. Anticipate that a flare will occur. Then you won't get caught off-guard when it does. By having a plan in place, you can reduce your fear.

FEAR OF PAIN

Nobody likes pain. And because pain is one of the most unpleasant problems associated with lupus, you may be fearful of it. If you do feel pain, you'll wonder when you're going to feel some relief. Each little twinge of pain may make you afraid that further deterioration of your condition will occur, or that additional problems exist or may develop. And even when you're not in pain, you may fear its occurrence.

What can you do about this fear? Try to accept the fact that some pain may be with you from time to time, but medication can reduce its intensity as well as its duration. Realize that each pain "cycle" will eventually stop, or at least ease up. The pain won't last forever. (For more suggestions on coping with pain, refer back to Chapter 9.)

FEAR OF MEDICATION AND POSSIBLE SIDE EFFECTS

Regardless of which medication your doctor prescribes, there may be frightening things about it that may upset you.

For instance, you may be nervous about the different medications that you have to take, even though you need them. You may be afraid of what they're doing to your body. Yes, it's true that virtually all medications have side effects (see Chapter 10), but you'll want to focus on the benefits of medications. Just keep reminding yourself about the damage lupus could do to you without medication! Your physician is aware of the possible side effects, but will still prescribe medication as long as the advantages of the medication outweigh the side effects, and the side effects are not as potentially dangerous as uncontrolled lupus.

What if you've had problems with your treatment? What if all the therapies you've tried haven't seemed to do any good? If it seems as if you experience unpleasant side effects with every medication you try, you may begin to fear that nothing is going to work. Unfortunately, there are some people who have more difficulty than others finding the right "formula." And it's possible you may not benefit as much as you (and your doctor, family, therapists, friends, and others) would like. But hang in there. New medications and techniques are being developed all the time. And who knows? More trial and error may result in a solution. Giving up will just make you more tense and uncomfortable anyway. So keep trying.

Deal with your fears regarding medication and treatment by asking any questions you need answered. Learn as much as you can. Speak to others who have experienced your prescribed treatment. Make sure you understand the purpose of the treatment, the potential for success, and the fact that there are often ways to minimize side effects. By anticipating what may happen, you'll be in much better shape to deal with the possible consequences.

FEAR OF DYING

Although the mortality rate for lupus has been greatly reduced, it still has not been totally eliminated, so being afraid of dying is understandable. When might you be most afraid of dying? Probably when you're in the middle of a flare, or when your symptoms are particularly intense. Beginning a new treatment or being involved in any of the ups and downs that remind you of your vulnerability can also cause these fears. When you feel the worst, you're more likely to fear the worst. However, being afraid of dying is not going to help you feel better or live longer. If anything, it's only going to make you feel worse! Being afraid of dying, therefore, falls into the category of fears that you can do little or nothing about.

How do you attack this fear? Research is constantly exploring new and improved treatment possibilities for individuals with lupus. So think positively. Others have had worse symptoms and still live comfortably. Do you see how you must work on your thinking? If negative thoughts make you more afraid, then positive thoughts . . .

FEAR OF NOT BEING BELIEVED

Are you in pain? Do you find it hard to let other people know about your pain? Maybe you're afraid that they won't believe you. "I can't believe that anybody would experience as many symptoms and as much pain as you do with lupus," you're afraid they're thinking. How can you have energy and be able to function one minute, and the very next minute be so tired that you can barely move out of the chair? It may seem strange, but you know it's true; however, it's frightening to think that other people just will not understand. You don't want to be labeled a hypochondriac!

What can you do? Talk to the nonbelievers. Share reading material with them. Try to explain lupus as best as you can. You've then done all you can. You can't crawl into someone else's head and change his or her beliefs. As long as you believe in yourself, you'll better deal with this fear.

FEAR OF DISABILITY

The thought of being disabled may be horrible. Because you know that lupus, in some cases, can cause severe physical restrictions, you may have this fear. But being "disabled" is a bad term, since it suggests that you can do virtually nothing.

Other than trying to take good care of yourself, what else can you really do? Take things as they come, but think more positively. If you look around you and think more objectively, you'll realize that a physical disability wouldn't make you any less of a human being. You would still have many, many capabilities. Numerous Olympic champions began their athletic careers to overcome physical disabilities. Beethoven wrote some of his greatest music after becoming totally deaf. There have been athletes playing professional ball despite having diseases such as diabetes, concussion syndrome, or even lupus. There even was a one-armed baseball player in the major leagues, and an *American Idol* finalist with Tourette's syndrome. Regardless of their conditions, these people all had one thing in common: the knowledge that they could overcome or at least compensate for a limitation in one area by developing abilities in another. So remember: You still have a lot of room for self-fulfillment.

FEAR OF THE REACTIONS OF OTHERS

Are you afraid that other people will not accept you with lupus? Do you fear they may shun you for physical reasons? You may fear rejection if you can't socialize the way you'd like to. Unfortunately, some people can be cold and unfeeling. They may be put off by the fact that you can no longer keep up with them. But don't try to, because pushing yourself can be a painful way to maintain a friendship. And who needs those kinds of friends anyway? Your true friends will accept you under any circumstances.

Other fears in this category can be even more frightening. "What if my spouse leaves me? What if all my friends stay away from me?" Fear of desertion can be horrible. If it's not happening now, you may be afraid of it happening in the future. You may be afraid that none of your friends will remain "in your corner." To reduce the chances of such rejection, you may hesitate to make plans with friends or family. This will only add to your feeling of isolation.

Naturally, you should aim to remain involved with family and friends. But be realistic. Remember that a change in a social relationship can occur for any reason, not just because of lupus! And since you can't change the way some people feel, try not to be too concerned with their reactions. Instead, be more attentive to your own needs and feelings.

Of course, if you feel that an important relationship is in jeopardy, you should try to figure out why, and what you can do to improve things. And if you feel that people are shying away from you, try to discuss this with them. Find out what they are afraid of. Maybe you'll be able to remedy the situation. Get counseling, if need be. But remember that you can do only so much. If your efforts don't work, at least you'll know that you did your best.

Finally, if you have been troubled by the reactions of others, you may find it helpful to get involved in a support group. You know that the people in these groups will not shy away from you or abandon you. Why? Because they're going through the same kinds of things that you are! And because of their own experiences, participants may even be able to give you some tips on dealing with family and friends. (For more information on dealing with others, see Part Four.)

FEAR OF OVERDOING OR UNDERDOING

You may not know how much you should be doing. You may be afraid of doing too much, but feel guilty about doing too little! How can you conquer this fear? Get advice from experts. You'll need professional guidance to come up with the best "mix" of rest and exercise. And you'll need to know which, if any, activities may be too strenuous for you.

Of course, even your doctor may not have specific answers for you. You may be told that the answers will become apparent only through trial and error. After all, experience is the best teacher.

So what should you do? Pace yourself. Change your level of activity gradually. Then tell yourself, as with so many other fears, that you're doing the best you can.

FEAR OF DEPENDENCE

If you are finding that lupus has placed some restrictions on your activities, you may be afraid of becoming too dependent on your friends and family. You may worry that you'll be too much of a burden on your loved ones if you ask for help. You may fear that you'll lose your ability to help yourself.

You can deal with this fear by concentrating on those things that you still can do. Graciously accept the help you may have to take from others, but don't view this as dependence. Instead, focus on the benefits you're receiving from increased interaction with family and friends! So don't let yourself give up—you'll be doing yourself a great disservice.

FEAR OF GOING OUT

Are you afraid to go out? You may think you're going to get tired or get sick. Maybe you're concerned about collapsing from weakness and not being helped. Jeannie planned a very pleasant outing to the city only to find that very shortly after she got there, she was no longer able to walk around! Are you afraid you'll get so tired that it will take hours to complete a simple chore? You may also be afraid of getting sick while you're out. You may be concerned about getting the help you would need if you fainted or couldn't move. You may also be concerned about how others will look at you or treat you. It is understandable to feel afraid of these things, but does that justify your staying home all the time? That won't help you get over these fears.

There are some things you *can* do to reduce your fears. If you plan ahead, you will feel more at ease. If you're concerned about your physical state, take someone with you when you go out, instead of going alone. Pace yourself. Plan your activities for times when you're the most rested, and don't try to do too much at once.

FEAR OF TRAVELING

People with lupus don't have to limit their travel, but traveling with lupus does present special circumstances and challenges. To some people with lupus, the preparation required to take a "relaxing" vacation can be overwhelming. And the thought of traveling far from familiar doctors and medical facilities can be downright frightening. Obviously, if you travel by car, this may not be as much of a problem. You're not going to be so far away that you couldn't get help if you really needed it. But you may not be sure you can walk as much as you'd like on your trip, or whether your destinations are conducive to your getting around.

Proper planning can ensure that you have a fun and *safe* trip—to almost every corner of the globe! (Refer back to Chapter 15 for guidelines that will help ensure an enjoyable trip.)

FEAR OF EMPLOYMENT PROBLEMS

Like many people with lupus, you may be concerned about the effect your condition will have on your job. You may want or need to work, but fear that you won't be able to. Your employer may be understanding at first, but you may worry about how long his or her tolerance will continue. And, of course, your need for money will be greater due to your medical problems! So if you can't work, the pressure can be tremendous.

What can you do? Talk to others who have been in the same situation, and see how they handled it. Speak to experts who can advise you on financial matters. Evaluate your vocational skills, and make sure you're equipped to do a job that you can physically handle. Remember, you'll work it out. (Refer to chapters 13 and 14 for more advice on dealing with job and/or financial problems.)

FEAR THAT YOUR CHILD WILL INHERIT LUPUS

The thought of transmitting lupus to your children may be so frightening that you may not want to have children. But even if you already have a family, you may be panicky. You don't want to live in constant fear of your child saying that a joint hurts or showing you a rash on that little face! Learn the facts. As discussed previously, a tendency toward lupus may be genetically transmitted, but the chances are very small that your child will develop the disease. Symptoms can occur in anyone, with or without a family history of lupus. Just because your child has one of the symptoms of lupus doesn't mean that he or she has the condition. Speak to your doctor, and relax. (You may also fear that lupus, or medications used to treat it, will increase the chances of miscarriage or birth defects. Make sure you discuss your concerns with your doctor. You can learn more about this in Chapter 17 on pregnancy.)

If your child is diagnosed with lupus, it need not be the end of the world. It's not your fault. Your child still "wanted" to be born and to be alive. Maybe you'll be able to help one another adjust. But don't resign yourself to the fact that your child is destined to get lupus until a diagnosis is made. Otherwise, you'll be blowing your fear all out of proportion. Remember: Treatment is improving and will likely be even better when your child is growing up than it is now. A diagnosis of lupus need not be a disaster.

FEAR OF NOT COPING

You may feel that you're barely handling your lupus. You may believe that any new problem that comes along will be enough to push you over the edge. And fear of falling apart can easily lead to panic: an out-of-control kind of feeling that can actually make this happen.

So get hold of yourself. Pinpoint those particular things you're having difficulty with, and get help in dealing with them. Don't wait, and don't project a false sense of bravado. If you feel yourself nearing the edge, get someone to help you steady yourself. Talk over your fears with someone. Once you have shared them, you may see things a little more clearly. You may be able to deal with problems with greater strength, knowing that you're not alone. And once you're back in control, your fear will disappear.

FEAR OF FEAR

The last fear in this section is the strangest, but also one of the most common. You may get to a point where your fear is no longer focused on anything specific. Rather, you're afraid of being afraid, of getting that fearful, anxious, panicky feeling that overwhelms your body and your mind. This is actually called a *secondary anxiety reaction*, meaning that you're anxious about being anxious.

So if you're not afraid of something specific, what can you do? Work on relaxation techniques, and do whatever you can to increase your feelings of control. After all, being afraid of fear suggests that you have little or no confidence in your ability to control this emotion. Remind yourself that you'll deal with any frightening thing that might come along . . . *if and when* it comes along, rather than letting this pervasive feeling of worry cause you to be afraid of being afraid. Any of these positive and proactive strategies, whether it be a relaxation technique, some type of exercise, or even an absorbing activity, helps you to directly counteract this out-of-control feeling, and shows you that there's less of a reason to be afraid.

When Are Antianxiety Medications Appropriate?

Many people are able to reduce anxiety through nonpharmacological methods such as those described above. However, because intense fear or panic may throw you out of control, you may require professional intervention—especially if these attacks have been occurring often. Don't feel that you are weak if you decide to consult a professional. After all, your goal is to feel better, right? So if you're having difficulty resolving some of these problems yourself, isn't it good to know that there are experts who can help you regain control?

Antianxiety medications can be an important, if not essential, part of your treatment. If medication seems to be part of the answer for you—and especially if your anxiety is very intense—there are three subcategories that may be helpful.

The first subcategory of antianxiety drugs are the benzodiazepines. The drugs in this group include Xanax (alprazolam), Valium (diazepam), Klonopin (clonazepam), and Librium (chlordiazepoxide hydrochloride). The latter two, although used to control anxiety, are not considered as effective for panic attacks. Benzodiazepines have few side effects, but can be habit-forming.

The second subcategory of drugs primarily used in the treatment of anxiety is the tricyclic antidepressants. Although primarily considered to be antidepressants, these medications were actually among the earliest ones found effective in dealing with anxiety, but are now used less often, since more effective medications have been found. The drugs in this category include Tofranil (imipramine hydrochloride) and Norpramin (desipramine hydrochloride).

The third subcategory of antianxiety drugs is the MAO (monoamine oxidase) inhibitors, also a category of antidepressants. Some consider this group to be the most effective for the treatment of anxiety and panic. However, of the three groups, this one probably requires the greatest care in following dosage schedules and other precautions in order to minimize side effects. For example, if you're taking an MAO inhibitor, it is important to avoid taking antihistamines or decongestants, as the drugs might be incompatible and cause further problems. Also, foods with high concentrations of tyramine or dopamine—aged cheeses, beer, and wine, for instance—should be avoided, as they may lead to hypertension (high blood pressure). Examples of drugs in this subcategory are Nardil (phenelzine sulfate) and Parnate (tranylcypromine sulfate).

As with the antidepressants mentioned in the previous chapter, it is important to check with your doctor to make sure the drugs you are taking are appropriate as part of your lupus treatment program. Be careful with dosages, reporting side effects, and mixing medications.

When using antianxiety medications, keep in mind that even when they are effective, they are really only blocking the anxiety. It is still important to deal with the triggers of the fears and anxieties, and to implement any changes necessary to resolve the problems that led to the anxiety in the first place.

A Fearless Summary

Although many different fears have been discussed in this chapter, we probably haven't covered all of the ones you have experienced. In addition, the coping suggestions offered certainly don't include all possible ways of dealing with fear. So what should you do?

Anticipate that you will be fearful of certain things from time to time. Some fears will return, but plan on riding through them rather than succumbing to them. Not only is it okay to be scared, it's normal. Also remember that the most important thing is to stay on top of these fears so that they don't overwhelm you or render you less able to cope.

You're working on recognizing your fears, right? For some of them, you're modifying your behavior. For others, you're modifying your thinking. Soon you will feel more in control. As this happens, you'll notice your fears begin to diminish. That doesn't mean that they'll all go away. But as you work on them and feel more in control, they'll at least lessen in intensity, and you'll feel better knowing that you can handle whatever comes along.

25.

ANGER

It was the day of the senior prom. Linda, a seventeen-year-old high school student, was sitting by her telephone waiting for a call from her doctor. She had not been feeling that well, but she was hoping that the doctor would tell her that she was healthy enough to go to the prom. The telephone rang, and Linda answered. Her doctor told her the results of her blood test; they showed that a lupus flare had begun. He said that she would be best off if she got plenty of rest and recommended that she not go out. Barely able to say good-bye, she slammed down the telephone and threw herself on the bed, pounding on her pillow. Was Linda angry? You bet she was!

Diane, aged thirty-one, was fed up with joint pains. Practically anyone who went near her received an earful of comments you wouldn't want your mother to hear! Everyone from her doctor to her family was a victim of this verbal assault. What made her even angrier was that she wanted to slam her fist down on her kitchen table, but she knew it would just make her pain worse. Diane was angry!

In general, people with any chronic medical problem may be angry. Because anger results in the buildup of physical energy that needs to be released, it is important for you to learn how to cope with it.

Just what is anger? When you have a desire or goal in mind and something interferes with your efforts to reach it, this can be very frustrating. A feeling of intense tension and hostility may result, which is what we refer to as anger.

Are There Different Types of Anger?

In learning to deal with anger, it can be helpful to discuss three different ways in which anger can be experienced. This will enable you to more easily identify anger when it does occur.

One type of anger is rage—the expression of violent, uncontrolled anger. If Diane was feeling upset about her lupus and a "friend" told her that her joints would still be healthy if she had taken better care of herself, you can imagine how angry Diane might become. Diane's anger might even lead her to say or do things that would certainly not enhance the prospects of a long-lasting, friendly relationship with this person! This is probably the most intense anger you can experience. It is an outward expression that results in a visible explosion. Often, rage can be a destructive release of the intense physical energy that has built up over time.

Another type of anger is resentment. This feeling of anger is usually kept inside. What if Diane listened to her friend's well-meaning comments, smiled, and said nothing, but was seething inside? This is resentment—a growing, smoldering feeling of anger, directed toward a person or object, but often kept bottled up. Resentment tends to sit uncomfortably within you and can do even more physiological and psychological damage than rage.

A third type of anger is indignation, a more appropriate, positive type of anger. Unlike rage, it is released in a controlled way. If Diane had responded to her friend's comments by stating that she appreciated the concern but would prefer no advice at this point, this would have been an expression of indignation.

Obviously, these three types of anger can occur in combination and in many different ways. Understanding the different ways of experiencing anger can help you identify and cope with it when it does occur.

What Causes Anger?

There are, of course, a lot of things that can make you angry. You may get angry waiting for your doctor to see you. You wouldn't be too thrilled if you had to cancel your plans at the last moment. You may also get angry if you are told you need yet another type of medication. You may get angry if you feel that your family is not understanding enough, or you may think that they are trying too hard to protect you.

Insults from other people, aside from everyday frustrations, can cause anger. "If you washed your face better, you wouldn't have those ugly splotches on your nose and cheeks." This is not the kind of comment that would make you feel warm and fuzzy! If you feel that someone is taking advantage of you or feel as if you have been forced to do something that you did not want to do, anger may result. Let's say that your friend says, "I'm going to a party next Saturday. You have such good taste in clothes, please come with me to pick out a dress. We'll go to only seven or eight stores." If you do not have the ability or confidence to say no when friends ask for a favor, this can create feelings of anger—especially if you are feeling too fatigued to complete even your own tasks.

Becoming more aware of why you are angry is an important step in learning to deal with feelings of frustration or hostility. You must, of course, become aware of anger before you can deal with it. Unfortunately, resolving your anger won't make your lupus go away. Nor should you say that you'd stop being angry only if your lupus is cured. As with other emotions we've discussed, this is not realistic.

One of the common questions that people with lupus ask is, "Why me?" This question suggests that what has happened shouldn't have happened— that it's unfair, or that someone or something is to blame. It's important to realize that in this case, anger is not helpful—that asking "Why me?" will not benefit you in any way. It's far better to ask yourself what you can do about it now that it has happened. And you can even say, "Why not me?" This shows that lupus happened, you didn't cause it, you don't want it, but you can't waste valuable energy looking to point a finger!

In learning to cope with your anger, you must realize that anger exists uniquely in the mind of each angry individual. Anger is a direct result of your thoughts, not of events. An event in and of itself does not make you angry. Rather, your anger is caused by your interpretation of the event—the way you think or feel about it.

How Does Anger Affect Your Body?

When you are angry, a number of physiological responses occur. Your breathing becomes more rapid, your blood pressure increases (you may feel like your blood is "boiling"), and your heart may begin to pound. Your face may feel hot and your muscles may tense. You may also feel stronger when you're angry. The more intense the anger, the greater is this feeling of power. In fact, you may be able to remember a time when you were so angry that you almost felt you had superhuman strength.

Anger is a form of energy. The more physical energy that builds up in the body due to anger, the more necessary it becomes for you to release it. The energy cannot be destroyed. So if it is not released in some constructive manner, it will eventually come out in another, less desirable way. Imagine the energy from anger as a stick of dynamite about to explode. If you get rid of it, it will explode away from you. It may cause some damage, but it will not hurt you inside as much as if you swallowed the dynamite to keep others from being hurt. Obviously, the ideal solution is not to throw the stick of dynamite and not to swallow it, but (are you ready for this?) to try to defuse the dynamite! More about defusing, soon.

Extreme anger usually passes quickly. If, however, the anger lasts for a long period of time, it can have physically damaging effects on the body. You've probably heard about some of the physical problems that can result from holding anger in, such as ulcers, hypertension, and headaches. Well, anger can also cause a stress response that may exacerbate your lupus. It's just not good for your body. So it's vital that you learn to deal with your anger, not just for your emotional well-being, but for your physical health, as well.

How Does Anger Affect Your Mind?

Anger is usually experienced as a very unpleasant feeling. However, it sometimes exists along with a more pleasant feeling of power or strength. Frequently, the unpleasantness of anger is related to its consequences— knowing what you do when you are angry, and not being happy about it.

Sometimes anger may become so extreme that you feel like exploding. You may feel that unless you are able to punch, kick, or hit something—to get rid of the anger in some way—you will lose control. Hopefully this angry energy can be released without causing damage to another person, property, or yourself. If, when you finally calm down, you find that you have done something destructive, you may become angry all over again. Or you may experience another negative emotion, such as guilt.

Is Anger Good or Bad?

You may wonder how anger could possibly be good or constructive. "Avoid anger at all costs," many people say, "because nothing good can come of it." But this is true only if you don't deal with the anger properly. Anger can, indeed, be dangerous if it's kept inside or released in inappropriate ways.

Remember that stick of dynamite? What an explosive example! If anger is released in destructive ways, it can cause problems in relationships—to say the least! It can also aggravate existing medical problems. Does this mean that anger can make your condition worse? Well, what if you're so angry with somebody—perhaps your doctor or an overprotective spouse—that you rebelliously refuse to follow your treatment program, or decide not to take proper care of yourself? For example, what if you are so mad at the world that you don't take your medication properly? Taking more or less than the prescribed amount can be harmful to your health. Or what if being angry with someone or something causes you to do more than you should be doing? "I'll show them," you say. Having lupus, you know that you may eventually have to pay the price for overdoing it. What if you're angry with someone who cares about you and normally helps you deal with your lupus symptoms? That person, if upset by your anger, may be less willing to help you. This may, in turn, make you feel even worse. So if you want your anger to be good instead of bad, try to turn it into something that can be helpful rather than harmful to you.

How can anger be constructive? First, it can give you an indication that something is wrong—something must be creating this feeling of anger, something that needs attention. Second, it can motivate you to deal more actively with life's problems. Anger can give you a very constructive, motivating feeling of power or strength, of confidence or assertiveness. You can become so emotionally charged that it will have a positive effect on your life. So anger can be good, and it can help you to solve problems. This is not to say, however, that you should slam your finger with a hammer, break a couple of dishes, or have someone slap you in order to make you angry enough to solve your problems!

In order for anger to be helpful, there are some very important things to keep in mind. First, don't let yourself become overwhelmed by the anger. Once that happens, it is much harder to do what you have to do. Second, don't be afraid of your anger. If you do fear it, you probably won't be able to release it properly. More than likely, it will come out in unhealthy ways, or you'll bottle it up inside. Third, be sure that the way you handle your anger is socially acceptable. You might get a kick out of knocking out someone's teeth, but would that person (or the dentist . . . or the police) approve? Try to be flexible enough to recognize an appropriate way of releasing your anger.

Some Different Reactions to Anger

Maureen, a twenty-eight-year-old teacher, was having a hard time with her husband. He was trying to show concern for his wife by not letting her do any housework. But, surprisingly, she *wanted* to clean the house because she believed she felt well enough to do it. His resistance was so persistent and he was so "saccharin sweet" that Maureen felt it was too much. She wanted to be treated like an adult, able to determine when she could be active. But her husband just wouldn't let up. She was running out of patience. Let's see how Maureen might handle the situation in different ways.

THE "JUST IGNORE IT" APPROACH

If you feel overwhelmed by the intensity of your anger, and fear that you may completely lose control, you may try to do whatever you can to avoid the experience. This might include pushing any angry thoughts out of your mind, no matter how important the issue.

So rather than making a fuss over household responsibilities, Maureen could try to get involved in other activities and not show her resentment. Or she could try to appease her husband and agree with everything that he says. This would be at least temporarily effective in helping Maureen cope. In the long run, however, you can see that this would not be the best way for Maureen to deal with her anger.

THE "TAKE POWER" APPROACH

Maybe you enjoy the flow of energy and strength that comes from being angry. You may find that when you're angry, you are best able to assert yourself and get things done.

Maureen knows that if she is smothered once too often, she will explode. She might love the feeling of power that this anger gives her. She might almost look forward to the chance to say, "Honey, if you treat me that way once more, I'll take this vacuum cleaner and . . . !" If you enjoy this feeling, it's possible that you may even provoke situations to make yourself angry. Perhaps you've heard of professional football players or boxers who psyche themselves up before a confrontation with an opponent. For them, getting angry is the best preparation for a successful performance.

THE "TAKE ACTION" APPROACH

It's possible to see anger as a necessary, though unpleasant, part of life. You know that there will be times when you'll be angry, whether you like it or not. But you can choose to deal with both your anger and the situation that's causing it as effectively as possible.

For example, Maureen knows that she's not happy being angry and might decide to speak to her husband so that he could better understand her emotional needs. In this case, even if Maureen failed to persuade her husband to let her assume her normal household responsibilities, she would at least have the satisfaction of knowing that she did something about her feelings.

Your own reaction to anger is unique. It may also change from time to time. There may be times when you accept anger and almost value it as a motivator. At other times you may attempt to push it away. Maureen might enjoy expressing her anger. But if she didn't want to hurt her husband or upset the rest of the family, she might choose to have a calm discussion rather than shattering everyone's eardrums with an explosive confrontation.

Of course, the way in which you deal with your emotions now is probably similar to the way in which you've dealt with adversity in the past. If you have always dealt with problems in a generally positive, constructive manner, you will probably deal with new problems in the same way. On the other hand, if you have had difficulty dealing with stress in the past, you may also have problems dealing with it now. But remember that you can learn how to effectively cope with anger, just as Maureen did in the third example. Let's learn more about this.

How Can You Cope with Anger?

You've now begun to realize that anger can be constructive. Hopefully, the information you've read so far has been encouraging. But what, specifically, can you do to cope with your own anger?

Because anger is such a complex emotion, and because so many things can lead to this feeling, there are no simple answers. (Sorry about that!) Does this mean that there is nothing that you can do about anger? Of course not. Many things can be done to reduce your feelings of anger and to help you handle them more efficiently, comfortably, and safely.

The first important step is to be able to admit that you're angry, and you must figure out why you're angry. Once you've pinpointed the source of your anger, you may be able to defuse it or, if that's not possible, to find an acceptable outlet for it. Let's take a look at each of these ways of coping with anger.

RECOGNIZE YOUR ANGER

There are two steps involved in recognizing anger: admitting its existence and identifying its source. Let's discuss these in greater detail.

STEP ONE: ADMIT THAT YOU'RE ANGRY

The first step in dealing with anger is to recognize that you're angry. As simple as this may sound, many people cannot admit to being angry. They may try to deny it or to rationalize their feelings or behaviors using other explanations.

Do you feel that being angry is a sign of weakness? If so, you may not admit that you're angry—perhaps not even to yourself. You may feel that there is no appropriate reason to be angry, and that anger is a childish reaction. But, as with anything else, in order to change something, you have to first recognize that it exists.

How can you tell that you're angry? If you feel very tense (jumping at the sound of the telephone), or if you find yourself reacting with impulsiveness (slamming down the phone when you get a wrong number and storming out of the house) or hostility (cursing at your neighbor for leaving a speck of garbage on your lawn), chances are that you're angry. Don't be afraid to recognize it, as this is the first step in dealing with it.

STEP TWO: IDENTIFY THE SOURCE OF YOUR ANGER

The second step in dealing with anger is trying to identify its source. Where did the anger come from? What is contributing to it? What events have led to these feelings of anger? Why do you want to break all the furniture?

For one thing, as mentioned earlier in the chapter, you may be angry because you have lupus. You may be angry with yourself for neglecting your condition. You may feel anger toward your physician, whether justified or not. You may be angry because you have to take medication. In some cases, the events leading to an angry reaction may be quite obvious. In other cases, however, it may be hard to pinpoint the cause. At such times, it can be helpful to probe deeply enough to find the source of the problem.

Take, for example, the case of Suzanne, a forty-seven-year-old homemaker. She was awakened one bright, cheerful morning to hear birds singing right outside her bedroom. Instead of feeling happy and carefree, she felt angry. She had just awakened, but she felt angry. Initially, she was unable to figure out why, on such a beautiful day, she might feel angry. But finally, after giving the matter a lot of thought, she realized that because it was sunny and bright out, her less than favorite cousins were going to come from out of town to visit, and she would feel obligated to entertain them—something that she did not wish to do.

Of course, much of this anger is irrational. But, like other emotional reactions, it must be worked through. It cannot just be pushed away. Simply telling yourself, "Don't be angry," is not enough. It's as effective as telling yourself, "Don't breathe!" You must learn to channel your anger more effectively.

Why is it important to identify why you are angry? Mainly, to decide whether the anger you are feeling is realistic. Analyze your reasons for being angry. If necessary, write down what you think is making you angry. Be honest when writing down your thoughts, regardless of how violent or profane they may be! Rich, colorful language can be helpful in getting your feelings out and will ultimately allow you to control your anger. Try to look at these thoughts objectively, the way someone else might look at them. If you recognize that your reasons are not realistic, this alone may help you deal with these feelings of anger. If, on the other hand, you can objectively say that your feelings of anger are rational, your next step will be to decide how you can best handle them.

Now, depending on the situation, you can either defuse your anger or find an appropriate outlet for it. Read on to see how each of these techniques can work for you!

DEFUSE YOUR ANGER

In the past, it was falsely believed that there were only two possible ways of dealing with anger: to keep it inside or to let it out. But what about a third possibility? Remember when we talked about defusing that stick of dynamite? Your anger is a result of the way you think! In your mind, you're interpreting events in a way that makes you angry. So if you can change the way you interpret things and reorganize your thinking patterns, you can actually stop creating the anger that you feel. Is this really possible? Well, if something happened that made you angry, would everybody in the world be angry because of it? No. You'd be angry because of the way you'd be thinking about, or interpreting, the event. Others might not be angry because their interpretation of the event would be different. For example, let's say you've made a doctor appointment. Ten minutes before you are ready to leave, the receptionist calls to cancel, saying she'll reschedule the appointment at another time. You might be furious because you feel you should have received more notice and because you really wanted to be seen. How aggravating! But others might not interpret it that way and might not get the least bit angry. So if we can learn to interpret events in a more positive, constructive, and calm manner, we can reduce feelings of anger. Let's look at some of the ways in which you can defuse your anger *before* it becomes a problem.

WATCH MENTAL MOVIES

An interesting technique that can be helpful in controlling anger is imagery, or "watching movies in your mind." When you become angry, you frequently have all kinds of pictures in your head—images of what's making you angry and of how you'd like to deal with your feelings. These "mental movies" can be a helpful means of defusing your anger.

For example, imagine that you are very, very tired. Your friend calls to tell you that her car has broken down. Could you please pick up her dry cleaning? When you tell her that you are too exhausted to go out, she says something about how she can never depend on you for anything. This is a friend? You become irate. At that moment, ask your friend to hold on. Then close your eyes and imagine all the abusive things that you would like to say to her. Then imagine the shocked expression on her face. By using mental imagery, you'll probably be able to complete the phone call without destroying a friendship. You may even smile or laugh as you think about the scenes playing through your mind. (Read more about imagery in the chapter on pain.)

Nora was quite fed up with her son, Pesty Pete. Whenever she asked for his help with normal household chores, his answers were fresh and abusive. Just before she was about to give him a haircut with a meat cleaver, she remembered the mental movie technique. She imagined herself strangling him—his eyeballs popping out and gurgling sounds coming from his throat. This helped to get rid of the intense, angry feelings that were making her crazy, and allowed her to deal with Pete more constructively. (No, she's not in jail.)

PICTURE A BIG RED STOP SIGN

Another technique that can help you to control anger is "thought stopping." Remember: It is the thoughts in your mind that are making you angry—the thoughts you have when you interpret an event. So when you find that angry thoughts have come into your head, picture a big red stop sign. Seeing that picture in your mind will serve as a momentary distraction. Then concentrate on something you enjoy. This can be a peaceful, relaxing scene, an activity that you enjoy, or a favorite movie or television program. Whatever you choose, you will divert your thinking and give your anger a chance to dissipate. You could also participate in a pleasant activity—such as reading a book or taking a walk, for instance. Any of these activities should help defuse your anger.

CHANGE YOUR REQUIREMENTS

At times, you may have specific requirements—particular ways in which you want certain things to occur. When these are not met, you may feel angry. Modifying your requirements can help you cope with your anger.

Let's say that you're not feeling well and you decide to call your doctor. The answering service tells you that she is not in the office and that you should get a return call within half an hour. After an hour, the doctor has not yet returned your call, and you are fuming. Why? Because your requirements were not met.

What can you do? Revise your requirements. Tell yourself that you would have liked a call within thirty minutes, but that your doctor may be tied up on another case, in transit, or simply unable to get to a phone. You'll be satisfied if you get a call at her earliest convenience. By modifying your requirements, you'll feel less angry.

Another way to benefit from this technique is to write down your requirements. Then try to revise them with new, more flexible desires. This may help you see your requirements in a more objective light.

PUT YOURSELF IN THE OTHER PERSON'S SHOES

One of the best ways of dealing with anger toward somebody else is to try to understand exactly what that person is feeling—what the person wants, or why the person is saying what he or she is saying. This will make you more aware of the reason for his or her behavior, and will also help you deal with it more constructively. Perhaps just as important, this technique can help you understand how that other person will feel if he or she is the target of an abusive release of anger.

Judy always got angry when her husband insisted that they go out for dinner when he got home from work, especially if she was in pain and the last thing on her mind was food. Judy knew that she had to find a better way to handle her anger. So rather than exploding, she imagined what her husband was feeling—how disappointed he was, because, after all, he loved trying new restaurants and going out with her. Judy's new understanding let her defuse her anger and explain why she couldn't always accompany him, even though she wished she felt like going.

LET YOUR ANGER OUT

We have now discussed a number of ways in which you can control your thinking and improve your ability to interpret events in ways that will prevent anger from growing. But these techniques might not always be successful. What if there are times when you remain angry? What can be done to deal with anger constructively when it can't be defused? Fortunately, there are a few possibilities. Let's see what these are.

TALK, DON'T BITE

Obviously, it is much more desirable to have a constructive discussion over an issue than an angry exchange of heated words that accomplishes nothing. In most cases, anger arises when you have a conflict or problem with another person. For this reason, it can be very helpful to learn how to get your point across constructively so that you can negotiate a solution. Remember that a heated argument—fighting fire with fire—is not the answer. Instead, you want to fight the fire by dousing it. In other words, you want to reduce the heat of the argument.

How can this be done? Try complimenting the person or looking for positive things in what the person is saying to you. This will work in two ways. First, it will probably surprise the person. How will this help? Well, part of what fuels the fire of anger is your anticipation of the other person's anger. So by catching that person off guard, and thereby preventing him or her from reacting with anger, you will reduce this fuel. Second, by focusing on words or thoughts that are more constructive, you will calm yourself, rather than letting your anger grow. And once you're calm, you'll be able to quietly state your feelings.

In the previous example, in which you were upset about your friend's demands to pick up the dry cleaning, instead of blowing up at her and telling her that she is so inconsiderate and just doesn't understand, tell her she's *right* in calling you. You're glad she thought of you. But then let her know that as much as you would like to do this favor for her, you don't have the strength to even get dressed. Keep looking for something positive to respond to regardless of what she says and continue to calmly indicate that you don't feel well. Eventually, you'll get the point across, and although she may not be too happy about it (she may even get angry), you will have been able to resolve a problem in a constructive way, with much less anger.

WRITE OUT YOUR ANGER

There are times when something or someone makes you so angry that you feel as if you're going to explode. You recognize the need to release these feelings because they're damaging to you, but either you don't trust yourself to speak to the person or you don't have the confidence to speak up. This would be a great time to write an angry letter. Writing such a letter can be a constructive way of defusing this intense anger, without damaging any relationships in the process. To whom should you write? You could write to your doctor, your partner, your neighbor, the medical profession, the "powers above"—virtually anyone, real or not, with whom you feel angry. (You could even write an angry letter to "lupus." You could write, "Dear Lupie . . . I hate you, you *#*@^%&*!!!") But remember that for this technique to work best, you can't let anyone see your letter! After you finish pouring your heart onto paper, destroy it. You'll be destroying some of your anger at the same time!

FIND A PHYSICAL RELEASE FOR YOUR ANGER

In general, one of the best outlets for releasing angry energy is physical activity. Because of lupus, though, this outlet may not be as available to you as you'd like. Besides being angry about something else, a very frustrating aspect of having lupus may be that you can participate only in reduced amounts of physical activity. And because you may be prone to fatigue and have less energy, this outlet may not be readily usable at all.

Interestingly, it has been found that physical energy from anger can be released by watching things. For example, by watching a sporting event, you may not be releasing energy through participation in the sport, but you may be able to release anger by "getting into" the activity you're viewing. Or you might want to try watching an emotionally draining movie. You may become so totally absorbed that your built-up energy is released through worry, fear, or excitement. A book that allows you to identify with the characters can be beneficial as well—especially if the characters themselves release anger.

Believe it or not, another common and very effective outlet for anger is crying. You've probably heard about the therapeutic effects of a good cry. However, this technique is not for everyone. For instance, you may think that it's immature to cry—although the number of people who unashamedly let their tears flow might amaze you. But if your anger has built up to the point of uncontrollable crying, this will be a great way to let it out. (Of course, you may scare the daylights out of your family. But just tell them you read about it here!)

Some people like to count to ten when angry. This may distract you from what is making you angry, giving you a chance to calm down and think about it more constructively. Try counting out loud and expressing your feelings through facial expressions and tone of voice. Count to a thousand, if necessary!

An Anger-Free Ending

As you learn to cope with your anger, it's important to remember that events alone do not make you angry. It is your thinking—your interpretation of these events—that leads to anger. And since it is your thinking that makes you angry, you are responsible for feeling this way. Therefore, you are just as responsible for changing your thinking to help yourself cope with anger—or, at least, to reduce it to a more manageable level.

The best way to handle anger is probably to be in control so that it doesn't build up in the first place—to restructure your thinking so that your emotions don't get out of hand. But if anger does build, remember that when it is channeled and released constructively, it can be beneficial. And when this isn't possible, you can defuse or release your anger in a harmless way.

26.

GUILT

Have you ever felt guilty? Many individuals with lupus say that they have. Certainly, guilt is a very unpleasant feeling. You may feel guilty if you don't stick to your diet or if you don't exercise as often as you should. You may experience feelings of guilt because of feelings you have toward other people—feelings of resentment, perhaps, or jealousy—because they don't have lupus. Or you may feel guilty because you're not the family member you want to be. Take the case of Laura, a thirty-four-year-old mother of three. She was very unhappy because she couldn't be the kind of mother she wanted to be. Why not? Well, because she couldn't participate in enough activities with her kids. She wasn't able to give them the amount of time that she wanted. Frequently, when they asked her to do things with them or to play with them, she couldn't because of her lupus. She wasn't able to accompany them on school field trips or take them to the beach. So having lupus made her feel guilty because she felt that she was being a bad mother.

It may not be easy to cope with guilt, but you don't have to let yourself become a victim of these feelings. Let's first take a look at what leads to guilty feelings and then explore some ways in which you can reduce your feelings of guilt. After all, you want to do everything possible to make yourself feel better, and it's hard to feel good when you're feeling guilty!

What Are the Two
Components of Guilt?

Feelings of guilt usually have two components. The first of these is the sense of *wrongdoing*—the feeling that you have either done something wrong or haven't done something that you should have done. The second component is the feeling of *badness* that results from the self-blame. It's this second component that's the true culprit! When you feel bad about doing something wrong, this is normal and understandable. But when you start telling yourself that you are a bad person, guilt follows.

Is the behavior that you are blaming yourself for really that terrible or wrong? Does it justify the feeling of badness that leads to guilt? In Laura's case, she felt guilty because she wasn't spending enough time with her kids. Is that a reason to be so self-critical? Did she really want this to be this way? Of course not. Laura might feel better, therefore, if she emphasized the quality rather than the quantity of time spent with her children.

What Causes Guilt?

There are lots of things you might feel guilty about, even though there's probably no validity to any of them. For example, maybe you're concerned about something you did to contribute to the development of your lupus. You may, for instance, feel guilty because you didn't take care of yourself properly, perhaps eating too many unhealthful foods and allowing yourself to become overweight. Perhaps you feel that if it weren't for certain actions—or lack of actions—on your part, you would not be in this situation. You may also feel guilty because you believe that you're complicating things for your family. Therefore, you blame yourself.

There are a lot of things related to your lupus that might make you feel guilty, even though there's probably no validity to any of them. For example, maybe you're concerned that something you did caused your lupus. You may, for instance, feel guilty because you didn't take care of yourself properly, perhaps waiting too long before going to the doctor. Or you may feel guilty simply because you are not able to find any rational reason for the disease. Therefore, you blame yourself.

You may also feel guilty if you think that you're complicating matters for your family as a result of your lupus. You may worry that you're not going to be able to do all that is expected of you. You may feel guilty about letting yourself down or about disappointing others, whether they are family, friends, or colleagues. Guilt may also result because you are jealous of others who do not have lupus.

Perhaps others have told you that your feelings of guilt have no rational basis—that you're not at fault. Unfortunately, this may not eliminate guilt. Why? Because your feelings may have nothing to do with what others say or think. Remember: Your guilt comes from your own belief that you are a bad person.

Obviously, guilt can be a destructive emotion. It can drain you physically and emotionally, and can undermine your efforts to cope successfully with lupus. Fortunately, there's plenty you can do to improve your outlook. In the remainder of this chapter, we'll look at the various techniques you can use to cope with guilt.

How Can You Cope with Guilt?

Regardless of the cause of your guilt—and regardless of whether it is a new or long-standing problem for you—there are a number of strategies that can help you reduce or eliminate this unpleasant and harmful emotion. Let's take a look at some of the best ways of coping with guilt.

FIND THE SOURCE OF YOUR GUILT

In order to successfully cope with guilt, you must first focus on what led to the guilty feelings in the first place. Sometimes just by pinpointing the source of this emotion, you can greatly reduce or even eliminate it.

Then ask yourself if you have actually done something wrong. If you feel you have, ask yourself if the behavior you're blaming yourself for was really that terrible. If you feel guilty because of your lupus, ask yourself if that makes sense. Did you make it happen? Of course not. So identify the cause of your guilt and examine the wrongdoing you feel you committed. You will probably find either that you are not responsible for the wrong action or that the action was really not terrible enough to justify your feeling so bad!

Sometimes people feel guilty about thoughts or desires, rather than specific actions or behaviors. Recognize the difference between feeling guilty over a thought and feeling guilty over an action. Then, once you've identified the thought that's making you feel like a bad person, change it. Learn to talk to yourself in a positive way. Look at thoughts objectively and constructively in order to reduce your guilt.

TURN YOUR THOUGHTS AROUND

Dora, a thirty-one-year-old woman with two children, said that she felt guilty because her sixty-four-year-old mother was spending so much time taking care of her and her kids. Dora felt guilty because she was not getting any better and did not know how much longer it would be necessary for her mother to take care of her, and because her father was complaining about the loss of time spent with his wife. Is it appropriate for Dora to blame herself and feel guilty because of a disease she could not control? Since she hasn't done anything wrong, Dora can feel better if she modifies her thinking.

Is there anything you can do about the negative thoughts that lead to guilt—those thoughts that make you feel that you're a bad person? One helpful thing to do is to try to restructure your thinking to make it more positive and guilt free.

For example, let's say that you feel guilty because you believe that you're not being a good parent. Ask yourself if you've ever done anything that a good parent might do. Just about every mom or dad can come up with something! This type of thinking will begin to eliminate your feelings of guilt. The idea is to turn your mind's negative thoughts into reasonable, positive ones. This way, the feelings of guilt will not take a stranglehold!

But what if you feel guilty and simply can't remember what you were thinking or doing that made you feel this way? How can you use all the great thought-changing ideas we're going to talk about if you can't identify the thoughts you want to change? Good question! In order to pinpoint these "target" thoughts or behaviors, you might want to keep a brief written log of feelings or activities that may be causing your guilt. Once you have written these down, you can begin to determine the root of the problem and then think about what changes might improve the situation.

Mary, aged thirty-nine, had been feeling increasingly guilty recently but didn't really know why. By keeping a log, she noticed that besides complaining of fatigue almost all the time, she had been arriving at work late on a regular basis. She wasn't aware of how frequently she had been late, and she had always been proud of her punctuality. The log helped her to see that she needed to improve her morning routine in order to be more punctual. As she worked on this problem, her guilt lessened.

If, despite your best efforts, you're still feeling guilty and don't know why, cut yourself a little slack. Call your own time-out and calm yourself down. Remind yourself that, living with lupus, you can't be perfect. You'll find that this will ease some of your emotional pain.

REEVALUATE YOUR EXPECTATIONS

Depending on the person, people with lupus may feel guilty about their inability to handle their children or about the lack of time they have to spend with their children, or their inability to advance in their careers or fulfill their job responsibilities the way they feel they should. Connie, a forty-two-year-old mother of three, had to stay home frequently from her job. As a result, she earned less money and couldn't provide all of the luxuries that she and her family had previously enjoyed. Feeling guilty, Connie tried to push herself harder to increase her earnings, which in turn made her feel worse physically. Obviously, Connie was not coping well with her guilt. Instead, she was allowing it to affect her health. How can you cope with these feelings?

Do you see a difference between the way you are doing something and the way you think you should be doing it? If so, you may really feel guilty! How do you work this out? Major union/management problems would be easier to solve! Can you work harder to do more? If you can, then do it. If not, try examining your day-to-day goals for working and living. Check to see if these goals are practical, considering what you cannot do because of your lupus. Try to take more pride in what you can do. Although most people hate hearing, "Things could be worse," this phrase is quite true. You might not be able to do anything at all. If you concentrate on the things you can do and place less emphasis on what you can't, your feelings of guilt will diminish. You'll feel a lot better. Changing the emphasis in your thinking will also help you to lessen the gap between what is and what ought to be. This is what led to the guilty feelings in the first place.

Does this approach work only for working men and women? No. It applies to anyone who feels guilty about falling short of expectations and desires. Barbara, a sixteen-year-old-student, was feeling guilty because she was unable to devote the amount of time to her schoolwork she used to, or because she couldn't spend as much time on it as she would have liked. She was more and more reluctant to go to school because she was so frequently unprepared for her classes, and she missed a number of school days because of lupus. The guilt she felt affected her schoolwork even more. How might Barbara cope with these guilty feelings? It might be beneficial for Barbara to speak to each of her teachers and explain how lupus was affecting her, cautioning her teachers that physical problems might restrict her from devoting the same amount of time to her schoolwork as she had previously and that her attendance might not be as good as it had been. At that point, it would be helpful to discuss possible methods for making up for this, such as extra projects that she might be able to work on when she was feeling up to it, or alternate arrangements for testing (to try to show her teachers that even with less time available for studying, she was still interested in succeeding in class). By working with her teachers and setting more realistic goals, Barbara could reduce the feelings of guilt related to having lupus and its effect on her schoolwork.

ELIMINATE YOUR "SHOULDS"

When evaluating your goals, you may find that among the most common causes of guilt are thoughts containing the word *should*. "Should" is a dirty word! Connie thought that she "should" have been able to work harder and earn more money. Other "should" thoughts might include: "I *should* have been able to finish that job today." "We *should* have that party. All our friends have entertained us this year." "I *should* have been able to finish cleaning that room today." "You *should* have let me do the dishes." "I *shouldn't* have any more pain." "I really *should* be taking my kids to the park today." These "should" thoughts imply that you must be just about perfect and right on top of everything. Naturally, you will become upset whenever you fall short of your "should." But *should* you blame yourself when "should" thoughts establish goals that are unrealistic—goals that you may not be able to fulfill? Of course you shouldn't!

Do you see a difference between the way you are doing something and the way you think you *should* be doing it? If so, you are probably feeling guilty!

So what steps can you take to stop feeling guilty about the things you *should* have done? For starters, reword your thoughts to eliminate the word "should." Use less demanding ones. Say, "It would be nice if I could finish that task today, but I can't," rather than, "I should finish that task today." If you have trouble changing the wording of your "should" thoughts, try asking yourself, "Why should I . . . ?" or "Who says I should . . . ?" or "Where is it written that I should . . . ?" This may help you decide whether you are setting up impossible requirements for yourself. It can also help you reduce your feelings of guilt.

Let's say, for example, that you are thinking of having a party because all your friends have invited you to get-togethers. Ask yourself why you should. Is it because the "Party Rulebook" tells you that your friendship license will be revoked? Is it because if you don't have a party, your friends won't invite you to their homes anymore? As you think of some realistic answers to these questions, you'll come to realize that you don't have to have a party. Although it would be nice, it would be more sensible to wait until you're feeling better.

ESCAPE FROM "ESCAPE" BEHAVIOR

Sometimes, people who feel guilt—and have failed to cope with this destructive emotion—act in negative ways to hide from their feelings. There may be a tendency to indulge in "escape" behaviors, such as drinking or excessive sleeping. Instead of dealing with these feelings head-on, they push them away.

Jill, a twenty-year-old secretary, felt guilty because she had stopped making plans with her friends. She had done this because she was embarrassed about how many times she had to cancel plans at the last minute because of her lupus. She felt that since she had had to cancel so often and would probably have to continue to do so, why should she even bother to make plans? As a result, she began to lose friends, and her guilt became more and more difficult for her to bear. She began drinking each day and going to bed right after dinner, in an attempt to "escape" and to forget her misery. This behavior did not help the situation, and it certainly didn't help her medical condition. In fact, it was downright dangerous. Not only did it compound the problem, but there was also the added danger of mixing alcohol and medication. Now Jill had something else to feel guilty about: her escape behavior. This could enforce her belief that she was a bad person and lead to even more guilt, creating a vicious cycle.

As you may have already guessed, the first step toward improvement is to look past the escape behavior and identify whatever is causing the guilt. Then consider what can be done to rectify the problem. At the same time, try to eliminate the escape behavior, recognizing that it is only a cop-out. It is possible, however, for there to be no clear-cut solution to the events or feelings creating guilt. If, for example, Jill's physical condition is keeping her from making plans with her friends, can she believe that the only way to make things better is to force herself to do things she physically shouldn't? Should she wait to make plans until her lupus "goes away"? That would be ridiculous. Don't give up because no complete solution exists. Look for partial solutions. These may not be as desirable, but they can still help to reduce guilt by reminding you that you are trying to improve the situation. Jill's lupus won't go away, but she could at least try to make small, undemanding plans with a few friends. And, she certainly could try to explain the problem to her friends so she'd be less embarrassed if she did have to cancel plans.

TALK IT OVER

It's very important to discuss how you feel about your condition with others who may be affected by it. Share your concerns and try to figure out solutions to any problems that exist.

Janet, a twenty-three-year-old woman who had been married less than a year, had enjoyed a very active social life before developing lupus. In addition to going out on weekends, she and her husband had played tennis with friends or had participated in other social activities at least two or three evenings during the week. Now, because of the way lupus was affecting her, she had to restrict her activities. She just couldn't go out as frequently. She couldn't even play tennis at all. Sometimes, she wouldn't want to go out even once during an entire week. Not only did she feel unhappy about her condition, but she also felt extremely guilty about holding her husband back. She felt that he couldn't have a good time because of her. It would be helpful for Janet to discuss alternatives with her husband. If she could arrive at a solution with her husband's cooperation, she could effectively reduce guilt feelings and improve her marriage.

A Final Guiltless Thought

Guilt is a very unpleasant, destructive emotion—one that can interfere with your success in coping with lupus. It can lower your self-image and exhaust your emotional resources. By becoming aware of how guilt develops, by pinpointing the source of your guilt, and by changing your thinking to be more positive and realistic, you should be able to decrease or eliminate this feeling, and, instead, use your energy to work on successfully coping with your condition.

27.

STRESS

S tress! Every time you turn around, you either read or hear about stress. What exactly is it? Stress is a response that occurs in your body. It is a form of energy—a normal reaction to the demands of everyday life. It helps mobilize your strength to deal with different events and circumstances.

Many things occur each day that require you to adapt. These are known as *stressors*. The changes that take place in your body when something (the stressor) provokes you are known as the *stress response* (more about the stress response later in this chapter).

We all know that stress can play a role in causing or exacerbating virtually any medical problem. And lupus is no exception. In fact, stress can certainly make your lupus symptoms worse.

Chances are you've been feeling a lot of pressure lately and would be a lot happier if you could lower your stress level. So let's learn more about stress—what causes it, how it can affect you, and, most important, how you can learn to cope with it.

What Are the Symptoms of Stress?

Your body will tell you when the stress you're experiencing is excessive. What might you feel? Physically, excessive stress can manifest itself as sweaty palms, heart palpitations, tightness of the throat, fatigue, nausea, diarrhea, or headaches—among other things. Emotionally, depression, anxiety, anger, frustration, or simply a vague uneasiness are just a few possible symptoms. As long as you tune in to your body and mind, you'll know when you can benefit from stress-reduction techniques.

How Does Stress Affect You?

The effects of stress—much like the effects of depression, discussed in Chapter 23—are not isolated problems. Instead, they are part of a complex response that can affect both your body and your emotions. Let's examine this in more detail.

HOW STRESS AFFECTS YOUR BODY

Stress is a natural survival response. It occurs within the body whenever you feel threatened by thoughts or external stressors.

Stress can manifest itself in many ways. When you are in a stressful situation, your circulatory system speeds up and blood is pushed rapidly toward different parts of the body—particularly those organs and systems necessary to protect you—raising your blood pressure. Because the blood supply has been diverted, the supply to the digestive system is usually reduced as well, making the process of digestion slower and less effective. Stress also constricts the blood vessels, increases heart rate, and produces other physiological manifestations—all instantaneously!

What else can occur? You may tremble or perspire. Your face may flush. You may feel a surge of adrenaline flowing through your body. Your mouth may become dry and you may feel nauseated. Your breathing may become more rapid and shallow. Your heart may begin to pound. Your muscles may become tight, leading to headaches or cramps. Sounds wonderful, doesn't it?

So when you experience stress, your body prepares itself physiologically to counter any threat to its survival. Why? Well, perhaps you've heard of the *fight-or-flight* response. You see, when an animal feels threatened, it prepares to either fight or run away. You will never see an animal standing there, scratching his head, and thinking about how he might best handle the situation! Even though we have the ability to think and reason, we also experience the fight-or-flight response, which causes the secretion of many different hormones and tenses the muscles in preparation for battle. If the response does involve physical action—fight or flight—the hormones are utilized as they are supposed to be, and the muscles are exercised, with energy being appropriately released. If there is no physical exertion, however—if you think, instead of taking action—the energy that was mobilized may not be released in the way expected. This may explain why, after a period of stress during which no action was taken, you feel exhausted just the same.

When does stress lead to physical problems? When your body is strong, it can fight off most foreign invaders, bacteria, and germs. When you can't respond to stress in a way that eliminates it, the stress continues unabated—and physical problems can result. An inability to do anything to relieve the stress may cause even more stress, creating a vicious cycle. And this can take its toll on your body. In fact, many researchers believe that prolonged stress puts such a strain on your body that your defense mechanisms may ultimately break down, making your body more vulnerable to the very problems you'd like to avoid!

HOW STRESS AFFECTS YOUR MIND

Your cognitive or emotional response to stress may not be as visible as your physical response. You may start worrying and fear the next "event." Your attention span may be reduced, and you may be less able to concentrate on the task at hand. You may have trouble learning something new. You may be afraid to do things. You may withdraw or feel nervous. You may lose confidence in yourself.

As you become nervous and upset, you may become more aware of any unpleasant physical responses you're experiencing, and this may make you feel even more stressed. For example, if you have responded to stress with shallow, rapid breathing or heart palpitations, your awareness of these physical responses may lead to feelings of panic. Most people respond to stress both physically and emotionally, although it is possible to respond in only one way. Don't you have your own "typical" reaction? Maybe you become too jittery and unfocused to concentrate on your job. Perhaps you feel physically ill, with extreme intestinal discomfort or a throbbing headache. Regardless of what you feel, it's important to learn strategies that will enable you to deal effectively with stress.

Is Stress Good or Bad?

By now, you've probably figured out that stress can be either good or bad. It is good when it gives you extra energy to do the things that need to be done during stressful times. In fact, a certain amount of stress is normal and necessary. Stress helps you to "get your act together" and prepares you to handle your life in the best possible way. But when left unchecked, stress can be highly destructive, draining all your energy and possibly worsening any existing physical or emotional problems. So while stress can be helpful, this chapter concerns itself with harmful stress—the kind that can hurt you if it goes uncontrolled.

Esther, a thirty-eight-year-old housewife, was under pressure. Her husband was bringing his boss home for dinner. She had just gotten over a flare, and because she knew she got exhausted easily, she carefully paced herself as she prepared the meal so she wouldn't get run-down. The stress she felt was tolerable; that is, until the phone rang. Her husband called to tell her that due to an emergency business meeting that evening, they'd be arriving two hours early! Esther's stress was no longer tolerable!

What Causes Stress?

A number of things can act as stressors. Work-related problems, marital disputes, family deaths, even some positive events—all can cause stress. But in this book, we're most concerned with the effects of lupus on your life, and this can cause stress in a number of different ways. Pain alone can cause stress. Your concern about how your disease will affect you can cause stress. Problems with medication are also stressors. And worries about being able to fulfill responsibilities may provoke a stress response, as well.

The Stress Response

Everyone has a unique way of responding to the world. Your pattern of response depends on a number of things. Your upbringing, your self-esteem, your beliefs about yourself and the world, the way in which you guide yourself in your thoughts and actions—all of these things help determine your stress response. The degree to which you feel in control of your life also plays an important role in this response. And the way you feel physically and emotionally—as well as the way you get along with people—is also a factor.

To sum it up, everyone's method of dealing with stress is as unique and individual as a fingerprint, and it depends on a complex combination of thoughts and behaviors. To keep things simple, though, we can view the stress response as dependent on the "chemistry" between two factors. The first factor is the stressor, or the outside pressure. In other words, what is going on around you that is creating a problem. The second factor is your interpretation of the event. It is the interaction of the stressor and your internal interpretation that determines your response to stress. (Sound familiar? Yes, it's the same "formula" that can be applied to anger, depression, and any other emotion.) So the "equation" for the stress response is as follows:

Stressor + Interpretation = Stress Response

This equation has important implications for coping with stress. Why? It shows you that stress is not solely the result of your environment, your illness, or any other factor around you. The way you interpret this stressor is of equal importance. Of course, some stressors would produce stress in anybody. What would happen, for example, if somebody aimed a knife at your throat? Calm acceptance or a stress response? Get the point? In most situations, though, you do have the ability to control your reaction to the stressor.

As you learn to cope with stress, it's important to remember that your mind responds to any thoughts of stress as though they are real and happening right now. Any thoughts or images in your mind that produce a stress response are perceived as existing in the present, as the brain and nervous system do not recognize the differences among past, present, and future. So it's easy to see that you contribute to your body's stress response with your own thoughts and images. This makes it even more important to feed your mind with the best, most beneficial, and most constructive information available.

Three Reactions to Stress

When a stressful stimulus occurs, you will most likely respond in one of three ways. You might respond immediately and impulsively without giving enough thought to a better response. You might not respond at all, and either try to ride it out or become so frozen that you are unable to respond. Finally, you may respond to stressors in a well-planned, organized, and effective manner. If so, you may not even need this chapter! But if not, read on!

How Can You Cope with Stress?

For a person with lupus, it is especially important that stress be controlled. Why? Although stress by itself does not cause lupus, it certainly may play a role in exacerbating your lupus symptoms. Because stress can affect the body and mind in so many ways, stress management is a very important part of any program for coping with lupus. The good news is that, regardless of how successfully you have dealt with stress in the past, you can learn effective strategies that will help you deal with it now. These strategies will make you feel more in control, lessening the feelings of panic and increasing your emotional well-being.

But before we look at how you should cope with stress, let's look at what you *shouldn't* do. Smoking, alcohol abuse, the use of inappropriate drugs, and overeating are all common but poor coping strategies. True, these activities will distract you and perhaps delay the effects of the stress, but they can also hurt you and prevent you from coping with stress in a constructive way.

So what should you do? Try to learn new, more appropriate ways of dealing with stress. Relaxation techniques and regular exercise can be helpful parts of stress-management programs. And by thinking more appropriate and positive thoughts, you can go a long way toward reducing stress as well. But be realistic and remember that while stress can be managed and controlled, it cannot be eliminated. Your focus, then, should be on using the following management techniques to help yourself deal better with both the physical and the emotional effects of the stress response.

USE RELAXATION TECHNIQUES

Because relaxation is incompatible with stress, the best way to start controlling stress is to use relaxation techniques. In fact, relaxation techniques alone—used without any other coping strategies—may help you to significantly reduce both the physical and the emotional effects of stress.

Relaxation benefits you in many ways. First, it can give your body a chance to rest and recuperate. And a stronger body can help you deal better with the ravages of stress—and life! Relaxation will also help you sleep better. Relaxation is also pleasurable and will increase your feeling of emotional well-being. And it can give you a powerful sense of reestablishing control over your life, despite the presence of a chronic medical problem.

There are many different types of clinical relaxation techniques, including meditation, autogenics, and deep breathing. Hypnosis and biofeedback can also be used to induce relaxation, although they have other uses as well. (See Chapter 9 for a full discussion of these and other relaxation techniques.)

One relaxation technique that is often successful in combating stress is imagery—a technique that can also be used to cope with pain, anger, and other problems. Imagery is the process of formulating mental pictures or scenes in order to harness your body's energy and improve your physical or emotional well-being. In this case, of course, you'll want to conjure up images that are relaxing and stress-free. Imagine not only the sights, but also the smells, the tactile sensations (touch), and the sounds. The more vivid your image, the more helpful it will be. Feel comfortable with whatever degree of clarity your image takes on. The degree of relaxation you'll experience is up to you and will benefit only you. You are in control. (Read more about imagery in Chapter 9.)

PINPOINT THE SOURCE OF YOUR STRESS

Now that you're more relaxed, you're ready to objectively identify your stressors. What, specifically, is causing you to feel stress? Maybe you're having a hard time with the symptoms of lupus. Maybe you're tired of sticking to your treatment program. Maybe you're concerned about medication. Maybe you fear another flare. Maybe you're having a hard time dealing with pain. Maybe you're concerned about the reactions of others. Or maybe you're just tired of thinking about lupus. Of course, there are many more possibilities.

What if you're not sure what's causing your stress? Try keeping a log of your daily stressors. This will allow you to more easily recognize the people, places, and things that have the potential to create stress in your life. But what if you can't pinpoint which of your many activities are the real culprits? As you keep your log, you might want to use a numerical rating scale, such as the Subjective Units of Disturbance (SUD) scale. Here's how it works. Ratings on this scale range from 0 to 100, depending on the amount of stress you're experiencing. Use 100 to represent the most extreme and disturbing stress, and 0 to represent no stress—total and complete relaxation. Then rate your activities, experiences, and thoughts. The ones with the higher SUD numbers are the ones causing you the most stress. (For example, loud music blasting from your neighbor's radio might be rated a whopping 85!) By being aware of the degree to which you're affected by a stressor, you'll be better able to prioritize the ones that deserve your attention.

IDENTIFY YOUR STRESS REACTIONS

Once you have begun identifying your stressors, you'll want to become completely aware of your responses to them. Are they more physiological or psychological? What parts of your body seem to be the most vulnerable? What kind of reactions does your body have? Does your attention span suffer? Do you get heart palpitations? Do you start losing confidence, or feel as if you're "slipping"? As you become more aware of these things, you will develop a complete picture of your own unique stress response. This picture will help you choose the coping strategies that will be most useful in dealing with your stressors.

ELIMINATE STRESSORS WHEN POSSIBLE

What's the next step? Once you recognize which stressors are causing the most trouble, try to determine whether you can eliminate them. Removing the source of stress is an obvious and logical way to manage it. For instance, if the task of managing your household expenses is causing you stress, you might have your spouse take over this chore. Taking a sledgehammer to that radio might be great, if you could lift the hammer! Obviously, different types of stressors would have to be removed in other ways.

CHANGE YOUR VIEW OF THE STRESSOR

What happens if you can't eliminate the source of your stress? In such cases, changing the stressor may be out of your control, but changing the way you react isn't. So you'll then have to work on your interpretation of the stressors. You'll have to work on the way you think and the way you respond in order to manage stress. You might want to use some of the suggestions already discussed. Or you might want to try systematic desensitization, discussed in Chapter 24.

Another technique that might help you cope better with stressors is *stress inoculation.* How can you be inoculated against stress? Well, you're certainly familiar with the use of inoculations to protect children from diseases such as measles. By exposing a child to a very mild form of the virus or other agent that causes a disorder, inoculations gradually strengthen the child's immunity to the disorder. Similarly, stress inoculation uses mental rehearsal procedures to help you confront and, gradually, tolerate stressful situations. As we previously discussed, because your mind responds to thoughts and mental images as if they were real and happening right now, thinking about something can be just as stressful as experiencing it. So by learning to cope with a situation in your mind, you can learn how to cope with it before it even happens.

Start your stress inoculation process by using whatever relaxation techniques you have found most helpful. Once you have achieved a comfortable level of relaxation, start imagining one of the stressors you've previously identified. As you imagine the stressful scene, recognize any physiological sensations or psychological changes that you may be experiencing.

Margaret realized that much of her stress was being caused by the fear that, during an office visit, her doctor would tell her that her kidney involvement was intensifying. Margaret's stress reaction—nausea and a tightening in her throat—would appear whenever she imagined this frightening scene. So she decided to use stress inoculation to gain control. Repeatedly she imagined herself in the very situation she feared. She visualized the doctor's office. She imagined herself sitting in the chair by the doctor's desk. She actually heard the words she was afraid of. As Margaret gradually increased her tolerance of this image, the symptoms of her stress lessened.

Like Margaret, whenever you use stress inoculation to visualize and mentally experience a scene, you'll increase your ability to handle that particular stressor, and your symptoms will decrease. In other words, your body and mind will be "inoculated," allowing you to tolerate that stressor. One added advantage of using this technique is that you will become more aware of exactly when these tension-producing situations begin to affect you. This will enable you to use your coping strategies sooner, before your body and mind begin suffering from the stress response.

If you have already read the explanation of systematic desensitization found in Chapter 24, you may realize that stress inoculation and desensitization are very similar. But there is a difference. In desensitization, the technique of imagining a stressful situation is alternated with the use of relaxation techniques. In stress inoculation, relaxation techniques are employed only at the start of the session. Experimentation will show you which method is best for you.

USE PHYSICAL STRESS RELIEVERS

Certain physical activities can be a great means of stress control. For example, some people relieve tension or stress by driving. Certainly, as long as you continue to observe safety rules—and as long as you enjoy this activity—driving can be very relaxing. But if driving isn't your idea of a calming pastime, there are a number of other activities that may be just the ticket.

EXERCISING

Exercise not only is a wonderful means of releasing stress but also, as you learned in Chapter 12, can be a very beneficial part of your lupus treatment program. Regardless of how lupus is affecting you, there is certain to be a type of exercise that will help you control your level of stress. Virtually any type of exercise is effective. Anything that gets the body moving, gets the heart pumping faster, and allows for a release of tension is ideal. Just be sure to get your doctor's approval before beginning any exercise program.

KEEPING BUSY THE FUN WAY

Hobbies and other leisure activities are often very effective ways to reduce stress. They can divert your attention from the stressful situation and direct it toward something more enjoyable. They may also help you to feel more productive—and a lack of productivity may be one of the stressors giving you problems in the first place! If you don't have a hobby, this is a great time to look into painting, model building, gardening—whatever suits your fancy. If you're already involved in a hobby, you now have the perfect reason to indulge yourself whenever you can.

CATCH UP ON YOUR SLEEP

Another technique for dealing with stress is sleep. Some people have difficulty sleeping when they're experiencing high levels of stress. But, when possible, catnaps or even prolonged periods of sleep may help you reduce stress to a more manageable level. After all, you need your rest, anyway!

A Stress-Free Summary

What are your goals? Are you trying to gain greater control over your emotions? Do you want to live life more fully? Whatever they are, if stress is keeping you from reaching them, then your stress response is negative. By learning how to control your stress—by eliminating the things that are stressing you or by modifying your reaction—you'll be far more likely to meet these goals. Just as important, you'll have a head start in coping successfully with lupus.

28.

OTHER EMOTIONS

The emotions discussed in the previous chapters in this section are not the only ones you may experience, of course. What other emotions might you want to learn to deal with better? This chapter will discuss four additional emotions that many people with lupus have found to be problematic: boredom, envy, loneliness, and grief.

Boredom

Hopefully, by this time, you are not so bored that you have stopped reading! If I've still got your attention, let's talk a bit about boredom.

What an empty feeling boredom is! It's one of the worst feelings you can possibly experience. It has been said that more problems and tragedies are caused by boredom than by any other single emotion. I bet you never thought of lupus as being boring. But it can be, primarily because of the restrictions your condition may impose on you. Some activities that provided enjoyment for you in the past may now be out of reach. You may not even want to bother starting something new, telling yourself that future activities will be restricted because of lupus.

Celia was too tired to leave her house. She couldn't go shopping, she couldn't meet friends for lunch, and she was fed up with the garbage on television. Was Celia bored? You bet she was! Her friend suggested that Celia go along with her to take a course in interior decorating, since Celia had a lot of talent in this field. But despite her enthusiasm, she decided not to because she didn't want to start something she felt she couldn't finish.

Olive hated the fact that her condition prevented her from knitting. She was tired of music, and she didn't want to read. Was Olive bored? Definitely! But did she have to be bored? No! Her family and friends suggested that she try new activities, and Olive was soon able to feel less bored.

Why are you bored? There may be no meaningful activity going on, no stimulation or excitement. Your life may seem to be going nowhere. Nothing is challenging you, and there's no incentive to do anything. Because you weren't born bored, you must have learned to be bored. You weren't always bored, and even now you are not always bored. There are still certain things that hold your attention from time to time. Right?

So what should you do? To begin with, don't let your condition cause you to give up on life. Distinguish between what you can do and what you can't. If you do have to curtail any activities because of lupus, you'll do so. If you have to drop an activity, you'll drop it. But you don't have to eliminate all activities simply because you may not be able to complete them. How else can you fight the boredom blues? Read on!

TRY NEW ACTIVITIES

If boredom is a problem for you, you'll certainly want to find ways to add some interest to your life. You may find that the activities you used to enjoy now seem artificial and uninteresting. You may no longer derive any pleasure from them. Don't feel that you must push yourself to enjoy these activities, as forcing yourself to be amused rarely works. Instead, try to find some new activities that will make your life more interesting. Remember that preferences change. Be open-minded, and try things that never appealed to you before. This time around, they may spark your interest.

LEARN SOMETHING NEW

One of the most effective weapons against boredom is learning. The mind is like a sponge, always thirsty to soak up information and knowledge. Select a potentially interesting topic you don't know much about. Try to go out and learn something about it. You may want to begin by going to the library and reading some books on the topic. Or read more about it online. Perhaps you'd like to enroll in an adult education course. Boredom often disappears once you become involved in something new. As an added benefit, your new pursuit may put you in contact with some interesting new people. And increasing your circle of friends is always a good way to fight boredom.

SET GOALS

Boredom often arises from plodding along with no purpose in life. So one of the best ways to fight it is to always give yourself something to look forward to—some goals (short-term *and* long-term). This doesn't mean that you'll never be bored. You may still have to give yourself an occasional kick in the butt to get yourself moving toward those goals. But the promise of some pleasurable activity will make it much easier to keep yourself going.

What kinds of goals might you set? They can be as simple as reading a chapter of a good book, writing a letter, making that phone call you've been thinking about, watching a television program you enjoy, or meeting somebody special for lunch. Try to schedule something to look forward to every day. This way, even if part of your day seems boring—for example, whether you're doing menial chores or just resting to build up your strength—you won't give the weeds of boredom a chance to take root!

Envy

You've heard the cliché, "The grass is always greener . . ." If you have lupus, you are probably envious of those who don't. This is understandable. You may also be envious of other people who are able to do more than you can. But envy is still a destructive emotion because it's a type of self-torture. It can be very painful. When you feel envious, you're constantly putting yourself down and comparing your own qualities with the seemingly better qualities of somebody else. You feel inferior. And this can lead to other negative emotions, such as anger or depression.

Why is envy a problem? Envy is often irrational. When you're envious, you want to be like somebody else. You want to have what somebody else has. Does this mean that the other person has a life that's happier than yours in every way? Stop and think for a moment. You may have lupus, but this doesn't mean that everything else about the other person's life is superior. I'm sure you can come up with some areas in which your life is better!

IS ENVY A POSITIVE EMOTION?

In general, emotions usually serve a purpose. Emotions such as anger and anxiety mobilize you to prepare to handle their sources. On the other hand, envy is a destructive emotion. It does not have the positive qualities that other emotions may have. But maybe you can find something positive in envy. If you recognize that you're envious, analyze the reason why. Try to change the way you feel by concentrating on yourself and your own attributes. Don't let envy get you down.

WHAT LEADS TO ENVY?

Basically, there are four conditions necessary for envy to occur. First, you must feel deprived in some way. You will feel like you can't have something that you want or need. I'm not talking simply about money, pleasure, or even health! Envy is an intense feeling that involves much more than this. It seems as if your feeling of need lies deep inside.

Second, to experience envy you must feel that somebody else has what you feel you're missing. Perhaps the person has a bigger house, for instance. Or perhaps the person does not need to take prednisone.

Third, you must feel powerless to do anything about this problem. You must feel totally unable to change the circumstances that have made you envious in the first place. This helplessness causes you to become more and more bitter. And this makes you even more envious!

Fourth, there must be a change in the relationship between you and the person whom you envy. You are no longer simply comparing yourself with that person; you now feel fiercely competitive. You may begin to feel that the only reason you don't have what you want is that somebody else has it.

There are two types of things that may cause you to feel envy. One type is tangible—jewelry, cars, homes, and so on. The other type is less tangible—friends, pleasure, or health, for instance. If you have lupus, you may still have many tangible things. You may still have a car and a place to live. You may still have a job. But your medical condition may cause you to feel envious over less tangible things.

MAKE THE BEST OF WHAT YOU HAVE

To get rid of this destructive emotion, concentrate on increasing those benefits and pleasures you *can* get out of life. Why worry about comparing yourself with somebody else? How is that going to help you? Sure, you may have lupus. Sure, your body may not be functioning the way it used to. But that doesn't mean that you can't get a lot of enjoyment from life. Set up reasonable goals for yourself, considering what you *do* have and what you *can* do. And recognize that you'll feel better when you stop comparing yourself with others. Remember that you are who you are. Make the best of what *your* life has to offer.

Loneliness

There is a difference between being alone and being lonely. Being alone simply means that there is no one else with you. This can be either good or bad. But being lonely is always negative. Loneliness is a sad, empty feeling in which you become upset by your awareness of being alone.

WHY ARE YOU LONELY?

Why might you feel lonely? You may feel left out if you can't spend time with others the way you used to—either because you're not feeling well or perhaps because you can't do what others want to do. Or you may feel lonely because you think that others don't understand your condition—and don't want to be with you. You may simply feel different. And you may decide to change some of your relationships just because you're having a harder time dealing with people.

It's hard to be lonely—and not just because loneliness is such a bad feeling. Unfortunately, loneliness doesn't just happen. It actually takes effort to make and keep yourself lonely. There are many opportunities to enjoy the company of others. As a result, loneliness often occurs out of choice rather than by accident. To be really lonely, you must purposely exclude everyone around you from your life. You have to always be on your guard, protecting yourself from the horrible possibility of making new friends!

DO YOU *WANT* TO BE LONELY?

Why might you want to be lonely? There are four possible reasons. First, deep down you may actually enjoy being lonely. (This may contradict your complaints to everyone else!) In fact, you may enjoy it so much that you refuse to do anything about it. Why? Because you may feel more comfortable when alone than when in the company of others.

Second, if you're lonely, you may be hard to please. You may feel that you don't want to even bother trying to create new relationships because no one meets all of your requirements.

Third, you may feel that you must be lonely. You may have resigned yourself to it. You may even tell yourself that this is an unavoidable part of having lupus!

Fourth, and probably most important, you may be lonely because you're scared. You're afraid to develop new relationships. You may be afraid of rejection. You may recall previous relationships that didn't work out the way you wanted and feel that they are not worth the hurt and pain.

END YOUR LONELY WAYS

Fortunately, whether your loneliness has been plaguing you for some time or is a relatively new problem, there is a light at the end of the tunnel! Recognize where your feeling of loneliness comes from. Admit to yourself that you should try to change this destructive emotion. Then do all you can to fight it.

Don't Be a Pusher

The first step in ending loneliness is to stop pushing people away. It's likely that you're giving off unseen signals—vibrations that tell people you don't want them around. These vibrations can reduce your number of acquaintances, adding to your feeling of loneliness. This must stop. You have to learn to give off positive vibrations—the kind that welcome people instead of chasing them away. Smile at people. Show interest in what others have to say. Let them know that you like being with them.

MAKE CONTACT!

Once you start giving off new, more positive vibes, you'll want to make more friends. How can you meet people? You can start by getting involved in some kind of organization. This type of activity usually attracts people who are interested in being with others who share a common goal. Because you have lupus, you may want to get involved with your local lupus organization. There, you'll meet other people with similar concerns. Besides relieving your loneliness, the members of your support group may also share some valuable coping skills. You may even find ways of helping others.

If support groups aren't your cup of tea, try getting involved in a new learning activity or hobby. Take adult education courses, for example. This may help alleviate loneliness as well as boredom. Invite people to your home. (Be sure to pace yourself, though!) Most important, be as receptive as possible to the people that you meet. Try to see the good in everyone. Don't reject someone simply because there are a few things about them that you don't like.

You may feel that you'll have a harder time breaking free of loneliness if you are homebound. But even if you can't get out of the house, you still have connections to the outside world: your telephone and the Internet. If you're feeling particularly blue, your close friends and loved ones are just a phone call away. Remember, the special people in your life want you to be happy, and they'll be there to support you—even if "there" is at the other end of the telephone line.

If you own a computer, then you can get connected through the Internet. You'll soon find that your online resources are endless! You can meet people who share your interests and concerns in online chat rooms and through social networking. You can even find support groups on the Internet (more about this in Chapter 34). Your doctor, other health care professionals, or your local lupus organization may be able to give you some good resource sites on lupus that can help you get started. (Check the Appendix for a number of websites that can keep you from being lonely!)

If you work at conquering loneliness, you'll feel much better about yourself and your life. This will make life more enjoyable, even with lupus. Give yourself and others a chance, and your feelings of loneliness will disappear, regardless of the limitations your condition has placed on you.

Grief

Feelings of the unpleasant emotion grief—or mourning over a loss—are common with people who have lupus, especially when they are initially diagnosed.

You may grieve the major changes in life necessitated by your lupus. Why do you grieve? Because you're aware that you have lost something that you value—in this case, your former lifestyle. The loss may be temporary or permanent. You may feel that you have lost some physical strength. You may not like yourself as much, and may grieve this feeling of lower self-esteem.

Grief may occur as you sense that your role in life has changed to one of lesser importance. If you are used to having one role within your family, and this role has been modified or significantly changed because of your having lupus, you may grieve this loss. Paul was a thirty-eight-year-old construction worker. He took pride in providing a good income for his wife and five children. But then, along came lupus. He was no longer able to work the overtime he had grown accustomed to. There was some concern about his continuing in the construction field at all, and where else he would be able to earn that kind of money. He recognized that his wife was going to have to work to supplement his reduced income. His role as breadwinner was being changed and he was miserable. This change in lifestyle happens frequently for the breadwinner with lupus because of a physical need to change jobs or to adjust to reduced earning capacities because of the condition. The person's role as breadwinner is reduced, if not eliminated. Some may grieve the loss of their former role.

WORK THROUGH YOUR GRIEF

What can you do about grief? Unfortunately, it cannot be avoided. Only by analyzing your grief and working through it will you be able to get back to the act of living. Paul had to face the realities of his situation and see how he might take on less demanding work. Only by focusing on the source of his grief and beginning to address these concerns could Paul begin to feel better.

CRY

How else can you combat grief? Crying can be helpful. That doesn't mean you should force yourself to sob, but if the tears start welling up, don't stop them. Let your feelings out. Think about what has changed and what will change. Talk about your feelings with the people you're close with. Don't avoid the fact that you have lupus or you won't be able to go through the grieving process.

Remember that grief is like a deep infection. The only way it can improve is to open it up and let what's inside come out, even if it means a good cry. This may be difficult, but eventually the wound will drain and begin to heal. Soon you will exhaust your grief. Then the healing will begin.

An Emotional Ending

Living with any chronic medical problem can involve a number of painful emotions. But it is possible to cope with these emotions—to learn strategies that will eliminate or lessen them, and help you live more comfortably and happily. These strategies are just what the doctor—and family and friends—ordered!

PART FOUR

Lupus and Relationships

29.

LUPUS AND RELATIONSHIPS: AN INTRODUCTION

You do not live your life alone—unless you're reading this book on a deserted island in the South Pacific! You interact with many people every day. So you'll certainly want to be able to deal with any difficulties you are having in your interpersonal relationships. For example, you might be worried about what others are going to think now that you've been diagnosed with lupus. How are they going to react? Are they going to ask questions? What kinds of answers will they listen to, and what answers will turn them away? These are some of the questions that may bother you.

Since you'll probably be with other people during a good part of your waking hours, it makes sense to be aware of how lupus can affect these relationships. Obviously, different problems exist in different relationships. But before we begin discussing all the different people who may be part of your life, here are a few general guidelines you may find helpful.

Do unto Others . . .

When you interact with others, try not to get too wrapped up in your own feelings. If you disregard the feelings of those around you, you will also prevent them from getting close to you. So make a conscious effort to be considerate of others, just as you'd like them to be considerate of you.

What does this mean? Just this: *You're not the only one who has to cope with lupus.* The important people in your life may also be having a hard time, simply because you mean a lot to them. Remember that. You might not realize that your problems affect those around you. You might think, "Why would they be upset? It's happening to me!" But if you give this some thought, you'll see that you're not being reasonable or fair.

Take your family, for example. A problem for you is also a problem for them. Of course, it may affect you in a different way. It's certainly true that you're the one who's experiencing the restrictions and the physical changes, as well as the apprehensions and anxieties. But your family doesn't like to see you suffer. You'll be better able to cope with these important people if you bear in mind that they are experiencing almost as much emotional turmoil as you are. In fact, this may explain why family members and friends might be unable to provide all of the support you want as quickly as you want it. Like you, they are probably going through a tough period of adjustment!

Then again, rather than being unaware of the emotions of others, you may feel guilty about the added burden you are placing on your family. This can be a hard feeling to cope with. Keep in mind, though, that you may be projecting this difficulty onto other people—and possibly adding to their problems in the process.

Change Yourself, Not Others

Do you feel that if you try hard enough, you'll be able to change the attitudes, feelings, or behaviors of others? Unfortunately, it doesn't work that way. Whether the people in your life accept your lupus or deny that you have any problem at all, you won't be able to change them unless they want to change. So it makes sense to use your energy to change the one person over whom you do have control—yourself. Spend more time working on yourself and less time worrying about others. In fact, once others see the changes in you, they may even alter their own attitudes. So help yourself. Be your own best friend.

Look Through the Eyes of Others

If you have an argument with someone, you may believe that you're right and the other person is wrong. If this continues, nothing will be resolved, and the other person's behavior may drive you crazy because it seems so unreasonable.

Take a moment and look at the situation through the eyes of the other person. What does he or she see? What might the other point of view be? Once you've done this, you'll be better able to explain how you feel in a way that he or she will understand. And then you'll be able to find a solution to almost any problem that might exist.

Pride, Yes; Revenge, No!

Revenge! There are times when you might think, "I only wish that _____ could know what it's like to live with lupus for an hour, a day, or a week, so that he or she could understand what I've been going through." But you know this isn't realistic, and you can't sit around waiting for it to happen. Besides, afterward you might not be too pleased with yourself for having such vengeful thoughts. So what might you do? Take pride in yourself. Concentrate on doing what's best for *you*. If you have to be a little more self-centered and a little less concerned about what other people think, just accept this as one more way of coping with your condition.

Learn to Accept a Little Selfishness

Perhaps you've been feeling rotten, but others seem to want you to do more and more. In the past, you may have had trouble saying no—either because you felt guilty, perhaps, or because you wanted to avoid disappointing the other person. But now things are a little different, and you really must curtail your generosity for the sake of your own well-being. Regardless of how much you want to be able to help others, and respond positively to the requests of others, there are times that it may not be in your best interest to do so. Yes, this may give you the appearance of being selfish. But as long as you don't abuse it, this selfishness can be positive for you. Do for yourself; think of yourself. You're Number One, and that's the way it must be. Only if you take care of yourself will you be able to deal with others. The reverse does not necessarily hold true. If you always take care of others first, this may actually make you less able to care for yourself.

Many people have a harder time saying no than any other word. But you can't always say yes. And sometimes you *shouldn't*. So what can you do? You can learn (and practice!) more comfortable ways to say no. For example, one of the easiest ways is to say, "I'd love to, but I can't right now." Sounds good, right? But what if even that doesn't work? Understand that those people who cannot accept your saying no, or give you a hard time for this response, are not truly looking out for your best interests. That may make it easier to deal with saying no to them in the future.

Open the Lines of Communication

You'll find it far easier to deal with lupus if you can rely on those closest to you, such as your partner, other family members, and close friends. This social network can give you added strength during the difficult period of adjustment to living with lupus. But right now, you may find it difficult to even talk to others. So how can you possibly ask for their support? Well, your first job is to get the lines of communication open. The best way to get the conversation rolling is to be open and honest about the way you feel. If you say anything that upsets or hurts someone, you'll deal with it then. But first, get your feelings out on the table.

Perhaps you're waiting for others to approach you and offer their support. But since you're the one with lupus, you may have to be the first person to talk about it. Some people may be reluctant to even mention the word in front of you. But if you bring it up and talk about it matter-of-factly, you may pave the way to more effective communication. Don't be ashamed to tell family and friends that you've been diagnosed or are living with lupus. It's a part of your life now. When others come to understand what you're experiencing, they will be better able to give you the support you need.

Janice, a thirty-eight-year-old mother of three, had recently been diagnosed with lupus. She had already broken the news to her family, but was unsure how to approach the topic with her friends. She decided to let a few of her friends know about her lupus at their weekly canasta game. As they sorted through their cards, Joy tentatively mentioned, "The doctor told me I have lupus, and I may not always have the energy I'm used to having." When she saw looks of concern on her friends' faces, she immediately added, "But don't worry—I'm really feeling all right, and the doctor said I will have no problem beating you at canasta for many years to come!" The light tone of her comments reassured her friends. Janice helped her friends handle the news by showing them that she could handle it.

What if you're afraid to share your feelings? Certainly, fear can make communication difficult. For instance, if you're fearful that what you say may make the other person uncomfortable, you may hesitate to say it. Or perhaps it's their fear that's stopping you. Fortunately, there's an excellent solution to this problem. Simply reach out and physically touch the other person. By holding hands or sharing hugs, you can quickly bring about a type of sharing that doesn't require words. And in the process, you'll reestablish the lines of communication.

ASK FOR HELP

Regardless of how independent and self-sufficient you are, there may be times that you can't do it all. Be able to reach out. Be able to ask others for help. Don't feel humiliated. Don't feel less than yourself. It takes a strong person to ask for help.

There are four very important things that you will find when you ask others for help:

1. More people than you would expect will be willing to help. In fact, many will be happy to be asked because they're glad to be able to do something for you.
2. There will be times that people say no; don't assume this has anything to do with you.

3. You're also setting a good example for others. By showing that you can ask, you're letting them know that they can ask, too, if they ever need to.
4. Remember, there is nothing wrong with asking somebody for anything, as long as you can accept the fact that they have the right to say no. So don't hesitate to ask.

Bring On the World

Now that we've introduced some general ideas, let's see how lupus can affect the relationships that make up your life. Of course, not every chapter in this section will apply to you. You may choose to read only those that are appropriate, or you may decide to read all of them. Regardless, you'll soon realize that problems exist in all relationships, but that you can learn to cope with them.

30.

YOUR FAMILY MEMBERS

Blood is thicker than water! Your family can be a critical factor in your successful adjustment to lupus. Why? You're probably with your family more than you are with anyone else. If you get along well with members of your family, you have a ready source of emotional and practical support.

The impact of your lupus on your family is sure to be profound. Family members may experience many of the same emotional reactions that you do—from anger and depression to fear of the future. Sometimes family members react more strongly and possibly even more irrationally than the person who's suffering with lupus. There may be more denial by a family member. There may be guilt, especially on the part of parents if they feel that they have somehow contributed to lupus in their child through genetics.

Any communication problems that exist within a family may be magnified by lupus. The fact that each person adjusts differently—and may find it hard to change—can also exacerbate family problems.

It seems that family members who are able to talk, share, cry, and hold on to one another during rough times have an easier time dealing with the problems posed by lupus. On the other hand, when family members experience the impact but are unable to talk to one another about it, the adjustment is much more difficult. Which of these families sounds like yours? If your family is like most, it falls somewhere in between these two extremes.

If you find it difficult to talk to loved ones about your lupus, treatment issues, or your feelings, don't give up. To maintain family unity—and to make sure you get the support you need—it's important that your concerns be brought into the open. This doesn't mean that all conversations are going to be pleasant. However, they should enable each person to share his or her feelings with the other members of the family.

Of course, different types of problems may pop up with different family members. So let's discuss how you can better deal with your partner, your children, and your parents.

Living with Your Partner

Lupus can certainly have an effect on your relationship. But this doesn't mean that your problems can't be resolved. There are very few problems that can't be resolved through better communication, understanding, and, if necessary, counseling. Let's discuss some of the ways in which lupus may affect your relationship and various ways in which its impact can be lessened.

CHANGES IN YOUR SOCIAL LIFE

Have restrictions caused by lupus forced you to cut back on some of the social activities you used to enjoy with your partner? You might not be able to do as much now as you used to. This can be hard to take, especially if you and your partner had active social lives before the onset of your condition. Because your partner does not have lupus, he or she may feel angry, frustrated, or helpless. You, on the other hand, may believe that your partner's social life has been put on hold, and it's all your fault. Or you may be angered by his or her seeming inability to accept these new restrictions.

Once you are better able to manage your lupus, you should be able to resume doing many things that you enjoy. Until then, try to engage in activities that are not too challenging or strenuous. Sometimes, it's fun and relaxing just to watch a video with a few friends.

If your social life is still on hold even after your condition has stabilized, you'll have to ask yourself if this is due to fear, depression, or other emotional problems. If so, be sure to refer to the appropriate chapters earlier in this book.

CHANGES IN FAMILY RESPONSIBILITIES

Lupus may create the need for temporary or permanent changes in each family member's responsibilities, as your spouse and children take over some of the functions that you performed in the past. This can surely be a potential source of friction between you and your partner, especially if he or she receives a heavy share of the load.

Sheila, a thirty-six-year-old mother of four, returned from a doctor visit and immediately called a family powwow. She told her husband that because she did not receive a good medical report, he would have to take over all of the household chores, including all of the cooking and cleaning (even washing the windows). Her two older children would have to do all of the grocery shopping and would have to take turns helping their younger brothers with their homework, bathing, and other daily routines.

Despite the fact that Sheila's family loved her and was concerned about her health, they were all understandably upset, especially her husband. Since he had difficulty boiling water, he certainly wasn't happy about his new assignment. The older children might also have a hard time dealing with their new responsibilities.

How can you make changes as smoothly as possible, without causing your partner unnecessary distress? First, make the changes gradually. Try to avoid overwhelming your partner—or other members of your family, for that matter. And be realistic in your expectations, keeping in mind that it takes time for *anyone* to comfortably incorporate new responsibilities into his or her routine.

How else can you help your partner adjust to a heavier burden or responsibility? Make sure you leave some free time for the pleasures of life. It's only when new responsibilities seem to be all-consuming that serious problems occur. Be sure to look at any changes through the eyes of your partner. Consider how you'd feel if the situation were reversed. Think how upsetting it would be if you no longer had time for the things you enjoyed because of added responsibilities and pressures. Discuss the needed changes reasonably, and be gentle.

IF YOUR PARTNER DENIES YOUR CONDITION

What can you do if your partner simply won't accept the fact that you have lupus? You might hear, "Oh, come on, you look fine. What are you complaining about?" You can, of course, try to "educate" your spouse, but try not to go overboard. If you're constantly badgering your partner, pointing out how things must change because of your condition, it may only cause further denial. Keep in mind that your partner will not accept your condition until he or she is ready to do so. In the meantime, concentrate on improving your own thoughts and feelings. Others' feelings may change, but they will do so slowly, and not necessarily at your urgings.

FINANCIAL PROBLEMS

Lupus can present added money problems, especially for your spouse. Money concerns are frequently a major source of friction in any marriage. If you are the breadwinner, your spouse may fear the unpleasant role of becoming more responsible for financial aspects of family management. If your spouse is the major income producer, pressure from the added costs of treatment and medication may be tough. Both you and your spouse will worry about whether all obligations can be met (and whether they can continue to be met). Your medical bills will compound the problem.

What can you do? Sit down with your partner and talk over your financial problems. Try to be realistic and to reach practical solutions. Admit that new problems may arise, but emphasize the fact that these frequently have a way of working themselves out. If not, you will deal with them as they arise. Be patient, be communicative, and—above all—be positive. (For tips on dealing with financial problems, see Chapter 14.)

HAS YOUR SEX LIFE BEEN AFFECTED?

Another important area in which lupus may affect a relationship concerns sex. Lupus can affect sexual relations. If this is a problem for you and your partner, or if you'd just like to learn more about the possible impact that lupus can have on sex, see Chapter 16. There, you'll learn how sexual problems can be worked out so that sex can remain an important and pleasurable part of your life.

IN SICKNESS AND IN HEALTH? SORRY!

Unfortunately, some relationships have ended because of chronic medical problems. Lupus-related fears, symptoms, restrictions, and side effects certainly have the potential to drive a wedge into what may have previously been a good relationship, replacing feelings of closeness and intimacy with coldness and distance. This can wash the "magic" right out of a relationship.

But it may not be all your partner's fault. You may be so apprehensive that you can't enjoy your relationship. Your sensitivity may cause you to be less patient. So breakups do occur. But realize that about 50 percent of all marriages end in divorce anyway, even when lupus is not involved!

Statistics aside, what do you do if your partner is frightened and "wants out"? Your partner's fear, your own condition, and your fears of abandonment may all be combining to create a horrible package of anxiety, depression, hopelessness, and panic. If communication has become a problem in your house, you may not be able to talk to your partner. You may find communication to be either nonexistent or counterproductive.

So what should you do? This isn't a problem one can—or should—handle alone. Get some help. The aid of a professional or an objective outsider may help to resolve some of the problems that you and your partner have been unable to work out yourselves. If your partner doesn't seem open to outside help, get some counseling for yourself. Regardless of the results of your efforts to save your relationship, any support you can muster will only improve your emotional well-being.

A MARITAL (CON)SUMMATION

Every relationship has its ups and downs, with problems that have to be worked out. Of course, lupus does make relationships more vulnerable to crises and arguments. But by giving added attention to your partner's feelings and needs, you will find that many—if not all—of these problems can be worked out over time. And isn't your relationship worth the added effort? Once problem spots have been smoothed out, your spouse may become your greatest ally in dealing with your condition.

Dealing with Your Children

It's hard enough for you to deal with lupus. But then you worry about how your kids are going to deal with your being sick. Children—regardless of how old they are!—may be especially vulnerable to the stresses and fears that occur when a family member has a chronic illness. Certainly, at this time, you may not be able to help them as much as you used to or spend as much time with them as you'd like. But you can surely use the time you do spend with them as productively as possible, and you can also help your children to handle any fears or changes that may be bothering them. How? Let's see how you can help your children better cope with your lupus.

ENCOURAGE QUESTIONS

When you talk to your children, make sure that you take the time to answer any questions they may have. Discussions, if handled properly, not only will be helpful for your children, but also can provide both you and your kids with a special feeling of closeness. Of course, you want to protect your children. But keeping your lupus hidden is not the answer. Keep your kids in the loop. If you don't answer their questions, they may actually fear that worse things are happening.

It is very important for parents to be united in what they tell their children. Decide together how you're going to do this. You want to also make sure that your efforts are not sabotaged by significant others in the family, or outside the immediate family, who might say things that interfere with what you're trying to accomplish. Anticipate this, and let these people know beforehand what you're trying to do so they can recognize that this is your responsibility and leave it up to you.

FIELDING CHILDREN'S QUESTIONS

How do you answer your child's questions? That depends on the age of your child and how detailed your child wants your answers to be. The best advice is to provide direct answers to their specific questions. Don't go into detail unless your child asks for more information.

The younger the child, the less of an explanation he or she will need. Anything that you tell a youngster will have to be explained simply. With very young children, for example, you might simply say, "I don't feel well, so I can't play with you right now. I'd like to, but I just can't." Unless you're noticeably affected, you may not have to say much of anything.

The questions of older children will probably be more direct and more specific, requiring a more detailed explanation. Resulting discussions, if handled properly, will be helpful for your children, and you will enjoy them. You'll also enjoy the comforting feelings of closeness that can result.

But what if your kids don't ask questions? Remember that if your children really don't want to, they won't, no matter how much encouragement you give them. But you should let them know that they can ask anything they want. Remember: Fears and anxieties can be very destructive if they're kept bottled up inside. Once your children know that they have the option of talking to you freely, they can decide what they wish to discuss.

Think, for example, about parents talking with their children about sex. Because of the delicate nature of the subject, and the discomfort or anxiety of the parent, more information than necessary is usually given. Have you heard the anecdote about the very young child who walked up to his mother and asked, "Mommy, where did I come from?" The mother started to tremble because this was the first time she had heard such a question from her child, and she wasn't prepared to answer it. After thinking for a moment, she nervously explained the various parts of the female anatomy and how the sexual act resulted in conception. She told how this ultimately led to the birth of the child. When she finished after about fifteen minutes, she breathed a sigh of relief and expectantly waited for her child's reaction. The child responded, "But Mommy, I didn't want to know all that. I just wanted to know what hospital I was born in!"

The message in this anecdote is clear. Try to determine exactly what your child wants to know. Some children may not even know what answers they are looking for. So just start answering and then ask if that's what they wanted to know. Continue from there.

Certainly, whenever you're speaking to your children about illness—especially if your kids are young—you should be careful not to frighten them. Remember that children have great imaginations, and often blow things out of proportion. You do want your kids to continue talking to you about your condition. If you show that you accept lupus and that you welcome questions about it, this will greatly benefit your relationship with them.

Keep this in mind if you're preparing to talk about how life may change. Assure them that there will always be fun and happiness in your lives, regardless of any of the changes that take place. Prepare your children for as many things as you are realistically able to prepare them for, such as doctor visits, hospitalizations, changes in physical appearance, new symptoms, or anything else that you become aware of beforehand. You know your children. You can probably guess the kinds of things that are most important to them—and what you'll need to discuss.

Be prepared to talk about whether lupus is contagious (as you already know, it's not!). But children may be afraid that they're going to catch lupus (especially if they're misinformed—or teased—by others) and then go through what you're going through. Of course, because there is a genetic predisposition to lupus, it is statistically possible that your child might get it. If that happens, you'll want to have another conversation explaining that genetics is the reason for their diagnosis, not that they "caught" it, or shouldn't have stayed close to you!

DEALING WITH THE "BIG" QUESTION

Of course, there's one question your children might ask that will be particularly hard to answer. Whenever children know that a parent has an ongoing medical problem, they may worry and may even ask if the parent is going to die. Be prepared to talk about this. You'll want to handle this very carefully. Children become petrified thinking about the death of a parent. So reassure them emphatically that you're not planning to die. Although these may seem like empty words, that's what they need to hear.

You know by now that lupus is not considered to be a fatal disease. But it may not be enough for you to tell your child that you will not die, especially if you're not sure yourself. Telling your children that you're not dying is obviously what they want to hear. But, despite that, there are times that this may not be very reassuring. Why? They may just not believe you. (Children are very perceptive; they'll recognize your fears.) Your body language may say otherwise. They may be so frightened that your words go in one ear and out the other.

Keep trying to talk to them. Find out exactly what's making them so afraid. For example, if they're concerned about the treatment you are undergoing, you can tell them that there are always times that your body needs a little tweaking in order to do better. Most people need some tweaking. For example, you can explain to your children that there are people who wear glasses to help their vision, or hearing aids if they have problems with their hearing, it does not mean they're going to die. Or if your children see you taking medication, remind them that many people take medicine to help them feel better or conquer symptoms. It doesn't mean they're going to die.

If you need more doctor visits, or even require hospitalization, this is, unfortunately, part of life with lupus. But it does not mean you're going to die. Explain that this is a way for the doctors to spend more time with you to help you to get better. There may be times that you want to take your children with you to your doctor visits. If this is the case, especially if your children are nervous about the possibility of you dying, you may want to call your doctor's office before the visit, explain what you're planning on doing and why, and ask them to be as comforting and as reassuring as possible.

What if your children cry? Recognize that this is an outward sign of them being scared . . . and sad. Don't feel that you have to tell them to stop, or try to stifle their tears. Rather, be encouraging and supportive. Keep focused on the positive, for your sake as well as theirs. It's okay if you cry as well. Letting them know that crying is okay will help them cope if they feel emotional, or if they're worried that their tears are a burden on you. Of course, many children feel more frightened if they see a parent cry. So make light of it, as best you can. For example, you might want to say, "Every now and then my faucets leak! So let's go and water some plants with our leaky faucets!" Yes, it is okay to make them laugh to help them "get it together."

Finally, if you're still having difficulty discussing your illness, or the answer to the question "Will you die?" (or any other difficult questions) with your children, it may still be a good idea to speak to a professional—your doctor, their pediatrician, a psychologist, or other mental health professional—and have him or her take control of the discussion.

Let's review some tips for providing basic information to your children:

- Be honest. But provide information on a need-to-know basis.
- Provide information that is suitable for the age of your children. Providing too much information for young children may be as inappropriate as providing too little for older children.
- Provide time for your children to ask you questions. Here, too, your answers should be on a need-to-know basis and age-specific.
- Make sure that the time that you have set aside to discuss lupus with your children is uninterrupted time.
- Be as reassuring as you can be in any comments you make to children.
- Show strength. The way you handle lupus will help determine how well they handle it. But don't feel like you always have to be strong. Be human, instead. By showing your children that you have emotions and are dealing with them, you're setting a good example for them. By your being willing to talk about things, you're sharing with them that they can talk about things as well.
- Say something if you see your children keeping their distance, being less emotionally or physically demonstrative with you. For example, if they're reluctant to hug you, they may be afraid of hurting you. Talk about this—and then grab 'em!
- Avoid giving false hope, or making empty or false promises. This can come back and bite you, and will cast doubts on how you are believed in future conversations.
- Prepare them for what other people may say, especially if others don't have the same constructive approach to lupus that you want to be the cornerstone of your family's communication.
- Prepare them for changes. You know that you may have to make some changes. Parents may have an easier time accepting this than children. So approach this issue gradually with your children.
- Keep the door open to future conversations.

FOCUS ON QUALITY, NOT QUANTITY

You may have a hard time if you're not able to do as much with your children as you would like. One of the hardest parts of coping with lupus is feeling as though you're disappointing them. You want to be a good parent. But what does that entail? Parents often believe that they must spend a lot of time with their children, always making themselves available to take them places and do things with them. If they don't do this, parents may feel guilty. But what about those times when lupus is restrictive and prevents you from doing a lot of what you'd like to do? Just remember that you have no choice.

How can you solve this dilemma? How do you explain to your child that you can't take him or her somewhere, or that you can't do what you had promised? Children don't want to understand when they're upset. They may express their unhappiness (and then may even feel guilty about that). This is an important area for communication. Try to come up with solutions together, discussing how all of you will deal with this. Making deals can help. Honestly explain to your children that, at times, you'll need to rest, and you may not be able to participate in the usual family routine. Come to an agreement with them about some enjoyable activity you can do together when you do feel better. You might say, "I really can't do this right now, but if we rest together, maybe we can do something you'd like when I have a little more energy." Or, "This is not something that I can do with you, but if you *really* want to do it, maybe we can ask your friend to do it with you." This arrangement will show your children that you're aware of their unhappiness and want to help.

Also, try to be less concerned with *quantity time*—the number of minutes and hours you spend with your kids—and more concerned with *quality time*—special time during which you share feelings and pleasurable activities. If your time together is well spent, with plenty of talking and laughing, you'll make up for any missed time. And as you share your thoughts with your children, you'll be helping them better handle your medical condition.

ADOLESCENTS

Although your adolescents are still your children, and they may have the same fears and concerns as younger children, coping with adolescents can be very different from coping with young children. Because adolescents are older and can read more complex material, they can read most of what has been written for adults. They can ask questions if anything they read is too complicated. However, the main difficulty in coping with adolescents is recognizing their special needs.

During adolescence, children begin to assert their independence. Look out, world, the future generation is coming! Adolescents want to start moving away from the family setting and its responsibilities. Even under normal circumstances, this creates problems in many homes. Add a parent with lupus to the picture, and the problem is compounded. Why? Because of your condition, your teen may have to help out more than usual around the house. At the same time, he or she probably wants to do less around the house and be away more.

How can you cope with this problem? Imagine how helpful it can be for you to be aware of your adolescent's feelings. Take the initiative and offer a reasonable compromise. Just showing that you understand will help. Maybe things won't seem so hopeless to the adolescent, after all. If you recognize that, in truth, you may not be able to change your teen much, perhaps you can learn to cope in a way that, at the very least, keeps you sane! Let's learn more about dealing with teens.

DON'T EXPECT MIRACLES!

First, realize that dealing with teens is quite different from dealing with younger kids—which you probably already know. As already discussed, teens are far more absorbed in themselves than in their families. Remember that they are going through quite a few difficult adjustments of their own. Of course, not all teens are alike. Some are less self-centered and more sensitive and compassionate than others. Certainly, you know your child better than anyone. But perhaps you now expect your usually insensitive child to rise to the occasion and enthusiastically pitch in with household chores. Be aware that you are probably setting yourself up for disappointment if you expect your child to change so significantly.

Of course, this doesn't mean that you shouldn't discuss lupus with your teen. Talk to your child candidly, treating him or her like an adult. This will probably provide the best chance for a positive response. Think about the concerns your adolescent might have regarding your lupus, and try to be reassuring. If your child feels comfortable talking to you about your condition, encourage discussion. But you should respect your child's wishes if he or she does not wish to talk about your illness.

ADOLESCENTS AND FRIENDS

Adolescents are usually less interested in spending time with family members and more interested in being with friends. It may be easier for your teenager to deal with your lupus if his or her friends spend little time at your house—that way, your adolescent need not explain your condition. Even if your teenager's friends don't know about your condition, your adolescent may be much more sensitive to the situation. Does this sound strange? Most adolescents want to impress their friends. Somehow, having a parent who has trouble walking doesn't quite "fit the bill." Of course, there are some adolescents who are more mature and open about it. The extent of their love for their parent and a sound family relationship minimize the problem. They may sometimes end relationships with those friends who cannot understand the situation. Unfortunately, this is not often the case.

Another problem for your adolescent is transportation (that means you!). Many adolescents count on their parents to drive them to friends' houses, parties, meetings, and so on. But you may not be available (or able) to chauffeur your teenager around as much. As a result, you may feel guilty because you believe you're not being a good parent. Your teenager, thinking less of you and more of himself or herself, can become upset or even angry. Recognizing this selfishness of feeling like too much of a burden, your adolescent may feel guilty as well. The best thing to do is to talk it out.

TALK TO YOUR ADOLESCENT

Understanding the needs of your adolescent can open the door to much better communication. However, if you want your discussions to be helpful, treat your adolescent like an adult. This will provide the best environment for interaction. Think about your teenager's concerns about your condition and be as reassuring as possible. If your adolescent feels comfortable talking to you about your lupus, encourage it. But remember to respect the rights of those adolescents who would rather not discuss it.

When You Need Your Teen to Pitch In

Because of your condition, your adolescent may now have to shoulder more responsibilities. But will your teen be willing to help out? That's the real question!

Fifteen-year-old Douglas felt guilty about not helping out more at home. However, he thought that giving in would be a sign of weakness. (Heaven forbid!) These mixed feelings caused Douglas a lot of anguish—which, of course, he didn't want to discuss with his parents. Because of the guilt he was experiencing, Douglas escaped by spending even more time than usual out of the house—and less time helping out! Douglas's parents sat him down, and together they worked out a compromise. Douglas would not have to spend all his time helping out at home, but he would make himself available when necessary. After reaching an agreement, both Douglas and his parents felt closer to one another—and Douglas felt a good deal better about himself.

As you can see, it may pay to take the initiative and offer a reasonable compromise. Just showing that you understand your teen's feelings may help. Perhaps things won't seem so hopeless to your child, after all.

Another tactic, too, may prove helpful. If your adolescent must take on some adult chores, consider that he or she may also be ready to enjoy a few adult privileges and pleasures—within reason, of course. Adolescents will usually be more willing to help out if they know that they will be treated and trusted in a more grown-up way.

Remember that you can go only so far in trying to get your adolescent's cooperation. You can't move mountains. Continue to be as constructive as you can, putting as little pressure on your child as possible, in order to keep the door open to good relations. As long as you know you've tried, you can hold your head up high.

Dealing with Your Parents

Parents often have difficulty coping with a child's illness—even if their "child" is an adult. Therefore, if your parents are alive, anticipate that they will have a rough time handling your lupus. This, of course, will make coping harder for you, too. Why? You don't want your parents to suffer. And you know how your parents feel, because you'd certainly be upset if your child were ill.

If your relationship with your parents is good, then you're among the lucky ones. But what if you normally have difficulty dealing with your parents? Having lupus won't help! Regardless of the type of relationship you've had previously, consider how your parents have treated you since your diagnosis. Have they ignored or minimized your condition? Or have they smothered you? Let's look at these two possible reactions and see how you can better cope with your parents.

THE IGNORERS

Elizabeth, a twenty-two-year-old secretary living with her parents, had lupus for two years. Since her diagnosis, her parents had been showing less and less concern about her condition. When Elizabeth was in pain, her mother just told her to take her pills. When she was tired, her father told her "staying in bed won't accomplish anything." If looks could kill, Elizabeth's parents would no longer be around! Other than making these insensitive remarks, Elizabeth's parents had little to say on the subject of her lupus. They certainly never asked questions about her condition. Even worse, when she did try to discuss it, they showed no interest at all.

Parents who ignore or play down your lupus often do so because they can't deal with it. They can't face the fact that their child is sick. Worse, many parents agonize over the possibility that your problem might have something to do with them. While this may not make any sense to you, your parents may be afraid that they did something to contribute to your illness or that you inherited the condition from them. To avoid these intolerable thoughts, they may try to deny that you have lupus, or they may minimize your illness, hoping it will go away.

Remember what we discussed in the previous chapter about seeing a situation through someone else's eyes? Don't you think that it holds true in this case? As you look through the eyes of your seemingly indifferent parents, you'll probably realize that this is the only way in which they can cope with the situation right now. Yes, their behavior may change over time, but the change will be gradual and not necessarily in response to your urgings.

THE SMOTHERERS

Since Alice developed lupus, her mother has visited her an average of four times per week. This would have been nice, except: (1) her mother lives thirty minutes away by car, (2) she has a heart condition, and needs her rest, and (3) Alice simply did not want to see her that often. You see, Alice was thirty-six years old, hadn't lived at home for seventeen years, and often disagreed with her mother—especially regarding what activities she should participate in and how much rest she should get. Alice certainly felt smothered.

Parents who smother believe that if you have any kind of problem, they must take care of you. Having lupus certainly fits this requirement. It doesn't matter what your marital status is or how old you are. The fact that you can take care of yourself doesn't matter. What matters to them is that they are your parents—they are responsible for your welfare. They'll call frequently, asking how you're doing. They'll want to know what they can do to help. They may come over as often as possible to make sure that you're okay. Whether they visit or not, they'll constantly bombard you with questions about your health and activities.

What can you do, short of moving out of town and taking on a new identity? Again, look at yourself—and your condition—through the eyes of your parents. How do you think they feel? They care about you. What do they see? They see a child who needs them! You may not agree with them, but understanding their point of view should help you better communicate with them and more effectively explain how you feel.

WHAT IF TALKING DOESN'T HELP?

If you've talked to your parents and haven't succeeded in modifying their behavior, at least you know you've tried. This, alone, may help you feel better! What else can you do? Concentrate on helping yourself feel better. If your parents are unhappy with you because you seem to be rejecting their well-meant intentions, so be it. If they are unhappy with you because you're making it hard for them to ignore your condition, that's fine, too.

By the way, if you're unhappy with parents who are ignorers, you'd probably love them to smother you for a while. And if you don't like smothering parents, the thought of being left alone is probably very appealing. (Yes, the grass is always greener . . . !) There's rarely a perfect situation or relationship, and no one gets along with everyone all the time. So instead of complaining about your parents' faults, try to look at the positives in their behavior. This may make you feel better and will certainly help you avoid going crazy over their actions.

HOW MUCH SHOULD YOU TELL YOUR PARENTS?

A common question of people with chronic illnesses concerns how much they should tell their parents about their problem. Have you worried about this, too? First, think about your parents. How do they usually deal with unpleasant situations? Then ask yourself what you want to share with them. Next imagine how they would react to this, and how you would handle their reactions. All these factors will help you decide how much you should tell them.

For instance, you might wish you could share your fears and worries with your parents because of the reassurances it would bring. It would certainly be nice to know that you don't have to face something unpleasant alone. But what if your parents couldn't readily accept your problems even if they wanted to? It might be more detrimental to tell them things that they couldn't handle. So don't impulsively blurt out your feelings. By spending a little time figuring out what's best, you can help yourself feel a lot better. You'll probably improve your relationship with your parents, as well.

Finally, keep in mind that it's sometimes easier to talk to one parent than to the other. Consider telling one parent what's bothering you, and letting that parent tell the other. For example, your mother may be able to get through to your father better than you can. This will make things easier for everybody.

A Familial Finale

As you learn to cope with lupus, your biggest ally—and an important source of emotional support and practical assistance—may be your family. By learning to deal with your family members in the best possible way, you'll not only make things easier for them, but also make them better able to help you cope with lupus.

31.

FRIENDS AND COLLEAGUES

Aside from family, you also deal with friends and colleagues on a daily, or near daily, basis. Are there any ways in which you can better deal with these important people? Of course!

Dealing with Your Friends

What reactions to your lupus have your friends had? How many of your friends really know what you're going through? They may have read about your condition, and, at first, they may have thought they knew all about it. But because they weren't physically affected, they might not have been able to really understand what you were experiencing. Then, of course, there are the special problems that may crop up because of your condition, such as activities canceled because of physical symptoms, or the need to ask for help. Some wanted to learn more about all of this; some wanted to forget what little they knew. How can you handle this? Read on!

BE PREPARED FOR DIFFERENT REACTIONS

Certainly you should be prepared for a variety of reactions to your condition. Some friends, for instance, may be supportive. Other friends may seem uninterested and distant. Why would a friend seem distant at a time when you need special support? Well, some people may not know what to say to you. What should they ask you? How should they talk to you? Should they even mention your condition? They may not want to run the risk of stirring up unpleasant feelings for you—or for themselves, if they don't know how to respond. Their doubts and fears may cause so much tension that they don't even want to be with you. Of course, some friends may be very supportive— perhaps *too* supportive! There may be times when friends keep asking you how you are, or offering help, when you'd rather be left alone.

Certainly, friendships can be hurt because of misunderstandings and uncertainties. Can anything be done to prevent these problems from undermining your friendships, or do you have to be a hermit for the rest of your life? Don't despair. There are things you can do to improve the situation.

Try to establish ground rules with your friends. If you're the kind of person who likes to be asked how you feel, let your friends know. If you'd rather not be asked, let your friends know that, too. If your preferences fluctuate (sometimes feeling talkative about your condition, but at other times reluctant to even think about it), let your friends know. Your changing feelings may be harder for friends to deal with, so let them know that they can talk to you whenever they really want to. You'll let them know if and when you're having trouble.

Clear up the question marks. If you tell your friends how you feel and what your needs and desires are, fewer unknowns will exist. The uneasiness about what to do or say, which can hurt friendships, will be reduced. Your friends will become more aware of your needs, and will feel closer to you and less afraid.

CHANGING PLANS

Don't you love having to change plans with a friend at the last minute because you're so tired that you can't even move? Probably not. So you can understand how your friends might feel if they were to have restrictions placed on their activities. This doesn't have to be so. As you learn to cope with lupus, there will most likely be times when you don't feel up to going out, or when some aspect of living with lupus takes precedence over your social activities. Good friends, those who understand or at least *try* to understand what you're going through, will probably be better able to accept these last-minute cancellations. Others may not hide their annoyance when you have to cancel plans.

Kelly hated when she and her husband made plans with friends and she had to bow out because of lupus. What made it worse was that her husband went ahead with the plans anyway! She had to stay home alone because no one else wanted to change their plans. So there was not only friction between Kelly and her friends, but increasing marital arguments as well. So what could Kelly do? She might suggest that they have two sets of plans, such as going out to eat, or bringing food in, so that a last-minute decision would depend on the way she felt. Or she might suggest that they go out to eat without her, but pick her up before going to a movie if she felt up to it.

So how can you remedy this situation? It's a good idea to sit down with some of your closest friends and work out a solution to the problem. You can even ask them for suggestions. Although you may not always get the understanding you want, you'll probably find at least one or two friends who will be willing to work on a solution to any problems you may have.

ASKING FOR HELP

As you learn to live with lupus, you may have a greater need to call on your friends for help. You may need help cleaning the house, getting places, taking care of children, or purchasing groceries, among other things. Are you becoming more selfish? No—although it may seem that way to you. You'd probably like to be able to do these things yourself, but it just may not be possible. The reality is that there are certain things that must be taken care of, and if you can't take care of them yourself, you must ask others to help you. So if you need help, reach out for it. That's better than pushing yourself too hard and suffering the consequences.

When planning to ask for help, keep in mind that older friendships tend to be stronger and more resilient. Long-time friends will probably be more receptive when approached for favors. Newer or more casual friends should probably not be burdened as much. Without giving a friendship a chance to become firmly planted on your hook, you may lose your prize fish—a good, long-lasting friendship. Don't come on too strong. You might think, "But can't they see that I need help?" The answer is, "Not necessarily."

Try to arrange for a proper fit when asking for help. For example, if your friend Myrna loves children, it would probably be better to ask her for help with the kids. If you know that Maureen suffers from "supermarketitis," requiring daily therapeutic visits to the local food emporium, then sending her for groceries shouldn't bother her at all. If Mario has a driving phobia, don't ask him to chauffeur you around. (By the way, no matter how old and dear the friend, once you feel up to it, it would be nice to show your appreciation with an unexpected gift or gesture.)

What should you do if your friends complain or show resentment when you request help? Back off for a while. In addition, try to talk it over with them. Discuss these problems when the conflict can still be resolved; don't let them build up until the friendship is destroyed. If your efforts to mend the friendship fail, remember this: Friends who can't understand your need for help are not very good friends, anyway.

For your own peace of mind, remember that needing help in certain things may be temporary. Hopefully, you will find out that the only thing permanent about lupus is the diagnosis! Everything else seems to fluctuate, including dependence and independence. At those times when you feel less independent, remind yourself that your needs at the moment may not necessarily be for the rest of your life.

LOSING FRIENDS

What if the people you thought were your friends don't call or visit? What if they seem reluctant to make any plans with you, preferring to "wait and see how you feel"? What if some seem to be "turned off" by your condition? Maybe they're afraid it's contagious! When friends seem to drift away, it's certainly sad. But remember that it was not your decision to end the friendship. And you don't want it to be your problem!

Why might this have happened? Maybe your friend felt uncomfortable being with you. Maybe he or she was "turned off" by the fact that you have a medical problem, or felt unsure of what to say or do. Whatever the reason, you've probably learned a hard, unpleasant lesson: You can't change someone else's feelings.

If a friend, or anyone else, cannot handle your condition, you may feel rejected. This can be devastating—especially if you fear that you won't be able to develop any other meaningful relationships! This is not true. You are still the same person you were before, except for the ways that lupus has affected you physically. Keep telling yourself this so that you can restore any confidence that may have been shaken by your friend's action.

Usually, if rejection occurs or if a relationship breaks up, it couldn't have been too strong to begin with. Many weak relationships have broken up because of medical problems. A sturdy relationship, even if it has to go through some rough times, will probably end up even stronger than before. Be reassured that most people who lose friends do make new ones. Anyway, you don't really want a "friend" who is uncomfortable around you. You want a friend who likes you for who you are—lupus and all! And there are plenty of wonderful, understanding people out there. So don't give up!

Dealing with Your Colleagues

If you work, you're probably spending a number of hours a week with colleagues. These people are likely to show a variety of reactions to your condition (if they know about it), as well as to any impact your condition may have on your work. You'll certainly want to feel comfortable around them. Let's discuss some of the ways in which you may better cope with your colleagues.

SHOULD YOU TELL YOUR COLLEAGUES?

Hopefully, if you're comfortable with yourself, others will be, too. Many colleagues will take your condition in stride, and won't even think about it. Might it be helpful to provide them with some basic information on lupus? It could be, although you should realize that this will not necessarily improve their attitude toward you or your condition. Unfortunately, knowledge doesn't always lead to understanding. However, just knowing that you've tried to help your colleagues understand might make you feel better.

Of course, unless nosy colleagues ask questions, you may decide not to even bother telling your co-workers about your lupus. Obviously, there is no requirement that you do so.

COOPERATIVE COLLEAGUE COMPROMISES

Elaine found it impossible to complete all her required work. She was afraid she'd lose her job. However, rather than giving up, she was able to make an arrangement with one of her colleagues who was willing to assist her in completing her tasks whenever she felt physically unable to do so alone. As a result, much of the pressure on Elaine's shoulders was removed.

Occasionally, you may find that you are unable to complete all of your work. If this happens, try to work out some kind of an arrangement with a colleague. What type? Certainly, it depends on the relationship between you and the other person, the type and amount of work to be done, and, of course, what is permitted by your company. You might, for instance, offer to pay your co-worker for completing your assignment. Or you might offer to perform a task for a co-worker at some later date.

This type of arrangement may seem strange—even uncomfortable at first—but it can result in even better relationships between you and your colleagues. You have nothing to lose. The worst your co-worker can say is no.

Whether you need to work or simply enjoy working, you'll certainly want to minimize any potential occupational problems your lupus has caused.

WHEN COLLEAGUES ARE RESENTFUL

Terry was a thirty-six-year-old bookkeeper who had worked in the same office for sixteen years. Because of lupus, Terry occasionally found it necessary to reduce her eight-hour-a-day work schedule to four hours. This plan was endorsed by her physician and employer, but was not accepted graciously by her fellow workers, many of whom would have preferred similar arrangements! This caused bitterness and strain between Terry and her colleagues.

If you have to curtail your working hours, or find that you must occasionally miss work because of lupus, you, like Terry, may encounter some resentment. As discussed above, at this point you may decide to explain your situation to your colleagues, or you may prefer to keep this information to yourself. Either way, accept the fact that some people just won't want to understand what's happening to you and why. Remember: You can't change another person. If a colleague—or anybody else, for that matter—can't handle or understand the effects of your disease, that's his or her problem. You can try to educate people about lupus, but you shouldn't make their attitude your problem. If you've got an employer with an open mind, you are very fortunate. Don't be as concerned about the attitudes of co-workers. Instead, concentrate on doing what's best for you.

Time to Punch Out

Whether you're dealing with friends or co-workers, always take one day at a time. Don't worry about problems that have not occurred yet, and, for that matter, may never occur. If your lupus does cause a problem, be precise in identifying exactly what the problem is. Then don't hesitate to employ the best strategies you know to resolve the dilemma and to restore good relations between you and the people you deal with in your day-to-day life.

32.

YOUR PHYSICIAN

How do you feel about your physician? (What a question!) Some people see physicians as gods. Others feel that they're cold professionals who make them nervous. You may feel that doctors don't really know what to do for you, and that you yourself know better than anyone else how you feel. Of course, there are other opinions. What are your thoughts? You may find that your feelings toward your physician—or toward physicians in general—have changed since your diagnosis. Some people with lupus don't have much confidence in their physicians, probably because they haven't been "cured." Others recognize that they should not expect miracles, and continue to rely on their doctors to offer the best treatment possible. Although physicians frequently bear the brunt of much hostility, and although they may occasionally feel as frustrated as you do, for the most part, they *truly do* want to help . . . and can.

Regardless of your opinions of the medical profession, your condition makes it impossible for you to stay away from your physician. You'll have to see your doctor more often than someone who is not chronically ill, so you'll want to make sure you have a good working relationship. Since lupus has the potential to be serious, it requires ongoing visits to your physician to keep your symptoms in check and to allow him or her to carefully monitor the medications you're taking. Your doctor will also provide guidelines for any lifestyle changes that may be beneficial or necessary. Medical visits will also determine if treatment is proceeding properly. So checkups are important to keep your condition under control. Although some patients deny the possibility of any problems and try to avoid regular checkups, the intelligent person is the one who sees the doctor regularly and as "prescribed."

Many people with lupus question which type of doctor should be responsible for their treatment. As you probably already know, the consensus is that your primary physician should be a board-certified rheumatologist. However, other specialists may also be involved, depending on your particular needs (more about this later in the chapter).

This chapter focuses on the importance of a good doctor–patient relationship and discusses how you can improve your dealings with your own physician. After all, you want to best utilize your physician's professional services, don't you?

Creating a Good Doctor–Patient Relationship

Your doctor must be someone in whom you have confidence medically. That's a no-brainer. But, just as important, you'll want someone with whom you're comfortable personally. This is especially important in helping you to understand what's going on with your lupus, monitor any flares and remissions, and treat any symptoms that require treatment.

A great many factors will determine your ability to feel comfortable with your physician, including your personality, your doctor's personality, your doctor's philosophy regarding treatment, and more. Remember that the chemistry between a doctor and each patient is unique. A physician who is "perfect" for someone else may not be right for you. You'll have to pick somebody *you* feel good about, so your relationship gets off to a good start and continues on track.

SET COMMUNICATION GROUND RULES

It's vital to set ground rules regarding communication with your doctor or any health care professional. In the past, physicians believed that patients with chronic illnesses wanted to know as little as possible, so they limited the amount of information they shared. Today, this is often not the case.

Many people with lupus want to be very actively involved in their treatment and to know all the facts. Regardless of how much information you want, be sure to clearly communicate your needs. Of course, this is a fairly simple matter if you desire as little as possible or want to be told everything. But what if you want your communication to fall somewhere in between? Be aware that there's nothing wrong with saying, "Doctor, I really want all the information about my case. But please remember that I'm very sensitive, so try to tell me things as gently as possible!"

ASK QUESTIONS

You are certainly well within your rights to question any aspect of the treatment that is prescribed for you. Some people, of course, prefer to not ask questions, but to simply follow the directions of their physician. This is also within your rights. But remember that you want to do everything possible to help yourself, so the more you know, the better.

Of course, you want to have confidence in your doctors—to believe that they know what they're talking about. This doesn't mean, however, that you must blindly accept everything your doctor says. If you don't like a particular medication or if it does not seem to be working for you, for example, speak up. Don't hold back. For the most part, physicians respect patients who ask questions. Disagreement doesn't mean that your physician will throw you out or even back down. But if you are unsure of why something is being suggested, question your physician. You do have the right to question. In fact, you have the obligation to question. Uncertainty will surely make you feel tense. And relaxation is so important.

Getting the Most from Office Visits

Most of your communications with doctors take place during office visits. You certainly want these visits to be as helpful and productive as possible. But as you may know, this is sometimes more easily said than done. Virtually everyone has come home from a doctor visit and realized that they forgot to ask an important question. Or perhaps you did ask the question and then promptly forgot the answer! Nothing can be more frustrating—especially since it is often so difficult to reach a doctor by phone! Fortunately, there are ways in which you can avoid this frustration. Let's discuss some of the easy things you can do to get the most from your office visits.

MAKE A LIST

Before each appointment, it's important to prepare a list of all the questions you want to ask the doctor. Don't wait until the night before your office visit to put your list together. Instead, prepare the list by jotting down notes whenever a question or piece of information pops into your mind.

Although making a list may seem elementary, it is an excellent way to obtain the information you need to understand your condition, properly take care of yourself, and guide your treatment. Don't be concerned that the doctor won't like you walking in with a list of questions. Most good doctors do appreciate this practice because it tends to structure the appointments more efficiently. However, if your doctor doesn't like it, ask yourself this: Whose health is on the line, anyway?

Besides those questions that occur to you, you may want to include concerns expressed by family members or close friends—even if you feel that their points may not be important. Your doctor will be able to tell you what is relevant, as well as provide you with the answers.

Many people worry that the questions they wish to ask are too trivial, or even foolish. Remember that the only foolish question is the unasked one! If you need further explanation about your treatment, feel free to ask and be as straightforward as possible. This will make it easier for your doctor to respond with the information you need.

GET THE ANSWERS

As your doctor answers your questions, be sure to listen carefully. You can miss some important information if you're looking at the next question, rather than listening to the doctor's response to the current one! If you're worried that you won't remember everything that goes on during your doctor visit, there are three ways in which you can aid your memory. The first is to jot down notes as each question is answered. The second is to bring a recording device. The third is to bring a family member or close friend.

It can be very helpful to go to the doctor accompanied by somebody important to you, because two sets of ears are always better than one. It's easy to miss what's being said because of the tension you may feel in the doctor's office. Having an extra listener will increase the likelihood that all important information will be retained. This will also take some of the pressure off you, helping you to relax and more efficiently listen and respond. Following the doctor visit, you and your companion will be able to sit down and compare notes about what was said.

If you do decide to bring someone with you, make sure that this person knows what you want to accomplish during the appointment. Discuss in advance the kinds of questions you want to ask and the information you hope to obtain. Your companion will then be able to jump in and ask any questions that he or she feels you've overlooked.

It's also important to speak up when you don't understand your doctor's answers because they're either too vague or too technical. Don't hesitate to question your doctor further. Perhaps he or she is used to discussing cases with other doctors and has become accustomed to using specialized, scientific terms. Perhaps other patients have been too intimidated to ask for clarifications! Whatever the reason, don't be afraid to speak up. And don't be embarrassed. Your goal is to talk more comfortably and intelligently about what's happening to you.

OTHER CONSIDERATIONS

What else can you do to make your office visits as beneficial as possible? Remember that you're the only one who really knows how you feel. If you think that there is something happening that your doctor should know about, be sure to mention it and make sure that you're heard. Don't think that any piece of information is unimportant, even if the doctor doesn't seem to be as impressed by a particular statement as you expected. Every bit of information that you give can and should help your doctor determine the best treatment course for your lupus.

It can be very frustrating when you're trying to explain the way you feel to your doctor and you're not being believed. It's even more difficult when you have a hard time putting into words the way you're feeling, and yet you know exactly how you're feeling! All of this is even more difficult if you're feeling something . . . and standardized medical tests come back showing nothing wrong!

Are you hesitant about speaking to your physician? Perhaps you're afraid of being put in the hospital if your physician finds out how you've really been feeling. You might be concerned that your physician will not like the way you're taking care of yourself. You might be afraid that you'll be labeled as a complainer who's "crying wolf," and then won't be taken seriously if an emergency occurs. You might be worried that your physician will increase your medication—or not increase it! Or you may be afraid that your physician, thinking that the symptoms you're reporting are "all in your head," won't believe what you're saying! Despite these concerns, you do want your physician to do the best for you. So try to be completely open and honest about the way you're feeling and what you're doing to take care of yourself.

While you are at the office, make sure you also have a clear understanding of any medication that has been prescribed during the visit. Be certain you know its actions, any foods to eat or avoid with the medication, and any side effects you might expect. (For more information on medication, refer to Chapter 10.)

By the time you leave the doctor's office, you will, hopefully, have had your questions answered and will have agreed on your treatment program. By all means, follow this program. But be sure to report any problems that may occur during treatment. And don't expect instantaneous results. It can sometimes take weeks for your body to respond to a new treatment.

Being Able to Reach Your Physician

Do you know what's really frustrating? How about when you call your physician and have to wait hours before your call is returned? This may be one of your criteria when searching for a physician. Make sure you feel confident that your physician will promptly return your calls.

One of the most important questions you'll want to ask your doctor is when to call about a problem. Which symptoms should be reported immediately? Certain symptoms, such as intense pain, seizures, a sudden reaction to a medication, and a high fever, may require you to contact your physician without delay. Other symptoms, such as minor joint pains, may not have to be reported as urgently. Ideally, try to obtain this information as early as possible in your relationship. Ask about the specific symptoms, events, side effects, or other problems that you should report, and also ask the best time to call. But when in doubt, check it out. Don't sit by your phone wondering if you should pick it up; just do so. Remember that if you are taking a new medication, how can you be expected to know exactly how your body will respond? The doctor has been through this many times, and can tell you that it wasn't necessary to call about this (and why!). And remember that experience is a great teacher. After you've lived with lupus for a while, you'll know when you should call and when it's not necessary.

Getting Second Opinions

Beth was frustrated. She loved her rheumatologist, but felt that she just wasn't making any progress. Her symptoms continued as always, despite the heavy-duty medications she was on. More and more of her friends were advising her to get a second opinion, but she was afraid of hurting her doctor's feelings. Finally, she picked up the phone . . .

Because you may not agree with absolutely everything your physician says, and because no physician knows it all, there may be times that you might want—or need—a second opinion. You should have a justifiable reason for seeking another opinion. However, many people are like Beth— worried about hurting their physician's feelings. Don't let that stop you. Think logically. Most physicians will accept your desire to get a second opinion. It will either confirm what they believe and are doing, or point out the need for further discussion. If your physician objects to your getting a second opinion, you should certainly question why. This does not suggest, however, that you should make a habit of going for second opinions. Nor should you continually shop around for the "ideal" physician. No such person exists.

WHOM SHOULD YOU CONTACT?

The physician you see for a second opinion should certainly have as much, or more, experience than your primary doctor. But how can you get an appropriate referral? You may start, of course, by asking your primary physician for a recommendation. If this doesn't work, you can then check with your local lupus organization or with the chief of the rheumatology department in a hospital in your geographic area. Or you can check with your county or state medical society, which is probably listed in your local telephone directory. You might also have to check with your health insurance provider, who can give you a list of participating physicians. And, of course, you may wish to seek recommendations from people you know—especially from others who are themselves being treated for lupus. Support groups are another good place to learn the names of physicians who specialize in lupus treatment.

THE SECOND OPINION . . . AND BEYOND

When you go for a second opinion, make sure that you carefully select and prioritize your questions. Keep in mind that you may not have to ask the same basic questions you asked your primary physician when you were first learning about lupus treatment. Remember why you're going for the second opinion, and focus on the information that you wish to obtain. Then let the conversation, as well as your written list of questions, guide the way.

If the second opinion significantly differs from the first, you might try to bring the various professionals together to discuss your treatment. Physicians often discuss their findings by phone. If this is not possible, however, and there are still unanswered questions, it may be in your best interest to seek a third opinion. Understandably, you may find this an unappealing option, both because of the pressure it places on you to find another qualified physician and because of financial considerations. Remember, though, that this is your life! So if a third opinion seems to be in order, by all means, get it.

You're Not "Locked In"

Some people are reluctant to change physicians. Others seem to change physicians more often than they change their socks! If you're not happy with your physician, you're not under any obligation to continue to see him or her. Don't continue to be treated by a particular physician if you feel you can't ask questions, if you feel intimidated, or if you feel that you can't call when there's a problem. Don't stick with your physician if you don't have confidence in the information you're being given or in the course of treatment that's being prescribed. Finally, don't continue seeing your physician if you feel that he or she doesn't care about you or doesn't have your best interests at heart.

However, before you start looking for another doctor, carefully examine *why* you want to switch. Are you changing because your doctor doesn't give you the appropriate information at the appropriate time? Are you changing because your doctor doesn't seem compassionate enough? Try to pinpoint the cause of the problem.

After you determine what you don't like about your doctor, attempt to decide if your grievance is valid. Be aware that virtually any person who is diagnosed with lupus will experience anxiety—anxiety that can spill over into the doctor–patient relationship, causing problems. Physicians may not always have the answers. Thus tensions may rise even higher. Is this tension affecting your judgment of your doctor? Or is there, in fact, a real problem that must be dealt with?

If the problem is valid, you have three options. Your first option is to continue seeing your doctor under the present (miserable) conditions. Your second option is to be more assertive and to discuss the situation with your doctor in the hopes of improving your relationship. Your third option is to simply change doctors, either without trying to salvage the relationship, or if your efforts to improve things were unsuccessful.

Obviously, your first option is not a good one. Staying with a doctor who makes you miserable is not going to contribute to your well-being!

The second option, however, is worth considering. Many people find that if they talk to their doctor about their concerns in a constructive, positive way, problems can be ironed out. When this is possible, you may change your mind about changing doctors.

How might you go about approaching your doctor concerning problems in your relationship? Don't try to accomplish this over the telephone or at the tail end of a regular examination. Instead, set up a separate consultation so that you will have the time to sit down and discuss your concerns. Once your doctor is made aware of the problem, you may very well be able to reach a mutually satisfactory solution.

But perhaps you don't feel comfortable approaching your doctor in this way. If you are afraid of being honest—or feel that your doctor simply can't provide you with the care you need—this relationship may not be the one for you. If so, the third option may be your best choice.

Finding a New Doctor

If you decide that you want to look for a new doctor, what factors should you consider? First, you'll want someone highly qualified to treat lupus. (Smart!) But, just as important, you'll want someone with whom you're comfortable personally.

Here are a number of questions you can ask your doctor or yourself about a doctor you are seeing for the first time to determine if this physician is right for you:

- Is the doctor an expert in lupus, and has he or she had a lot of experience in treating people with it?
- How many lupus patients are regularly seen?
- Do patients receive referrals to other specialists when necessary?
- What treatment techniques are used and what types of treatment is this doctor most comfortable prescribing?
- Is the doctor's office located close enough to your home to enable you to visit easily at those times when you're in pain or are having difficulty arranging transportation?
- What are the office hours? Are they convenient for you? How long does it take to schedule an appointment?

- How long will it take the doctor to call you back when you phone with a question? Also, will you always receive a return call from your own doctor or will you sometimes have to talk to an associate?
- What are the anticipated fees? What are the doctor's policies regarding insurance?
- How supportive and cooperative is the doctor's staff? (You may find this question surprising. However, many people change doctors simply because of difficulties encountered with the office staff!)
- Does the doctor seem genuinely concerned about you as a person?
- If you have an interest in complementary or alternative treatments, what is the doctor's opinion (open-minded versus closed-minded and opposed) and knowledge on this subject?
- Is the doctor willing and able to answer your questions in a comfortable and understandable way?
- Does the doctor employ other professionals (such as a nurse practitioner or clinical nurse specialist) who will also work with you?

Of course we all want the perfect doctor—the one with the best credentials, the most experience, the most impressive reputation, and the warmest bedside manner. (And, of course, the office should be right around the corner, right?) But accept the fact that you probably won't be able to find a doctor who meets all of your criteria. Determine what you feel is the most important. For instance, you may be willing to accept a doctor with excellent qualifications whose treatment recommendations are your first choice, even if lacking in bedside manner. Use your best judgment, and make the decision with which you feel the most comfortable.

When You're Seeing Several Doctors

It is possible that, during your treatment for lupus, you may need to consult a physician in another specialty. Remember that your primary physician should be the "hub" of the wheel. He or she will—hopefully—be your advocate in determining which treatments are best for you, both now and in the future. He or she will also help coordinate the efforts of any other physicians who may be involved in your care.

How should you proceed? First, whenever you are referred to someone for the first time, be sure to contact the offices of your present doctors and request that copies of your records be forwarded to the new physician. Then, be sure to take your own personal cumulative, anecdotal records, dating back to the time you began dealing with your condition. What should you have in your records? Include all relevant information about your symptoms. List every doctor that you have seen—along with specialty, address, and telephone number—any diagnoses that have been made and treatments prescribed. Also include a list of all the diagnostic tests that you've received, the dates, and the results. Detail all prescribed treatments, describing the results, including both the benefits and the side effects. Also record any medications prescribed, including the name, dosage, length of time you took them, and side effects, if any. Any other details you feel are important may, of course, also be included.

Keep on updating this information on your computer, so that whenever you see a new doctor, you can quickly produce an easy-to-read copy. As time goes by, this information may prove to be invaluable!

It can be frustrating if there are communication gaps among the different professionals who treat you. Even though some of your physicians may work together and try to keep one another informed, there is always the chance that something will be lost in these communications. Is this a hopeless situation? Absolutely not! When communication gaps exist, either you or, more ideally, your primary physician can become the intermediary—the one who makes sure that each professional involved has all the necessary information.

Many people become uncomfortable when they have to be the "messenger," conveying information from one physician to another. This is even more difficult when the two physicians disagree regarding medication, tests, limitations, or any other component in your course of treatment. If this happens, insist that your doctors consult directly and reach a consensus as to what is best for you. Then you can have more confidence in implementing the agreed-upon treatment.

A Treatment Topper

Your goal in life may not have been to become an expert on lupus. Nor is it likely that your goal was to keep ongoing records of your medical history or to sharpen your communication skills. But you'll find that your efforts will pay big dividends when dealing with doctors—the biggest dividends being greater health, management of symptoms, and an improved ability to cope with lupus.

33.

SUPPORT GROUPS

Jane was having trouble dealing with her lupus symptoms. At her doctor appointment, she emotionally described how hard things were for her, and how no one seemed to understand . . . or care! Her doctor suggested she attend a support group meeting (good doctor!).

Jane's reaction? "Are you kidding? I don't need that!"

This is a common, but surprising, reaction, given how beneficial support groups can be. So what's the story with support groups?

It's so hard when living with lupus if you feel that no one understands, or if you feel different or isolated. Feelings of isolation often have more to do with your attitude than with your disease, your symptoms, the way you're functioning, or any other practical issues. Have you heard the saying, "You can be in a crowded room, and still feel alone"? One of the problems with isolation is that when you feel that way, you may feel less inclined to do anything to try to "fix" it. You feel that this is the way it is, and this is the way it's going to be, therefore why bother. This can hit you between the eyes at virtually any time, from when you were first diagnosed, to anytime during the course of your disease.

Unfortunately, this feeling of isolation is very common—few people really know what you're going through, and you may believe that they really don't have the patience to deal with your experiences, questions, or concerns. This feeling of "disconnect" can be very upsetting, can add to the feelings of isolation, and can even cause depression. But it is up to you how isolated you feel and continue to be. Support groups can be one of the most valuable ways to deal with this and with many other issues involved with living with lupus.

Are your social relationships dwindling? Do you ever feel shunned or ignored by others, or fear feeling this way? Groups can give you a feeling of belonging. There are people that you can be with—people who share a common bond—because they, too, are living with lupus. You'll know that you're not alone. You'll find other people out there who understand what you're going through, and, just as important, are willing to help you to better deal with your own experience with lupus.

Members of support groups all have a common goal: to learn how to live as best they can, and to do as much as they possibly can. You'll see how others handle problems, some of which may be the same as, or at least similar to, your own. Learning how other people cope can be a tremendous source of support, especially if you really want to cope better but are not always sure how to do it. In groups, any topics you'd like to talk about can be discussed. You may begin to share feelings more openly when you hear others talking about subjects you were previously reluctant to bring up yourself. As a result, a feeling of closeness—almost like family—develops.

Many times, members of groups dealing with chronic illnesses discuss feelings of hostility toward the medical profession. A person alone with these feelings may have a hard time dealing with physicians and trusting them. Talking about these feelings in a group can hopefully facilitate a more positive, constructive relationship with the medical profession.

The most important purpose of belonging to a group, however, is the sharing of ideas designed to help you cope. Methods of coping and techniques for helping yourself feel better are shared, suggestions are offered, and social relationships can develop. Participants offer encouragement, coping strategies, resources, guidance, advice, tips, and practical insight, any or all of which can help you live a better life with lupus.

Support groups can have clear agendas or they can be very informal and focus on whatever topics or issues are brought up by the participants. They can be led by a lay person, or by a professional facilitator.

Benefits of Support Groups

There are many benefits from participating in a support group. Let's summarize some of the more important ones:

- You'll feel less alone or isolated. You'll meet people who have "been there, done that."
- You'll get input and advice—answers to questions that you might not get anywhere else. This can be very different from what you may hear from family members, friends, or even doctors. (Remember: We're not talking about medical advice here! Yes, you may get information and suggestions, but professional advice should come only from a professional!)
- You'll find a place where you can be yourself and take as much time as you need to participate in conversation—or simply enjoy participating by being a listener.
- You'll feel safe, because everyone there wants to be there, wants to give as well as receive, and knows that meetings are confidential, so privacy is protected.
- You'll meet people who experience similar manifestations of the disease, or go through similar life experiences or changes because of lupus. It can be very helpful to talk and interact with these people.
- You'll learn from others how to better deal with people who do not know, or are not sympathetic to, what you're going through. This includes how to discuss lupus with family members, friends, colleagues, even your doctor.
- You'll learn more about living with lupus, from others who have walked (or are still walking) in your shoes. This includes the stress of lupus, how it can affect you emotionally, and how others deal with depression, anxiety, or any other negative emotions that can be so debilitating.
- You'll learn to have more control of your life and feel empowered, based on the experiences shared and input from others.
- You'll be participating in a "self-help" group, in which you can learn beneficial coping strategies, ones that have worked for others and can work for you.

- You'll have the opportunity to be honest and open about your feelings and experiences, and you'll feel less of a need to burden, and potentially upset, those who are closest to you.
- You'll get additional information about lupus, as well as recommendations for resources, professionals, or other materials.
- You'll be exposed to a lot of information from people who have gone through this and are happy about sharing. This includes learning more about the symptoms of lupus, dealing with pain and fatigue, medication and its side effects, treatment options, research, and the experiences of others.
- You'll share, share, share (if you want, want, want!).

What Will You *Not* Get from Support Groups?

As wonderful as support groups are, don't expect them to do everything. There are certain things not to expect from a support group:

- *You won't get group therapy.* Support groups are not the same as group therapy, which is led by a professional who uses therapeutic strategies to help participants deal with their own particular problems. Support groups, as you know, involve people with a problem or condition getting together in an informal setting, led by a facilitator, to discuss experiences, and to receive encouragement, compassion, strategies, and support.
- *You won't get a 12-step program.* There are some, by the way, who will tell you the only important step is the *first* step . . . getting there!
- *You won't see and hear only positive things.* You may meet people who have serious symptoms, or significant problems dealing with lupus. Don't assume, however, that you're going to experience the same things. Learn, try to help others, and focus on what you need to help yourself.

Irene had been very reluctant to attend a support group meeting. She was terrified that she would see someone with a serious manifestation of lupus, which would make her even more pessimistic about her own life with the disease. Finally, her husband talked her into it. She walked timidly into the meeting room . . . and the first thing she saw was a woman sitting in a wheelchair. Without looking any further, she turned, grabbed her husband, and ran crying out of the room. What she didn't know, and ended up learning when the support group facilitator talked to her, is that the woman in the wheelchair did *not* have lupus—she was there to accompany her husband, who did! The moral of the story? Don't fear the worst. Take what you see, hear, and learn in stride, and just remind yourself that your goal is to do everything you can to successfully cope with lupus.

Getting Started on Your Support Group Journey

How do you find a support group? Speak to people. Ask your doctor, other health care professionals, clergy, friends, or family members, or even your librarian, virtually anybody you know. Check with local lupus organizations. These organizations bring patients and families together, and provide lots of beneficial information about lupus and its treatment. You may also want to contact sources such as local hospitals or clinics, local schools of psychology, social work, or mental health counseling, religious organizations, or libraries. You can also look for support groups online.

Make sure any group you join is legitimate. You want to make sure they're truly offering support and ideas, and not trying to sell some magical cure. You can have confidence in reputable organizations such as the Lupus Foundation of America or the Lupus Alliance of America. Established national organizations have facilitators who are trained to run groups effectively, constructively, compassionately, and supportively.

Here are examples of some of the questions that you may want answered in deciding to join a particular group:

- Is the primary focus of this group what I need it to be?
- Are the schedule and the location of meetings convenient?
- Is the group professionally facilitated, or peer-led, and am I comfortable with this?
- Will the activities and discussion of the group be confidential?
- Does the group have appropriate ground rules?
- Do the content and focus of the group meet my needs?
- Is the facilitator reachable if I ever have questions or concerns?

It may be hard to obtain answers to all of these questions without attending a few sessions of the group to learn what it's all about. In fact, most good group facilitators encourage participants to come to two or three meetings before making a decision that a group is not for them.

Here are some of the things that may raise a red flag about a particular group:

- Does the group promise to cure your lupus?
- Does the group seem to emphasize the sale of products or services?
- Does the group seem to emphasize "doctor bashing"?
- Does the group require payment of fees?
- Does the group have a leader who often makes strong recommendations that go against your medical professional's treatment protocol?
- Does the group have participants who make you uncomfortable?

Once you decide to join a group, don't feel like you're locked in. The focus and makeup of the group may change, depending on the facilitator and participants, and your need for the group may change as well, if your medical and practical situation changes.

This chapter is primarily focusing on in-person groups. But there are also telephone groups or Internet-based groups. These special support groups can be very valuable if it's difficult for you to get out to a local group, or if there are no local groups available. Internet support groups are not the same as participating in social networking (see Chapter 34). Internet support groups usually involve the same or similar people coming online at the same time to "meet" on a regular basis. Social networks are different in that you're limited to whoever happens to be online when you choose (or need) to be online, and you're exposed to many people in diverse settings.

If you're participating in online support groups, be careful about:

- Revealing personal or medical information.
- Assuming conversations are confidential.
- Providing any personal or financial information that might make you vulnerable to identity theft.
- Being pressured to purchase products or services.
- Aggressive suggestions for you to change your lifestyle, or the people with whom you spend time.

Support Groups for Family Members

Support groups can be as beneficial for members of your family as they can be for you, giving spouses, partners, children, parents, and others a chance to get some support of their own. And since one of the best ways to be in control of your emotions is to have a supportive family behind you, you should most certainly encourage their participation.

Support groups for family members give them the opportunity to learn more about lupus, how it's affecting you, what they can do to help, and how they can deal with their own issues, without it being a burden on you. Unfortunately, there are fewer support groups out there specifically for family members than there are for patients. Keep looking, though. And if you can't find family member support groups for lupus in your area, remember that family members are usually welcome in patient support groups. But you do have three other options: look for family member support groups for other illnesses (there are similarities in coping, after all, and this can be beneficial), look into online support groups, and consider starting your own family member support group!

Some Final Supportive Thoughts

There are many people who believe that the support group is one of the best inventions since the discovery of sunblock! But don't feel that you *must* be in a group. If you're really uncomfortable with the idea, or you really don't think it's necessary because you're involved in other support activities, that's okay. Just make sure that you're honest with yourself. Don't feel that you have to share your emotional reactions with others. It's not necessary to talk them out, despite the potential benefits. But do realize that these emotions need to be recognized and worked through. That's really the only way to make progress.

34.

SOCIAL NETWORKING

One of the most important components of successful coping with lupus is the support that you get from others. Why? Living with lupus is a roller-coaster ride. Physical symptoms, as well as emotional reactions, go through so many ups and downs that it can make you dizzy. Often the support of others can be just the stabilizing force that you need.

When we think of support, we think of the support we get from family and friends. But what if you can't get the support you need from them? Or what if you're tired of burdening the people you know? The previous chapter talks about support groups, such as those run by well-known organizations, and how they can meet a critical need. But what if there are no support groups in your area? Or what if you are less able to get out and meet others? Why might this be? Your symptoms may prevent you from going out. Or you may not have the energy to get out. Or when you want or need to interact with others, you may not find convenient accessibility, to people, places, or time.

What's the solution to this problem? The Internet! The Internet is not only for informational purposes. It is also extremely valuable for social interactions, now called *social networking*. You've heard of Facebook, Twitter, or MySpace, right? Well, these are some of the most popular social networking sites. Let's talk briefly about what social networking is, and then discuss how it can help you cope with lupus.

What Is a Social Network?

Virtually everyone is part of a social network. Anytime you regularly interact with someone—a family member, friend, colleague, neighbor, physician, postal worker, mechanic, or just about anyone else—that person is part of your social network, a group of people who interact with one another because of areas of common interest or concern, or because of their relationships. You already have a social network related to your lupus: the family members, friends, acquaintances, health care professionals, and so on, whom you interact with due to your condition. But what if you want to expand this social network? For example, you might want to interact with more people dealing with similar symptoms or experiences so you can get some additional support, insight, or resources. And what if you are limited as to how many people you can meet? After all, how many people might you meet and get to know in a local lupus support group? Five? Ten? A few more?

Online social networking expands your opportunities to meet more people—exponentially! Now, instead of possibly adding up to a dozen or two new people to your own "face-to-face" social network for lupus, you have the opportunity to meet hundreds, if not thousands, of people who may be helpful to you! This is the power of the Internet! Sure, most of these connections will be less personal, and perhaps more superficial, than those people you spend time with in person. But this is often more than compensated for by the numbers of new people you can meet, and what they can add to your coping experience.

So what are the benefits of social networking for people with lupus? You'll be able to obtain valuable information from others, interact with people, and get support. Questions can be asked and answered, resources can be discovered, and new friendships and relationships can be formed. Social networking brings scores of people right to your desktop (or laptop!). Let's talk about this in a little more detail.

Obtain Valuable Information
from Others

Obtaining information through social networks is very important. Obviously, the ideal source of information about your symptoms and/or treatment is your medical doctor. But what if you want or need additional information? There may be facts that you don't need to get from your doctor, or are unable to get because you don't want to call every time you have a question. Social networking can be an excellent alternative (if used with caution . . . more later).

What are some of the things that you can learn from people online? You might want to learn more about:

- What others look for in a good doctor.
- How others make the most of their doctor visits.
- Experiences people have had with different medications.
- Side effects and how people have dealt with them.
- Health insurance, and other necessities you might need.
- How to deal with disability frustrations.
- How to prepare for an upcoming hospitalization.
- What books others would recommend for you to read.

Everything is not always easy. Be careful of the type and quality of information that you obtain from social networking. Information that comes from other patients, with their own personal preferences or experiences, may seem like strong recommendations for you to try what works for them. You may read information that looks credible, but may be just one person's opinion. Physicians have become accustomed to answering questions from patients about what they have "learned" from social networking. For example, "Dr. Smith, someone told me that their symptoms went away if they ate cereal mixed with orange juice three times a day. Why didn't you tell me that?" (Not true, of course!) Take all information with a grain of cereal.

Interact with People

For some people with lupus (for example, those in a flare, unable to get out, or physically limited), online social networks can be a great opportunity for social interaction. Before the Internet, the only way you could reach out to anybody if you were homebound would be by telephone. Obviously, this seriously limits the number of people you can speak with at a time (unless you're doing a conference call!), and the person you'd want to speak to would have to be available! Now, with social networking, you can connect with many people virtually 24/7.

Social networking can be valuable simply because it provides you with something to do. And you can do it easily in the comfort of your own home, at times of your own choosing. You don't need to follow (or depend on) somebody else's schedule or location.

Get Support

Support through social networking can help with a lot of the feelings of loneliness and isolation that we discussed elsewhere. Not only can you feel encouraged by spending time with others online, you can learn some valuable information as well.

What are some of the beneficial things you can learn from people online?

- How people with lupus deal with family members, friends, work environments, school environments, or any of the myriad issues that people with lupus may experience. There's so much to learn. Isn't it great that you can learn from others' experiences—as well as their mistakes?
- How to communicate better with others (whether it be people with lupus, health care professionals, family members, employers, friends, or colleagues). You'll always be talking to people. Learn how to make it count from others who have been there.

- How to deal with emotional ups and downs. Whether it's depression, anxiety, anger, guilt, or more, others have gone through it, too. Learn what they've done that worked for them.
- How to better comply with your treatment program. The support you get, as well as the accountability you have to others as you connect with more and more people living with lupus, can help you take better care of yourself.

Although these and many other benefits are available to you in face-to-face support groups, it's nice to know that there are many online options available for people who want all of these benefits, but can't take advantage of in-person services. But remember, as often as possible, the availability of social networking, message boards, chat rooms, forums, and other online options, cannot and should not eliminate the need for direct social interactions. Don't let the people you meet online, your so-called "virtual friends," replace or eliminate your effort to enjoy seeing real friends.

Risks

Yes, social networking can be extremely valuable, if used correctly and with care. Once again, though, things aren't always easy. There can be dangers, big ones. Let's discuss some of the most important ones.

HACKING AND IDENTITY THEFT

People have become a lot more comfortable and, as a result, less self-protective, using online sites. Many are more willing to share personal information because they see so many others doing the same thing. Be careful. Be protective of your confidentiality. There may be aspects of your life with lupus that you do not want to discuss with strangers. (Of course, social networking sites often brag that you will become friends with people that you connect with online, so that "strangers" is not a word that they want you to think about regarding their site.) But you have every right to be concerned about privacy and confidentiality.

One of the risks of using social networking sites is that others may take advantage of what you have said and who you are. An example of this is identity theft. Some social networking sites require you to give password information (such as your name, age, and geographical location) in order to join. Many others, though, don't require any personally identifying information. If you give financial information, such as your Social Security number or credit card number, to register on a particular website, a "hacker" or other unscrupulous individual might use it for illegal purposes.

Some sites provide information with no strings attached; there is no obligation, for example, for you to sign up. Others require you to register so that you can gain access to the site or receive information. There may be nothing wrong with doing this. However, make sure that you read any disclosure information provided by the site before you sign up for anything. For example, you want to be assured that your e-mail address will be kept private, confidential, and not distributed anywhere else.

What can you do? Protect yourself. Use caution and common sense. Don't give any personal information unless you're absolutely sure it's safe. Don't give out or share information that you don't want strangers, or even acquaintances, to have—they might be lured into doing something illegal with your information. Change your passwords regularly. The more well known the sites, the more likely that there are identity-theft safeguards in place, but be prepared and be careful.

AN INAPPROPRIATE AGENDA

Make sure the sites you go to are credible. Know where the information comes from, who the participants are, and whether there are any risks associated with these sites. The more highly recommended a site is, the more confidence you can have.

Be aware of social networking sites that seem to be too heavily sponsored by organizations with an "agenda." Although some truly are legitimate, others may have their own ulterior motives (such as building up their own mailing lists to sell materials, or accumulating e-mail addresses to sell to spammers). Be careful!

Some of the sites may have affiliations with health care organizations (such as pharmaceutical companies) that might slant information in their direction. Or if you see a lot of advertising for products that are questionable, or not FDA-approved, think twice about continuing to participate on such a site. An exception: If you are readily able to disregard the advertising and solicitations, or if you like a site because of the information or opportunity to meet far more people than those you might otherwise interact with in your own community, you may decide to stick with the site. But be careful, and be a smart consumer.

FALSE HOPE

Do you find yourself drawn to people who talk about success stories and what they have done to achieve success (for example, "My lupus was cured by . . .")? Yes, this can be motivational, and you may learn some valuable strategies, but be smart about what you read, and, more important, what you believe.

OTHER RISKS

There are many more risks to social networking, such as being stalked by people you don't know, exposure to viruses or dangerous software programs, phishing (scam artists trying to get information from you, such as user IDs or passwords), and other dangers that can be so anxiety-provoking that some people stay totally away from social networking. Just remember: There are tremendous benefits that can come from participating in social networks. But to be able to participate, benefit from, and enjoy social networking, be a careful, cautious consumer, and make sure you minimize your risks. The best motto for dealing with social networks: "It's better to be safe than sorry."

Getting Started

So let's say you want to get into the social networking experience. You want to meet more people and get more support. How do you start?

Start by looking into joining one, or more, of the popular Internet-based social networking websites. They provide a great meeting ground for people who want to share their interests, activities, or just their presence, and are the safest way to get started. The best-known social networking sites are Facebook, MySpace, and Twitter, but there are other popular ones. (See more information about social networking sites in the Websites section of the Appendix.) Some of them have more specific subsites that can help you in your efforts to cope with lupus. And many of the more popular social networking sites have special pages or support groups already established for people with lupus. If you're looking for additional sites and like researching on your own, you can do an Internet search, using Yahoo!, Google, or one of the other search engines, and look up "lupus support groups" for additional links.

Once you've found a site, do some exploring. (There are things to be careful about as you get started. More about this important matter soon.) If the site is a discussion group or forum that has posts (comments) from different people, look to see how frequently new posts appear. It is often preferable to join sites that have more frequent posts and greater interactions. This will help you look forward to responses to your own posts. Sites that have very infrequent posts may be beneficial for information but will be less beneficial to you as an interactive, social networking site.

Look at examples of the types of conversation that occur on a particular site. Consider the types of questions that are raised and, more important, the types of answers that are being given. You'll get a sense if answers are what you like, or "off the beaten path" and possibly too esoteric for your needs.

Some online sites are moderated. This means that there are individuals who monitor the information being posted, in order to verify its accuracy and to make sure it "fits." Although this monitoring does not guarantee accuracy and safety, especially if the moderators are not medical professionals, you can at least have a little more confidence in the information provided on these sites. This, however, should not replace your own efforts at self-protection. Sure, there are often methods to "report" any violations or concerns, but by then it might be too late. Of course, if you are using any unmoderated site, you just have to be that much more careful. If you learn anything that seems potentially beneficial for you, make sure you run it by your doctor.

Approach any new sites slowly. Take your time. Don't feel, for example, that as soon as you join a new site, you must immediately share your entire life story. Start by being a good listener. In other words, read what other people have to say. When you decide you want to step in and start interacting, you may want to mention some very brief information about yourself and then include a question. Often, the responses you get to your initial question will indicate whether or not this is a site you want to continue to visit.

Discuss social networking with your physicians. They may be aware of specific sites that have produced positive experiences, and their comments can help you decide whether to participate in a particular networking site.

Children and the Internet

Years ago, one of the best "nonhuman" babysitting options available for parents was television. Encouraging children to watch their favorite television show enabled parents to do something else while the children were distracted. Children now have other distractions to keep them busy. One of the most popular, despite being controversial, is social networking. More and more children, especially older children, are spending hours of time participating in social networking. In some ways, it can be very beneficial. For example, it can be fun, socially enhancing, and good for shy children as well as children who are living with lupus, who can experience isolation just like adults living with lupus. Remember the importance of peers and friendships during the formative years of childhood and adolescence. If lupus limits the possibilities for friendship, connections through social networking sites can be even more beneficial. But beware. The risks of social networking need to be considered for children as well. Online hackers, predators, and scam artists are lurking out there. You need to protect your children from them. This is an important area of communication between parents and children, and it must be approached carefully. Why? Children may resent parents intruding on their desired activities.

Making the Most of Your Social Networking Experience

If you have attended support group meetings, you may find that many of the ground rules or group "etiquette" for face-to-face support groups hold equally true for online social networks. For example, be pleasant and constructive anytime you are on a site. When you post to an online site, make sure that your posts are concise, constructive, appropriate, relevant, and respectful. Try to make sure that your posts are not lengthy, off the beaten path, inappropriate, irrelevant, unethical, long-winded, or insulting! Hostility toward other people on the site should be avoided. Being selfish, or trying to get everybody to focus on you, is also inappropriate. You don't want to monopolize a site. Sites should truly be give and take. When people become known as takers, others stop wanting to give.

Online sites are often rich in information, and chats often include suggestions. Most people who use these online sites truly are good-hearted souls who want to help. But you usually cannot be sure of another member's identity or agenda. Remember that people who use these sites are there for their own reasons. Even when people are there just to provide support for others, they're still getting something out of it. If they weren't, they wouldn't continue to visit, would they? So make sure that you check out anything that you learn with your doctor. (Yes, I know you've heard this before. But repeating it shows how incredibly important it is.)

The key to beneficial social networking is sharing. Sharing can include both good news and bad news. Sharing can include suggestions and ideas. Everything shared, however, should be carefully considered, rather than blindly followed.

Remember confidentiality. Respect the confidentiality of others, and make sure that you protect your own. Be aware that anything that you post online is now "out there"; anybody can read it and it may stay online forever. If you decide you want to retract something that you've said, you may not easily be able to do so. So if there is something that is private to you, and you don't want strangers to read it (now or in the future), don't post it. Use discretion. And be very careful about identifying yourself or others.

Don't "doctor bash." It can be embarrassing, even risky, to give your opinions about particular doctors. It would be better to discuss what you or others look for in a good doctor than to mention a doctor specifically by name. There may be others who do mention doctors' names (or, for that matter, violate some of the other sensible online rules). Don't let that encourage you to do the same.

There are opportunities online for individuals to interact directly with health care professionals. Of course, be careful about health care advice from a professional who does not know you!

Be aware of how a particular site is being funded. There is a cost to running and maintaining a site. Some sites are funded through advertising. Some may be funded by companies that have something to gain as a result of sites publicizing their information. For example, pharmaceutical companies may host sites to give information about the conditions treated by their medications. Don't feel that you have to avoid these sites, however, because a lot of that information can be very valuable. But you should know what you're getting into. Information about the funding should be clearly posted on the site. You may be more skeptical about posted information if that disclosure is not readily available.

Time to Log Off

It may seem like there's a lot to be concerned about in using the Internet. Actually, you're just being careful, and using good common sense. Keep your eyes open and use good judgment. Approach the Internet with intelligence and caution. Although there are many benefits to be gained by using the Internet, as with anything else, there can be both good and bad. You wouldn't go to a doctor without making sure the doctor had the proper credentials to treat you, would you? Should you? So focus on the best the Internet has to offer, and browse on.

35.

COMMENTS FROM OTHERS

As Ralph Kramden of *The Honeymooners* would say, "Some people have a *BIG MOUTH!*" You may agree with this when you think of some of the comments you hear from people around you. They may know you have lupus, but that doesn't mean they know how to talk to you about it or what to say. They may say things that they feel are true, witty, intelligent, or even sympathetic. But you may think otherwise! There are times when a certain comment might make you want to implant your knuckles into the speaker's teeth! Or a comment might make you wonder if you're talking to a graduate of the Ignoramus School of Tactlessness.

As you now know, you cannot change other people. You cannot make them more sensitive or teach them how to be more tactful. But you can learn to cope with some of the ridiculous comments you hear.

You're probably eager to learn a few coping strategies. But before we discuss the techniques that will help you cope with annoying comments—and the annoying people who make them—it's important to realize that most people say things out of sincere concern. They're trying to find the right things to say; it's with the right intent. They may be trying to make you feel better, to show their support, or to show an interest in you by questioning how you're feeling. However, if you're not feeling good, you may not interpret their comments that way. Despite the good intentions behind these comments, it may not always be possible to respond to them politely and thoughtfully. For example, hearing the same questions over and over can get on your nerves.

Initially, you may try to gently respond to comments and questions, or try to politely change the subject. But this may not always work. That's why it's okay to respond using more humorous comments to the people who frustrate or upset you. It's all about coping, right?

Certainly, some people with lupus avoid unwelcome comments simply by not telling others about their condition. If your lupus is noticeable, however, or you've had it for a while and people are aware of it, certain comments may be directed toward you anyway. For the purpose of this chapter, though, let's assume that we're discussing those comments that you can't avoid, made by people who haven't yet learned to tune in to your feelings. If you've never experienced any comments of this nature, that's great! But read on anyway. You never know when a tip might come in handy!

How Should You Respond?

Many of the things that people say to you may be legitimate comments, but may bug you just the same. Others may not even deserve answers. Still others may be said without any consideration of your feelings. But it doesn't matter why a comment is inappropriate. What's important is that you handle these comments in a way that makes you feel comfortable.

How might you respond to an annoying comment? There are three ways of responding that might work—that is, that might prevent you from getting more frustrated, while making you as comfortable as possible. The first way is to ignore the comment. This is not always easy, especially if the person persistently waits for your answer or seems genuinely insulted by your lack of response. How do you get the person to stop asking, short of buying a muzzle? If you are able to change the subject or walk away, you may get that person to stop asking questions.

The second way of responding is to answer in a rational and intelligent way, explaining how you feel or what you sincerely want to communicate to the other person. This may satisfy the person so that he stops making remarks or asking questions. But now you may feel like you're banging your head against a wall. What if you just can't convince the other person of what you're trying to say? There's a limit to the number of times you can explain something, especially if what you're trying to say isn't being understood or accepted. (And head-banging certainly isn't good for your physical health!)

As you see, you may not always be able to cope by ignoring a remark or responding to it rationally. So what can you do when these two approaches fail? You can respond humorously. Why would this work? Well, if someone says something that is really unanswerable, you'll accomplish very little by ignoring it or trying to reasonably explain your feelings. So you're going to have a little fun with your response, and humorously let that person know that his or her remark may have been somewhat inappropriate. One name for this technique is *paradoxical intention*. Let's use the remainder of the chapter to explore this further.

HANDLING THE "BIG MOUTH" SYNDROME

What might you hear? And how can you handle it? Remember, ideally, the best response is one that will educate the "commenter." You'd like to explain your situation nicely, in a inoffensive, sincere way. But you're only human. So how can you respond when you get fed up? Read on to see how you can answer the unanswerable—without losing your sanity or saying things that you might later regret.

"But You Look So Good . . ."

You've awakened in the morning after a full night's sleep, but you still feel tired. You have a lot to do to get ready for your day's activities, but you don't feel like doing much of anything. Your partner walks into the room and asks you if you are ready to get up. You respond that you're not ready yet; you'd like to rest some more because you feel really lousy. Your partner looks at you and says, "How can you feel lousy? You look so good."

Don't you wish you had enough energy to express how you really feel? One of the hardest parts of living with lupus is that the most common symptoms are pain and fatigue, and neither of them is observable. So when people say that you look good, they really don't know what you're feeling. Anytime that you don't feel well, it can be very frustrating to be told that you look good. This is one of those statements that's hard to ignore, but it's just as hard and impractical to try to explain rationally how you feel. So how can you respond to this statement humorously? You might say, "Yes, I know I look good. You can call my plastic surgeon and thank him." Or you can say, "I know I look good. Now put on your glasses and take another look." Or you can say, "Yes, I look good. Wait until you see me without my mask on." Notice that in all three cases, you are agreeing with the person first, and then you're saying something humorous. You could even say, "Isn't it amazing how many symptoms of lupus I have to live with and still look so terrific?" Isn't that better than saying, "How can you say I look good when I feel so awful?"

"YOU LOOK AWFUL!"

On the other side of the coin, it can be just as upsetting when somebody says, "Wow, you look lousy!" You may feel lousy, but you certainly don't want to be reminded of it. You surely don't want to think that the way you feel is so obvious to others. You'd like to believe that you at least look okay to those around you. Even if it's said sympathetically, this remark may be insulting. So what can you say? You might respond, "Thank you, so do you!" Or, "Good! All my hard work has paid off." Or if you're in a really cynical mood, you might say, "I know I look lousy. That comes from hearing people tell me I look lousy all the time!" Of course, you could always say, "That makes sense, since I don't feel so hot, either!"

"WHY DON'T YOU GET UP AND DO SOMETHING?"

Consider what you would do if you were in the following situation. You're sitting in a chair relaxing because you really feel exhausted and want some peace and quiet. Somebody comes over to you and asks what's wrong. You try to explain that you're feeling very tired and are trying to gather some energy. Obviously trying to show his or her concern for you and to be helpful, the person says, "You're spending too much time thinking about yourself. Just get up and do something. Soon you won't even remember that you're not feeling well!"

How would you react to that? Do you jump out of your chair? Of course not. If you had the energy to get out of your chair, you wouldn't have been slumped there in the first place. Should you sit there and try to explain that you are feeling lousy? No, because this person is obviously convinced that you're feeling fine. So how do you respond humorously? You might say, "I would like to get up, but somebody put fast-drying glue on the chair, and I'm stuck forever!" Or you might respond, "I'm trying to set a Guinness World Record for the most time I can spend in this chair." Or you might say, "Do you know how much energy it takes to remain in the chair, when what I really want to do is to get up and knock your block off?" Obviously, the type of response you use would depend on how angry or irritated you feel.

Remember: For this approach to work best, you want to keep your tone of voice as light as possible. This will show the person making the comment that you're fine, but that you simply don't appreciate what's being said.

"Aren't You Overdoing It?"

This comment implies that others know what "doing it" is all about! They may have their own views of what people with lupus should be doing. Sure, they may care, and not want you to do too much. But whose decision is it? It's hard enough to deal with the physical discomfort of having lupus; it's even harder to deal with the frustration that comes from dealing with people who don't let you do what you feel you can. So how do you handle that? You might respond, "I'd rather be overdoing it than underdoing it." Or, "How about if we talk about understanding instead of overdoing." Or you might respond, "When I hear comments like that I feel as though I'm overdoing our relationship."

"Stop Seeing So Many Doctors"

Let's say that a friend finds out that you have still another doctor appointment, and remarks, "You're just going to too many doctors. Why don't you stop going all over the place and just do what you have to do?" How would you respond to this? You might respond by saying, "No. I'd rather keep going to different doctors until I exhaust my bank account." Or you might say, "I like to go to a lot of doctors. The smell of the antiseptic waiting room excites me!" Or, "Do you realize how many of the doctors' children I'm putting through college?"

"What Did You Do to Yourself?"

Some people are convinced that whenever something goes wrong, it's a result of personal neglect. Let's say you're having a lot of pain in your legs.

As a result, when you try to walk, you're moving much more gingerly and uncomfortably than usual. You meet a friend in the street who says, "What did you do to your leg?" This kind of question usually does show genuine concern, so under some circumstances, you might simply want to explain a little about how your pain is keeping you from walking normally. But if this is the twenty-fourth time you've heard the same question, it may be hard to respond calmly. What could you say that would not be cruel, but which would still allow you to feel better about the way you handled the situation— and hopefully end the question-and-answer session? How about, "This isn't my leg. This is a piece of wood that I borrowed from Home Depot!" Or, "Normally I walk better than this, but I just finished a marathon dance contest." Or you might say, "I'm making a fashion statement." Or even, "I'm injured from kicking people who keep asking me what I did to myself!" This does not suggest that you be unfeeling in your answers. However, if you need to let the commenter know that you don't appreciate these questions, this'll do it!

"You're Not Handicapped—Why Are You Parking in a Handicapped Parking Space?"

One of the problems with not *looking* sick is the angry looks you get from others if you park in one of those cherished spots. Some people believe that anybody who parks in a handicapped parking space must *look* handicapped! It's frustrating to feel that you have to justify your lupus, or justify your need to park in a handicapped space. Sometimes you can just ignore the situation, but sometimes a comment is in order. So what can you say? Depending on your mood, you could say, "I like it here. Smell the fresh air." Or you could say, "Here's my rheumatologist's telephone number; why don't you call to get an explanation as to why I'm parking here?" Or if you're really frustrated, you could say, "You're right, you should probably be parked here, because you're showing you're *intellectually* handicapped by making that comment." Of course, you might simply want to carry a cane with you, even if you don't need it. For some reason, carrying a cane still elicits more understanding and acceptance of a disability than walking without one. (And no, don't use it as a weapon!)

"How Can You Stand So Much Pain?"

In response to this profoundly sympathetic expression of curiosity, you might want to ask, "What pain? The pain in my joints or the pain I get from these dumb questions?" Or you might want to point out other feelings, such as, "I've grown rather accustomed to not being able to move!" Or you might simply say, "I don't stand it. I usually have to lie down!" People will get the message. You may not like the pain of lupus, but at least you're working to cope with it.

"What Happened to Your Face?"

Unfortunately there are times when lupus may cause rashes, some of which may be more visible if they appear on your face. As you now know, the malar, or butterfly, rash is one of the more common symptoms of lupus, especially if you're in a flare. You may not have the patience, however, to explain this to someone who asks that question of you. You might want to respond, innocently, "Gee, I don't know, what happened to it?" Or, you might want to say, while reaching to your face with mock fear, "I don't know, it's still here, isn't it?" If all else fails, you might say, "Whatever happened to my face is nothing compared to what's going to happen to yours!"

"I Heard That _____ Cures People with Lupus"

You may choose to initially respond by saying that you appreciate that they're sharing with you what they've heard. You may want to tell them that if there were such a cure, you're sure that you would've heard about it from your doctor, or at least on a television network's evening news. You might explain that you keep a folder with all of the different ideas that people have shared with you so that you can discuss them with your doctor. If they seem to be waiting for an acknowledgment of how grateful you are for their comments, you can express your appreciation for their thinking of you, and tell them that you will consider what they had to say. But what if your frustration has built? What if people won't leave you alone, or are sarcastic about your lack of enthusiasm about their "cure"? You might respond, "Could you send me an e-mail? I consider all of these ideas every Saturday morning."

Or, if you're really frustrated, you could say, "I've heard that _____ cures people with ignorance. How about if you try it instead of me."

"I Heard That Lupus Is Caused by Stress"

You can provide a medical explanation that stress can exacerbate virtually any medical problem. You could explain that, as part of your treatment program, you're working to reduce your stress. But do you always have to be so straightforward? Of course not! You could humorously respond by saying, "If that's true, why are you stressing me out by telling me that?"

"I Never Heard of Lupus"

How do you respond if somebody says, "I never heard of lupus"? You might say, "Let's forget you even brought it up. Then you can keep your streak going!" Or you could say, "I never heard of it either. How's the weather?"

Remember: You really don't want to hurt the person's feelings by being sarcastic. If the question is a sincere desire for information, then you can try to give them the basics as simply as you can. Some people always have a supply of brochures about lupus with them to give out if it comes up. But you have to be in the mood to do this. If you're having difficulty communicating with someone, try to look at this through their eyes. Ask yourself why they're having trouble communicating with you. Try not to look at it defensively or with anger because of the difficulty you're having with them. This will help you to improve communication.

Should you *have* to explain to others? No, this is never obligatory. It is up to you to choose when you want to say something, and when you don't. Coping with comments from others can be one of the more frustrating things about living with lupus, especially if you just want to be left alone. There are times when being gentle and tactful with others is less important than helping yourself to handle comments without becoming aggravated.

So if someone asks why you sound sarcastic, you can explain that you're not trying to be that way. But the comment you just heard was so ridiculous that you figured the person was trying to be funny. So you decided to have some fun, too! But if the person really wants to know how you feel . . .

OTHER LOVABLE COMMENTS

What are some of the other comments that you may hear? How many of these have come your way? "Is lupus contagious?" "Is lupus a form of cancer?" "Why don't you quit your job?" "You should exercise more!" "Are you sure you can walk up those stairs?" "Go sit in the sun for a while!" "Rest. Don't do anything." "What did the doctor say?" "What are you using that cane for? You're giving in to the disease." "What is the prognosis?" "Wow, have you changed!" "You must miss the way things used to be." "What's the matter with you?" "Can I help you?" "I certainly don't envy you." "If you would eat right, you'd feel better!" "I feel so sorry for you." "Why don't you try my doctor?" "Your having lupus is the worst thing I ever heard!"

IS THAT ALL?

It would fill volumes to include all of the comments that you might hear from "well-meaning" friends or relatives. Hopefully, by reading the previous examples, you've gotten a good idea of how you can respond in a humorous way. Perhaps you'll be able to come up with some additional goodies. Remember that you don't necessarily want to be sarcastic or cruel. Rather, you want to show the speaker that you're feeling well enough to respond with humor and spirit. And you want to show that you can certainly do without this person's "helpful" bits of information and "words of encouragement"!

Perhaps you're thinking, "I could never say those things. It's just not my style." Well, you don't always have to. But you can at least *think* these comments. Even that may help you feel better! And keep in mind that even if you don't want to use this type of response all the time, you may want to use it occasionally—when it seems appropriate for you. As you learn to respond more comfortably to these comments, you'll find that you can handle them more calmly and with less stress. Then you'll be able to minimize the sarcasm and respond with more humorous and enjoyable answers. You'll keep people on your "friend" list rather than on your "you-know-what" list.

Remember, the purpose of this chapter is not to prepare you for the "Mean Person of the Year" award. Rather, it is to give you additional tools to use when you get frustrated at the comments others make about lupus or your symptoms. Increasing your confidence in handling other people is an important goal. You can achieve it by using different techniques like humor, ignoring the individual, offering a brochure, or biting your tongue. And, of course, don't forget how important it is to educate family, friends, colleagues, co-workers, and even health professionals that lupus is a serious disease that affects a *lot* of people.

The Last Word

One of the most common and yet most irritating comments has been saved for last. Imagine somebody who is supposedly sympathetic turning to you with eyes full of compassion and concern, saying, "I heard of someone who died from lupus!" As you turn to walk away, you respond, "I heard of someone who died for telling someone with lupus what you just told me!" You walk away, head held high and a smile on your face, leaving the astonished well-wisher behind you.

36.

CARING FOR SOMEONE WITH LUPUS

A chronic medical condition such as lupus doesn't affect just the person with the disease. It also affects everyone who's close to that person. Those who are in the inner circle are affected most profoundly. They are also in the best position to help the person who is living with lupus. This chapter is for you, the person who lives with, and cares for, someone with lupus.

Illness can create changes in relationships. No kidding! If you live with someone who has lupus, you may have a number of concerns. You may now view that person—and even yourself—differently. Maybe you see that person as being more fragile. Maybe you are reminded of your own vulnerability. You may feel guilty about his or her condition or about your feelings regarding the condition. Maybe you had been dependent on that person, but now you have to shoulder more of the burden. What if you feel anger toward this person, not because of anything that was done, but because of the fact that lupus has created changes? This is normal, but may still produce guilt. Why? Because this anger is directed toward somebody who, at the present time, is vulnerable and unable to defend himself or herself.

What does all this mean? Although you share the concerns of the individual who has lupus, you also worry about yourself. You may also feel concerned about the future and possible financial problems. And while you want to do everything you can to support that person, there may be times when it's very difficult for you to contribute. If you have difficulty dealing with your loved one because of lupus, you're not alone. Illness in a loved one often creates a lot of ambivalent feelings.

The Long Versus the Short of It

If a loved one has an acute problem, such as a heart attack, a specific treatable illness, or a broken bone, it's a lot easier for friends and relatives to rally around and to provide support and understanding, taking over the responsibilities for the patient while rehabilitation and healing are taking place. Sure, there is a period of time when lifestyle has to be reorganized and responsibilities reassigned. But once these changes start to take place, and healing occurs, things can go back to "normal." Life goes on.

But adjusting to a chronic condition such as lupus can be harder than dealing with acute problems, and even many other illnesses, because lupus is cyclical. There are times when your loved one may not be able to do much of anything and you will have to help out. At other times, during remission, for example, the person with lupus can do a lot more, so the family now has to readjust to different roles—roles that may be similar to those everyone had before the diagnosis of lupus. These cyclical changes can create major problems. Because there is no definite time when the patient is going to get better, you may have a difficult time dealing with changes in his or her condition. "This roller coaster is going to go on forever," you may think disgustedly.

How can you cope with problems caused by the chronic nature of lupus? Once again, work on your thinking. Long-range worries lead to long-term unhappiness. So instead of thinking about the future, do what you can each day to support your loved one and to make that person's life and your own as full and as happy as possible. Have faith in your ability to rise to new challenges if and when it becomes necessary to do so.

This chapter offers some suggestions to help you take care of your loved one *and* yourself, as you both learn to cope with lupus. (By the way, throughout this book I have purposely avoided calling the person with lupus a "patient," simply because I believe in emphasizing the person rather than the condition. However, for the sake of convenience and because repeating "your loved one" can become tedious, in this chapter I will occasionally refer to the person with lupus as the patient.)

What Can You Do?

If you are close to someone with lupus, you have an important job on your hands—a job made up of many components, the most important of which is the need to be understanding and supportive. This is very important, whether you live in the same house as the patient or are simply a relative or friend. Remember: People with lupus do not have it easy, but they'll have a much harder time if they feel alone and isolated. So what exactly is your job, and how can you best accomplish it? Read on!

BECOME A LOYAL LEARNER

A great way for you to help is by learning as much as you possibly can about lupus and its treatment. Do you enjoy worrying? You may have unnecessary worries if you don't know things about lupus treatment that the patient does. By understanding the patient's program, you can better provide support and understanding . . . and worry less.

You can help your friend or loved one simply by learning as much as you can about lupus and its treatment. The knowledge you obtain will allow you to provide support and true understanding—both can offer tremendous comfort to a person with lupus. Knowing the facts may help you, as well, as it may reduce your fears of the unknown and help decrease your confusion over symptoms, treatments, and side effects.

KNOW WHEN TO LET GO

As a family member or close friend, it's very important to be attuned to the needs of your loved one. Don't assume that you must be overprotective or underprotective simply because that's the way you would want others to act if you were ill. Be sure to find out what your loved one needs, and try to act accordingly.

Don't smother the person who has lupus. Sure, you want to help. When your loved one is tired, for instance, you can help out by taking over some of his or her chores. Try and anticipate ways that your friend or loved one may need assistance. Be specific in your suggestions and offers. But make sure to give the person enough space to regain control over his or her life. How? When your loved one is no longer tired, be sure to let him or her return to a normal routine. Don't insist that the person rest! Have faith in your special someone. That person will rest when he or she really doesn't feel well. And don't be uncomfortable if your attempt to help is rejected. Leave the door open for helping out another time.

What about accompanying your loved one on doctors' visits? If he or she asks, you may want to go along for the ride. Or at least you can suggest it. As discussed in Chapter 32, it's an excellent idea to have four ears, rather than two, listening when the doctor explains about lupus itself, medication, or other aspects of living with the disease. However, if the person wants to go alone and feels strongly about it, don't try to tag along.

What's the bottom line here? You should work with your loved one to set ground rules. Talk about your interest in being as supportive as you possibly can, and ask what you can do to help. Things will move more smoothly once you know what to do and when to do it. Even if no clear-cut answers emerge, at least you'll have shared some constructive communication. This will help you handle future problems. Perhaps most important—and, possibly, most difficult—try to respect his or her decisions regarding how he or she wants things handled.

ENCOURAGE, DON'T PESTER

There are many ways in which you can help your close friend or family member manage lupus, without being perceived as a "nag." You can show your support by participating in some aspects of his or her treatment program. For example, you can be an "exercise buddy" and jog, walk, swim, or bike along with your loved one. This will help your friend or relative stick to his or her exercise program. It might just do you some good, too! Also, if your diet consists mainly of nutrient-poor, high-fat foods, you may want to modify *your* eating plan—it can't hurt, right? Try choosing nutritious and delicious meals that your whole family can enjoy together. You may even find some new family favorites! This way, your loved one won't feel "different," or believe that he or she is being deprived of tasty foods.

Try to become aware of what can trigger a flare, so you can help your loved one avoid these situations. Let's say, for example, that you have decided to go to the beach. If you know that the person with lupus cannot take sun exposure, don't rub it in. Either don't go, or go without calling so much attention to yourself that he or she feels uncomfortable. By all means, don't say things like, "Oh, why don't you go, you'll be okay!"

Yes, encourage adherence to proper management routines and medication needs. But don't badger. If your loved one is not taking proper care of himself or herself, there is a limit as to how much you can do to change things. Screaming usually doesn't help (and it can hurt your vocal cords!). Should you tell the physician if your loved one is not taking care of himself or herself? That's a hard question to answer. You don't want to overstep your bounds, as this may lead to resentment. At the same time, you don't want to sit back and allow unnecessary problems to develop. This is especially true if your loved one doesn't seem to care.

So what should you do? Play it by ear. Voice your concerns. Explain that you're afraid his or her problems will become worse due to lack of proper treatment. Then listen carefully to his or her response before you contact the physician.

PROVIDE SUPPORT, NOT PITY

Living with lupus can be difficult. You may sympathize with your loved one. The sympathy you feel may help you to provide beneficial support. But going overboard with pity can be destructive.

At times your loved one may be too fatigued to do anything. When this happens, do not insist that he or she "get up and do something." That won't help the situation! Instead, try to help out by taking over some of your loved one's responsibilities. This can reduce some of the pressure that he or she may feel to get things done. At the same time, don't relieve your loved one of all responsibilities. In general, if the person is capable of doing something— even if it takes time—let the person do it. If you feel your loved one is malingering, have an open, honest discussion about this behavior. Your goal is to try to make life as normal as possible for the person with lupus.

MAINTAIN NORMALCY

When spending time with your loved one, try to behave much as you always have. Try to minimize any changes in your interactions. This isn't meant to suggest that you should ignore, through word or deed, that he or she has lupus. As we will discuss later on in the chapter, it's vital to be open about feelings and to honestly discuss any problems. Just try not to dwell on your loved one's condition.

Why is it so important to maintain normalcy? Well, living with lupus is difficult enough. By keeping life as normal as possible, you'll help to compensate for the many changes that must take place, and give your loved one a stronger sense of security.

PREVENT ISOLATION

People with lupus usually have to face many different types of problems. These problems can be even harder to handle when that person feels alone and isolated. Yet, in some cases, even a person with many friends can fear becoming isolated as a result of lupus. Why? Many people may be uncomfortable around someone with a medical problem. As a result, they find every excuse possible to avoid contact, rationalizing this behavior by telling themselves that there are so many people around that they don't have to visit or call. Still others don't intentionally avoid the person with lupus, but they make no special effort to see the person with lupus when symptoms restrict participation in activities.

Fortunately, in your position, you may be able to help. Do what you can to preserve the connection between your loved one and his or her friends and relatives. Speak to those people who seem to have vanished. See if there is anything you can do to reestablish these important relationships.

In some cases, relationships may become stronger than ever. Friends and family members may provide much-needed emotional support, as well as practical help. This is a wonderful blessing. But don't take advantage of others' generosity. Make sure that nothing happens to burn out these invaluable relationships.

KEEP TALKING

What's the best way to talk to your loved one? Unfortunately, because everybody's different and because needs change along with moods and circumstances, there's no way to know for sure. At certain times, you may feel that it's best to respond with sympathy and understanding. At other times, it may be best to ignore the situation and walk away. You'll have to play things by ear, remaining attuned to your partner's needs as much as possible.

However you decide to talk to your special someone, by all means, keep trying to talk! The key to maintaining harmony is communication. Why is this so valuable? Because communication will help you learn how your loved one feels, both physically and emotionally. And you'll be better able to help when you know how he or she feels. This doesn't mean that the conversations will always be pleasant. Talking about pain, other lupus symptoms, depression, or fears isn't very enjoyable, especially if you don't have any solutions. However, the feeling of closeness that results from shared experiences and concerns will overshadow any difficulties.

As much as you would like to talk to your loved one, there may be times when he or she will not be willing to respond. When this happens, it's fine to reassure the person that you're aware of this. You'll be there to listen when he or she is ready and needs a sympathetic ear.

TAKE CARE OF YOURSELF, TOO!

Although you've learned a great deal about coping with lupus from reading this book, so far little attention has been paid to the problems that lupus poses specifically for close friends and family members of the person who is ill. You may experience many of the same emotions and changes in lifestyle experienced by your loved one, but feel more helpless because everything is happening *around* you rather than *to* you. You may experience depression, anxiety, or anger. Or you may feel guilty if you have trouble adjusting to new chores and responsibilities, or a new daily routine. You may find that you are so focused on your loved one that you're neglecting yourself. You may not even be aware that you're doing so because you are so focused. But there are some warning signs to suggest to you that you may be a bit overwhelmed, and need to address this for your own sake:

- Do you usually feel tired?
- Are you feeling irritable, frustrated, and stressed?
- Are you eating properly? Do you notice changes in your eating patterns?
- Are you experiencing significant weight changes, either losing or gaining a lot of weight?
- Have your sleep habits changed? Are you sleeping too much, or not sleeping enough?
- Are you often feeling depressed, apathetic, or less interested in the things you used to enjoy?
- Are you feeling more anxious than usual?
- Have your physical activities changed? Are you getting enough exercise?
- Are you feeling less interest in spending time with other people?

Answering yes to any of these questions suggests that you are experiencing increased stress. Now you have to be aware if living with, or caring for, your loved one with lupus is part of the problem. Does this mean that you have to distance yourself from your loved one? No! Rather, you want to deal with the stress more effectively, so you can be more supportive of your loved one—as well as for yourself.

So what can you do to deal with your stress? Here are some tips:

- Learn as much as you can about stress in general, and specifically the stress caused by living with and caring for someone with lupus, and what you can do about it. Be aware of these warning signs so that you can head them off.
- Don't try to be perfect. No one is. You may feel worse if you try to be perfect and are not. Keep telling yourself that you're doing the best you can.

- You may want or need to ask others to help. Make a list of the things that you have to do. Remove the ones you know are your responsibility, then ask others (particularly those closest to you) if they might be willing to help you with any of them.
- Carve out time for yourself. This is not a luxury; it's a necessity. There should be some time every day where you are doing your own thing. Make sure that the time that you purposely set aside for this is time spent doing something that you enjoy. It can be as simple as resting, reading a book, listening to music, taking a bubble bath, talking to a friend on the phone, or anything else that will recharge you and, ultimately, help you to be a better family member or friend.
- Join a support group. You'll feel less alone, and can gain valuable insight into how to help your loved one.
- Maintain your own health. Don't allow yourself to get run down. Recognize the warning signs before the stress becomes overwhelming. Keep regular doctor appointments, and continue to maintain proper self-care activities.

A Caring Conclusion

True, lupus is not affecting *your* body. But it is certainly affecting you in other ways. There will be times when your loved one needs a helping hand, a sympathetic ear, a shoulder to cry on. Naturally, you want to provide all of this and more for your special someone. But you can't be strong for others if you don't take care of yourself, as well. So remember to take some time out for *you*. Don't feel like you're being selfish by taking care of yourself. Accept that it's okay to feel the way you do, but don't allow the feelings to linger. Change your thinking. Remind yourself that you are doing what you can to help your loved one. Don't forget that you also need—and deserve— nurturing attention. Don't be afraid to reach out and get it. The more you do to take care of yourself, the healthier you will be, and the better you'll be for your loved one.

PART FIVE

Hoping . . . and Coping!

37.

RESEARCH AND CLINICAL TRIALS

L et's talk about hope! The field of lupus research has been growing by leaps and bounds.

Many scientists are trying to learn more about what causes lupus and how best to treat it. Three of the most important areas of research in lupus are the cause, the development and exacerbations of the disease, and new treatments. The goal is not only to learn more about what goes wrong in lupus, but to learn better ways of making it right.

Questions that are the cornerstone of many of the current studies into lupus include: Exactly who gets lupus, and why? Why are 90 percent of the people with lupus women? Why is there such an ethnic disparity in people diagnosed with lupus? Why does the immune system malfunction? What genetic factors are involved and can anything be done about them? Which immune system cells are the primary problem in lupus symptoms? What can be done to control them better? How can medicine more efficiently fix the functioning of the immune system? How can the cells that play a pronounced role in the onset and development of the disease be more effectively targeted? How can the medication that is currently used to suppress the immune system be reduced (since a systemic impact can often lead to other serious side effects)? What new treatments can improve the physical, cognitive, and emotional manifestations of lupus? There are many other questions being explored by researchers. You probably have some questions of your own!

Laboratory studies are focusing on many medical aspects of lupus.

Learning more about genes and the roles they play in lupus, both in onset and exacerbation, is a high priority. Possible genetic defects that may lead to cell malfunction are being investigated. Other genetic problems that may lead to an overproduction or underproduction of cells that are critical in healthy immune system activities are also being explored.

In addition to genetics, scientists are studying other factors that may predispose an individual to develop lupus. Environmental factors are being investigated in order to determine which factors trigger an immune system malfunction that may lead to the onset of lupus, and why the same factors do not trigger that malfunction in others who may also be genetically predisposed to lupus. Research continues to explore the hormonal connection, especially because of the high female/male ratio of people with lupus.

A hot area of research is the search for biomarkers, indicators of disease process, flares, or other critical components of the course of the disease. Research into such biomarkers, examples of which include proteins, enzymes, or other types of molecules, is looking for ways to help physicians treat patients preventively in an effort to avoid flares and resulting tissue or organ damage. It also leads to the identification of symptoms earlier on, in turn leading to more rapid and successful treatment. One area where much biomarker research is taking place is kidney disease in lupus.

Scientists continue to study a number of drugs and treatments that have been effective in helping other conditions or symptoms, but have not received approval from the U.S. Food and Drug Administration (FDA) for lupus. When a medication is used for a purpose other than that specified in its FDA approval, it is said to be used "off-label." Before FDA approval of Benlysta, the only drugs approved for lupus were aspirin, corticosteroids, and Plaquenil; most of the other main medications managing lupus are being used off-label. Examples of off-label drugs or treatments that have been studied are Rituxan (rituxamab) and IVIG (intravenous immunoglobulin).

Research into medications for lupus is moving away from immunosuppressants, and more toward targeted therapies or biologics. Biologic agents that attempt to kill bad cells or block specific parts of the immune system, rather than suppress total immune system function, are being investigated. For example, studies have been targeting, among others, B cells, T cells, cytokines, and type 1 interferons. Some of the new agents are designed for people with mild disease, some for those with moderate disease, and others for those with more severe disease.

The recently approved Benlysta is an example of these new targeted therapies (read about Benlysta in Chapter 10), and its approval has been a "shot in the arm" for the whole field of lupus research.

It is an exciting time! More lupus research is taking place than ever before. You can learn about some of the innovative research taking place online. An example of an organization that has been doing a lot of ground-breaking research in lupus is the Lupus Research Institute. You can read more about their work at www.lupusresearchinstitute.org. Many new drugs are in the pipeline to see if they can be helpful in lupus treatment. And that leads to our discussion of clinical trials, the process by which new medical treatments are investigated using human volunteers.

Clinical Trials

The effectiveness and safety of any new lupus drugs are investigated in clinical trials. These are controlled, scientific experiments in which individuals with lupus participate in the investigation of new treatments. Human clinical trials usually take place after lab research on animals suggests that a new medication may possibly be effective in achieving its goals. The goal of lupus clinical trials is to answer two questions: Will this drug help people with lupus? And, Is the drug safe to take? There are no guarantees of a significant improvement, or even a benefit from the drug being investigated, and there may be some risks, since these treatments have not been approved by the FDA.

A number of treatments are currently being studied in clinical trials. It is possible that by the time you read this book, some of these trials may be discontinued, either because treatments have become FDA approved, or rejected as ineffective. But by then, there will most likely be new clinical trials taking place. So if progress in clinical research is something that interests you, periodically look into the latest clinical trials that are under way.

THE FOUR PHASES OF CLINICAL TRIALS

There are four phases of clinical trials:

Phase 1: These are the earliest human studies on a new drug. This preliminary phase is used to evaluate the proper dosage, and safety, of a new drug. The number of participants involved in Phase 1 is relatively small (often ranging from 20 to 200).

Phase 2: In this phase, safety continues to be addressed. But the primary focus now is whether or not the new treatment is effective. Does it work? Does it do what it's hoped it will do? More participants are included in this phase (often ranging from 100 to 400).

Phase 3: Phase 3 trials take place only after phase 1 and phase 2 have been successfully completed. At this point, the data suggest that the drug is beneficial, and it seems to be relatively safe. Experimentation at this point attempts to demonstrate the benefits and advantages of this drug, as compared to currently existing, approved treatment protocols. In other words, if other treatments work, what about this treatment makes it worth considering? The number of participants usually is in the thousands in this phase. In order for the FDA to approve any drug for treatment, testing must be successfully completed through these three phases, and rigid FDA requirements must be met.

Phase 4: This phase occurs *after* a drug has been approved. Research is now focusing on the long-term effectiveness and side effects of the approved drug.

WHY DO PEOPLE PARTICIPATE IN CLINICAL TRIALS?

Do you like the idea of being in at the beginning of something potentially exciting for lupus treatment? Do you want to play a more active role in your own health care? Do you want to help others by playing a critical role in the development of new treatment methodologies? Are you so frustrated with your lack of progress with existing treatments that you'll jump at the chance of trying something new (even if it hasn't yet been approved by the FDA)?

Are you excited about the idea of free treatment using state-of-the-art methods? These are a few of the reasons people participate in clinical trials. There may even be additional benefits. You may like the idea of working with experts, often in leading facilities, during the trial. You may be paid for expenses associated with your participation in the trial, such as travel expenses, and for your time.

IT'S NOT ALL ROSY!

Because any drugs that are part of clinical trials are relatively new, unproven, and not yet approved, scientists cannot be sure what side effects may occur. They may be significant or unpleasant. And, after all is said and done, the medication may not work as hoped! Rather than looking at this lack of success as a waste of time and being frustrated, it's still an important piece of scientific evidence. Scientists may then try to figure out how to tweak the treatment to make it work, or go back to the drawing board.

Another risk of participating is that you may not even know if you're getting the "good stuff"! Often, in phase 3 trials, a "double-blind" method of study is used. What this means is that neither the researchers, nor the individuals taking the drug, know if they are in the experimental group (in which they're actually getting the drug being investigated), or in a control group getting a placebo "drug" (something that has no medical value at all). In other words, both the investigators and the participants are "blind" as to who's getting which drug. This can be frustrating if you're really hoping that you will get some medical benefits from participating in the study.

Finally, you need to be aware of exactly how much is involved in your participation. For example, you may find that the number of visits you need to make to the clinical site exceeds your scheduling availability. All of this information will be explained to you by the professionals involved in the studies. You need to know all about this before you decide to participate. You have to sign an informed consent agreement to participate. Everything is spelled out in these agreements.

For your added protection, and in order to protect the safety and privacy of all participants, every clinical trial must be monitored by a professional review board. This is an independent committee comprising physicians, nurses, and other members of the research team, to make sure that everything is aboveboard and appropriate.

By the way, keep in mind that just because you decide that you want to participate in a particular clinical trial does not mean you will be accepted. Each study has specific participant characteristics that they are looking for (called *inclusion criteria*) as well as factors that might make an individual inappropriate for the study (called *exclusion criteria*). Factors that may be considered in either of these two sets of criteria include the person's age, gender, ethnic group, symptom manifestation, current treatment, and other medical history.

WHAT DO YOU NEED TO KNOW?

If you've found a study that looks interesting, and you're considering participating, make sure you know as much as you possibly can about the study before going any further. Questions you may want answered include:

- What exactly is being studied?
- What is the purpose of the study?
- What is the composition of the participants in the study?
- What are the procedures, tests, and specifics of the study?
- What are the potential benefits—to you and to others?
- What are the possible side effects and other risks?
- How will the experimental method complement, or interfere with, your current treatment?
- What impact will the study have on your daily life?
- How long will the study go on?
- Will you need to be hospitalized as part of the study?
- Are there any costs that you will have to bear?
- Will you be reimbursed for any of your expenses? (If so, which ones?)
- What kind of follow-up to the study will be necessary?
- What professionals will you be working with?

Many of these questions may be answered as part of the informed consent. But make sure you know what you're getting into, and make sure you've discussed participation with your physician. Once you have signed up for a clinical trial, you can stop at any time. However, a lot of time, money, and resources are put into these clinical trials. So please carefully consider the implications of your possible withdrawal. Of course, all factors should be carefully considered when you're thinking about participating in the clinical trial in the first place!

GETTING STARTED

If you're interested in learning more about clinical trials, what do you do? You'll have to do some leg work to find ongoing clinical trials, but the information is out there. There are so many trials going on these days that there could very well be something being investigated not far from your home. A good starting point would be to speak to your physicians, check with major hospitals in your area, or call a local chapter of the lupus organizations near you. You can also obtain extensive information on clinical trials, including an up-to-date list of lupus trials at www.lupustrials.org. Much more information is available at the FDA website (www.FDA.gov). As with just about everything else, make sure you discuss all of this with your physician!

A Research Recap

Perhaps by the time you read this, some drug or treatment may have proven itself to be more successful than ones currently available. It remains to be seen which new developments can improve your life with lupus. But at least people are working on the problem. It's nice to know that research continues to investigate ways of learning more about lupus and improving the effectiveness of treatment.

38.

A COPING REVIEW

Well, you've just about finished this book. We've covered a lot of information about lupus. Hopefully, you're already coping better and living well! People who are doing the best job of living well with lupus are those people who concentrate on what they can do and what their abilities currently are. This is so much more effective than dwelling on what they used to be able to do, and may currently be unable to do.

Research and experience have shown that the people who cope best with lupus have certain qualities in common. See how many of these apply to you. And then work to make them part of who you are!

You may be coping well with lupus if:

- You try to always be hopeful. Having hope enhances a positive attitude.
- You are able to constructively and beneficially deal with your emotions.
- You keep going. You persist and persevere. You accept the inevitable obstacles that befall you. You accept that some things have changed, but focus on what you still have, and what can make it better.
- You spend more time focusing on ways that you can improve your life with lupus rather than just accepting the status quo.
- You think outside the box. You are a creative problem-solver, always looking for a solution. You believe that a problem or obstacle is not necessarily personal.

- You are your own best advocate. You do the things you need to do to help yourself. You are an active participant in treatment.
- You have a good relationship with your doctor and other health care providers, are able to reach out when you need to, and won't hesitate to ask questions when necessary.
- You consistently follow the medical treatment program that has been prescribed for you, including medication and other components.
- You are assertive rather than passive. You speak up when you need to, rather than letting other people tell you what to do without any response.
- You are a person who has lupus, rather than a lupus patient, or, even worse, a victim.
- You believe that having lupus does not mean that you are sick. It means that your body is not running as smoothly as it should, or as you would like. You will continue to still live the best life you can live.
- You acknowledge that there may be limitations imposed upon you with lupus, and you deal with them effectively.
- You don't consider yourself sick unless you are in bed, unable to move or think. Other than that, you consider yourself like most other people in the world, able to function, with a few obstacles to deal with and adjustments to make.
- You focus on what is in your world, rather than what isn't.
- You try to minimize those unpleasant or energy-draining situations in your life.
- You accept the fact that you have lupus more than you try to deny it.
- You accept yourself as you are, rather than always wishing to be someone else. Self-acceptance helps you to better deal with the lack of understanding from others. You don't need validation from others to feel good about who you are.
- You believe in yourself, that you are just as capable as the next person in doing whatever needs to be done.
- You communicate effectively. Lack of communication increases feelings of isolation. Communicating increases the support that you can receive, and minimizes misunderstandings.
- You look for ways not only to improve your own life, but to pass this along to others.

- You have a strong support network of people you can lean on when you need to and can enjoy when leaning is not necessary. These support people have your trust, for you can always tell them the truth, guide them, point out their mistakes, and help them stay focused.
- You are able to reach out and ask others for help.
- You're able to talk to somebody when you feel the need.

Of course, you may be having difficulty coping if:

- You've lost interest in things you used to enjoy.
- You're not as interested in spending time with friends.
- Being with others is seen more as drudgery than stimulating.
- Your mood seems to be fluctuating more than normal.
- Your energy has decreased.
- It's hard for you to experience pleasure.
- You're feeling more tired than usual.
- You're not taking care of yourself.
- You notice changes in your appetite.
- You notice changes in your sleep patterns.
- You're consistently feeling emotionally down.
- You feel apologetic and guilty more than usual.
- You have difficulty with your thinking, concentrating, decision-making, memory, or other cognitive functions.
- You often feel agitated, frustrated, or angry.
- You feel worthless and helpless.
- Your former optimism has given way to pessimism.
- You have major concerns about the future.
- You are sad and may even cry too often.
- You feel out of control.

There are other indicators for coping problems as well. And, of course, there may be other explanations for these changes. Some of them may be direct physiological consequences of the lupus itself. But you're the one who knows best how you're feeling. You'll know, therefore, if you want to work on these things to improve your coping ability. If any of these apply to you, it's time to go back to the relevant sections or chapters of this book so you can resume being a "successful coper."

Some people consider coping to be an act of resignation. They feel it suggests that there's nothing you can do about the problem, therefore you might as well resign yourself to the fact that you have it. But coping is far from an act of resignation. It is a very positive, constructive, proactive way of dealing with your circumstances.

Not an Ending . . . a Beginning!

Although it would be impossible to include in this book every possible problem that might be caused by lupus, I hope that what you've read will help you develop your own strategies for coping. Because things change and something that troubles you one day may not trouble you the next (and vice versa), you can use this book as a resource. Whenever you have questions about how to cope with a certain aspect of lupus, consult these pages. If you have any comments—information you feel is important—or additional questions, feel free to write to me at the following e-mail address: drphillips@ coping.com. I'd be happy to hear from you.

I continue to hope that within the near future, research will discover a cure for lupus. Then, this book, along with any other book or article written on the subject, could happily be thrown into a shredder. I look forward to a day when it is no longer needed because lupus no longer exists.

And so, as I said at the very beginning of the book, until such time as there is no longer a medical condition called lupus, keep on coping the best you can. Look brightly ahead, act proudly, and enjoy life as best you can. Remember that despite lupus, you can *always* improve the quality of your life!

APPENDIX

For Further Reading

The following books written for consumers may help you cope better with various aspects of living with lupus. They provide more information on the material presented in this book and focus on other topics, as well. But by no means should you limit yourself to the books listed below. Many other publications also examine lupus treatment, the challenges of living with chronic illness, exercise, nutrition, and other subjects that may be of interest to you. Don't hesitate to take advantage of all the information available at your local library or bookstore, from professional associations and support groups, and on the Internet.

BOOKS SPECIFICALLY ABOUT LUPUS

Aladjem, H. *Challenges of Lupus: Insights and Hope.* New York: Avery, 1999.

Blau, S., and D. Schultz. *Living with Lupus: The Complete Guide*, 2nd ed. Cambridge, Mass.: Da Capo Press, 2004.

Butler, B. *The Monster Under the Bed.* St. Louis: Lupus Foundation of America, Missouri Chapter, 1989.

Del Rio, A. *Lupus: A Patient's Guide to Diagnosis, Treatment, and Lifestyle.* Munster, Ind.: Hilton, 2007.

Dibner, R., and C. Coleman. *Lupus Handbook for Women: Up-to-Date Information on Understanding and Managing the Disease Which Affects 1 in 500 Women.* New York: Simon & Schuster, Fireside, 1994.

DiGeronimo, T. *New Hope for People with Lupus.* New York: Random House, Prima, 2002.

Gorman, S. *Despite Lupus: How to Live Well with a Chronic Illness.* Four Legged Press, 2009.

Hanger, N. *The First Year—Lupus: An Essential Guide for the Newly Diagnosed.* New York: Marlowe, 2003.

Lahita, R., and R. Phillips. *Lupus Q&A: Everything You Need to Know.* New York: Avery, 2004.

Moore, S. *Lupus: Alternative Therapies That Work.* Rochester, Vt.: Healing Arts Press, 2000.

O'Loughlin, W. *What's Lupus, Mama?* CreateSpace, 2010.

Phillips, R. *Control Your Pain: 144 Sure-Fire Strategies for Reducing the Pain of Lupus.* Balance, 1996.

―――. *Living Well . . . Despite Lupus! 204 Sure-Fire Techniques for Taking Charge of Your Life.* Balance, 1996.

―――. *Successful Living with Lupus: An Action Workbook,* rev. ed. Balance, 2005.

Pratt, M., and D. Hallegua. *Taking Charge of Lupus: How to Manage the Disease and Make the Most of Your Life.* New York: New American Library, 2002.

Wallace, D. *The Lupus Book,* 4th ed. New York: Oxford University Press, 2009.

Books About Related Topics

Donoghue, P., and M. Siegel. *Sick and Tired of Feeling Sick and Tired.* New York: W. W. Norton, 2000.

Fennell, P. *The Chronic Illness Workbook: Strategies and Solutions for Taking Back Your Life.* Oakland, Calif.: New Harbinger, 2001.

Joffe, R., and J. Friedlander. *Women, Work, and Autoimmune Disease—Keep Working, Girlfriend!* New York: Demos Medical Publishing, 2008.

Kushner, H. *When Bad Things Happen to Good People.* New York: Anchor, 2004.

Lahita, R. *Women and Autoimmune Disease: The Mysterious Ways Your Body Betrays Itself.* New York: Regan Books, 2005.

Lockshin, M. *Guarded Prognosis: A Doctor and His Patients Talk About Chronic Illness and How to Cope With It.* New York: Hill & Wang, 1998.

Northrup, C. *Women's Bodies, Women's Wisdom: Creating Physical and Emotional Health and Healing.* New York: Bantam Books, 1994.

Pitzele, S. *We Are Not Alone.* New York: Workman, 1986.

Pollin, I. *Taking Charge: Overcoming the Challenges of Long-Term Illness.* New York: Times Books, 1994.

Spero, D. *The Art of Getting Well.* Berkeley, Calif.: Hunter House, 2002.

Books Related to Part Two

Achterberg, J., B. Dossey, and L. Kolkmeier. *Rituals of Healing: Using Imagery for Health and Wellness.* New York: Bantam Books, 1994.

Anderson, J. *Alternative Medicine: The Definitive Guide.* New York: Celestial Arts, 2002.

Balch, P. *Prescription for Nutritional Healing,* 5th ed. New York: Avery, 2010.

Bauer, J. *The Complete Idiot's Guide to Total Nutrition.* New York: Penguin, 2003.

Challem, J. *No More Fatigue: Why You're So Tired and What You Can Do About It.* Hoboken, N.J.: John Wiley & Sons, 2011.

Clever, L. *The Fatigue Prescription: Four Steps to Renewing Your Energy, Health and Life.* Berkeley, Calif.: Viva Editions, 2010.

Fanning, P. *Visualization for Change.* Oakland, Calif.: New Harbinger Press, 1994.

Friedberg, F. *Fibromyalgia & Chronic Fatigue Syndrome: Seven Proven Steps to Less Pain and More Energy.* Oakland, Calif.: New Harbinger, 2006.

Gliksman, Y. *Biofeedback. You Are In Control.* Lulu, 2008.

Kassan, S. *Chronic Pain for Dummies.* Hoboken, N.J.: John Wiley & Sons, 2008.

Lavin, J. *Special Kids Need Special Parents: A Resource for Parents of Children with Special Needs.* New York: Berkley Books, 2001.

Lazarus, A. *In the Mind's Eye.* New York: Guilford, 1984.

Lehman, T. *It's Not Just Growing Pains: A Guide to Childhood Muscle, Bone, and Joint Pains, Rheumatic Diseases, and the Latest Treatments*. New York: Oxford University Press, 2004.

Napier, K. *Power Nutrition for Your Chronic Illness: A Guide to Shopping, Cooking and Eating to Get the Nutrition Edge*. New York: Perseus, 2000.

Reinagel, M. *Nutrition Diva's Secrets for a Healthy Diet*. New York: St. Martin's Press, 2011.

Rossman, M. *Guided Imagery for Self-Healing*. Tiburon, Calif.: HJ Kramer, 2000.

Taylor, S., and R. Epstein. *Living Well with a Hidden Disability*. Oakland, Calif.: New Harbinger, 1999.

Teitelbaum, J. *From Fatigued to Fantastic!* New York: Avery, 2007.

Turk, D., and F. Winter. *The Pain Survival Guide: How to Reclaim Your Life*. Washington, D.C.: American Psychological Association, 2005.

Wallace, D., and J. Wallace. *All About Fibromyalgia: A Guide for Patients and Their Families*. New York: Oxford University Press, 2002.

Willet, W. *Eat, Drink, and Be Healthy*. New York: Free Press, 2005.

Wolf, P. *I Still Dream Big: Stories of Teens Living with Chronic Illness*. Bloomington, Ind.: Author-House Press, 2010.

Zukerman, E., and J. Ingelfinger. *Coping with Prednisone and Other Cortisone-Related Medicines: It May Work Miracles, but How Do You Handle the Side Effects?* New York: St. Martin's Press, 1997.

Books Related to Part Three

Burns, D. *Feeling Good: The New Mood Therapy*. New York: Harper, 1999.

McLaren, K. *Language of Emotions: What Your Feelings Are Trying to Tell You*. Boulder, Co.: Sounds True Inc., 2010.

Meyer, J. *Managing Your Emotions: Instead of Your Emotions Managing You*. Fenton, Mo.: Warner Books, 1997.

Orloff, J. *Emotional Freedom: Liberate Yourself From Negative Emotions and Transform Your Life*. New York: Three Rivers Press, 2009.

Spradlin, S. *Don't Let Your Emotions Run Your Life*. Oakland, Calif.: New Harbinger, 2003.

Books Related to Part Four

Agnew, P. *How to Talk to Your Doctor: Getting the Answers and Care You Need*. Sanger, Calif: Linden, 2006.

Donoghue, P., and M. Siegel. *Are You Really Listening? Keys to Successful Communication*. Notre Dame, Ind.: Sorin Books, 2005

Gottman, J., and J. DeClaire. *The Relationship Cure: A 5 Step Guide to Strengthening Your Marriage, Family and Friendships*. New York: Three Rivers Press, 2001.

Matthews-Simonton, S., and R. Shook. *The Healing Family*. New York: Bantam Books, 1984.

Porter, R. *Coping with a Loved One's Disease: A Guide for Caregivers*. Port Orchard, Wash.: Windstorm Creative, 2005.

Books Related to Part Five

Hackshaw, A. *A Concise Guide to Clinical Trials*. Hoboken, N.J.: BMJ Books, 2009.

Speid, L. *Clinical Trials: What Patients and Volunteers Need to Know*. New York: Oxford University Press, 2010.

Resource Organizations

There are many organizations that can provide you with more information on lupus or related conditions or diseases, as well as suggest helpful books and videos, direct you to support groups, and inform you of other valuable services. The following groups are representative of many of the resources that are available to you online. Feel free to contact these organizations and benefit from their expertise.

NATIONAL LUPUS ORGANIZATIONS

Lupus Alliance of America
3871 Harlem Rd.
Buffalo, NY 14215
866-415-8787
www.lupusalliance.org

Lupus Foundation of America, Inc.
2000 L St., N.W., Suite 410
Washington, DC 20036
202-349-1155 or 800-558-0121
www.lupus.org

LUPUS RESEARCH

Alliance for Lupus Research
28 West 44th St., Suite 501
New York, NY 10036
212-218-2840 or 800-867-1743
www.lupusresearch.org

Dorough Lupus Foundation
P.O. Box 11069
Palm Bay, FL 32911
321-474-2346
www.doroughlupusfoundation.org

Lupus Research Institute
330 Seventh Ave., Suite 1701
New York, NY 10001
212-812-9881
www.lupusresearchinstitute.org

REGIONAL LUPUS ORGANIZATIONS

Many such organizations exist; only the larger ones are included.

Lupus Foundation of Mid and Northern
   New York
P.O. Box 139
Utica, NY 13503
315-829-4272
www.nolupus.org

Lupus Foundation New England
40 Speen St., Suite 205
Framingham, MA 01701
508-872-5200
www.lupusne.org

Lupus Foundation of Northern California
2635 North First St., Suite 206
San Jose, CA 95134
408-954-8600
www.lfnc.org

Lupus LA
8383 Wilshire Blvd.
Beverly Hills, CA 90211
310-657-LOOP (5667)
www.lupusla.org

S.L.E. Lupus Foundation
330 Seventh Ave., Suite 1701
New York, NY 10001
212-685-4118 or 800-74-LUPUS
www.lupusny.org

INTERNATIONAL LUPUS ORGANIZATIONS

Lupus Australia, Queensland, Inc.
P.O. Box 974
Kenmore, Queensland 4069
07 38789553
www.lupus.com.au

Hope Foundation (Barbados)
www.hopefoundationbarbados.org

Lupus Canada
3555 14th Ave., Unit #3
Markham, Ontario L3R 0H5
905-513-0004 or 800-661-1468
www.lupuscanada.org

European Lupus Erythematosus Federation
(ELEF)
44 1708 73 12 51
www.lupus-italy.org/elef/index.html

Lupus Europe
www.lupus-europe.org

Lupus Trust of New Zealand
P.O. Box 249
Silverdale, Auckland, NZ 0944
09-817-2060
www.lupus.org.nz

Lupus UK
St James House
Eastern Road
Romford, Essex RM1 3NH, UK
44-0-1708-731251
www.lupusuk.org.uk

RELATED ORGANIZATIONS

Abilities! National Center for Disability
Services
201 I.U. Willets Road
Albertson, NY 11507
516-465-1400 or 516-747-5400
www.ncds.org

American Association of Kidney Patients
3505 East Frontage Rd., # 315
Tampa, FL 33607
800-749-2257
www.aakp.org

American Autoimmune Related Diseases
Association (AARDA)
22100 Gratiot Ave.
East Detroit, MI 48021
586-776-3900 or 800-598-4668
www.aarda.org

American College of Rheumatology
2200 Lake Blvd. NE
Atlanta, GA 30319
404-633-1870
www.rheumatology.org

American Diabetes Association
1701 North Beauregard St.
Alexandria, VA 22311
800-DIABETES (800-342-2383)
www.diabetes.org

American Hair Loss Council
30 South Main
Shenandoah, PA 17976
www.ahlc.org

American Heart Association
National Center: 7272 Greenville Ave.
Dallas, TX 75231
800-242-8721
www.heart.org

American Liver Foundation
39 Broadway, Suite 2700
New York, NY 10006
212-668-1000
www.liverfoundation.org

American Lung Foundation
1301 Pennsylvania Ave. NW, Suite 800
Washington, DC 20004
202-785-3355
www.lungusa.org

American Thyroid Association
6066 Leesburg Pike, Suite 550
Falls Church, VA 22041
703-998-8890
www.thyroid.org

APS Foundation of America (Antiphospho-
     lipid Syndrome)
P.O. Box 801
LaCrosse, WI 54602
www.apsfa.org

Arthritis Foundation
1330 W. Peachtree St.
Atlanta, GA 30309
404-872-7100 or 800-283-7800
www.arthritis.org

Asthma and Allergy Foundation of America
8201 Corporate Dr., Suite 1000
Landover, MD 20785
800-727-8462
www.aafa.org

Celiac Disease Foundation
13251 Ventura Blvd., Suite 1
Studio City, CA 91604
818-990-2354
www.celiac.org

Chronic Fatigue & Immune Dysfunction
     Syndrome Association of America
P.O. Box 220398
Charlotte, NC 28222-0398
704-365-2343
www.cfids.org

Crohn's & Colitis Foundation of America
386 Park Ave. South, 17th Floor
New York, NY 10016
800-932-2423
www.ccfa.org

Eyecare America
415-447-0385
www.eyecareamerica.org

Fibromyalgia Network
P.O. Box 31750
Tucson, AZ 85751-1750
520-290-5508 or 800-853-2929
www.fmnetnews.com

Food and Drug Administration
Office of Dietary Supplements
301-827-6242
www.fda.gov

Headcovers Unlimited (Hair)
214 S. Iowa Ave.
League City, TX 77573
800-264-4287
www.headcovers.com

The Kidney School
608-833-8033
www.kidneyschool.org

Kidney Transplant/Dialysis Association, Inc.
P.O. Box 51362 GMF
Boston, MA 02205-1362
781-641-4000
www.ktda.org

Lighthouse International
111 East 59th St.
New York, NY 10022-1202
212-821-9200
www.lighthouse.org
www.lighthouse.org/about-low-vision
  -blindness/amsler-grid

Macular Degeneration Partnership
6222 Wilshire Blvd., Suite 260
Los Angeles, CA 90048
310-623-4466
www.amd.org

National Center for Complementary and
  Alternative Medicine (NCCAM)
888-644-6226
www.nccam.nih.gov

National Family Caregivers Association
10400 Connecticut Ave., Suite 500
Kensington, MD 20895-3944
800-896-3650
www.nfcacares.org

National Fibromyalgia Association
2121 South Towne Centre, Suite 300
Anaheim, CA 92806
714-921-0150
www.fmaware.org

National Foundation for Celiac
  Awareness (NFCA)
224 South Maple St.
Ambler, PA 19002
215-325-1306
www.celiaccentral.org

National Headache Foundation
820 N. Orleans, Suite 411
Chicago, IL 60610
312-274-2650
www.headaches.org

National Hypertension Association, Inc.
324 East 30th St.
New York, NY 10016
212-889-3557
www.nathypertension.org

National Institute of Arthritis and
  Musculoskeletal and Skin Diseases
  (NIAMS)
1 AMS Circle
Bethesda, MD 20892-3675
301-495-4484 or 877-22-NIAMS
www.niams.nih.gov

National Institute of Neurological Disorders
  and Stroke
P.O. Box 5801
Bethesda, MD 20824
800-352-9424
www.ninds.nih.gov

National Kidney Foundation
30 East 33rd St.
New York, NY 10010
800-622-9010
www.kidney.org

National Library Service for the Blind and
  Physically Handicapped (Eyes)
Library of Congress
Washington, DC 20542
202-707-5100

National MS Society
733 Third Ave., 3rd Floor
New York, NY 10017
800-344-4867
www.nationalmssociety.org

National Organization for Rare Disorders
P.O. Box 1968
55 Kenosia Ave.
Danbury, CT 06813-1968
203-744-0100
www.rarediseases.org

National Osteoporosis Foundation
1150 17th St. NW, Suite 850,
Washington, DC 20036
202-223-2226
www.nof.org

National Pain Foundation
300 East Hampden Ave., Suite 100
Englewood, CO 80113
866-590-PAIN
www.nationalpainfoundation.org

National Sleep Foundation
1010 N. Glebe Rd., Suite 310
Arlington, VA 22201
202-347-3471 or 703-243-1697
www.sleepfoundation.org

National Stroke Association
9707 E. Easter Lane, Suite B
Centennial, CO 80112
800-787-6537
www.stroke.org

National Women's Health Information Center
U.S. Dept. of Health & Human Services
800-994-9662
www.womenshealth.gov/contact/faq.cfm

Patient Alliance for Neuroendocrineimmune
Disorders Organization for Research &
Advocacy, Inc.
255 Alhambra Circle, #715
Coral Gables, FL 33134
305-441-1591
www.pandoranet.info

Platelet Disorder Support Association
133 Rollins Ave., #5
Rockville, MD 20852
877-528-3538
www.pdsa.org

Raynaud's Association, Inc.
94 Mercer Ave.
Hartsdale, NY 10530
800-280-8055
www.raynauds.org

Renal Support Network
1311 North Maryland Ave.
Glendale, CA 91207
Hopeline: 800-579-1970 or
        866-903-1728
www.rsnhope.org

Scleroderma Foundation
300 Rosewood Dr., Suite 105
Danvers, MA 01923
978-463-5843 or 800-722-HOPE
www. scleroderma.org

Service Dogs America
P.O. Box 29
HVNP, HI 96718
808-291-0429
www.servicedogsamerica.org

Sjögren's Syndrome Foundation
6707 Democracy Blvd., Suite 325
Bethesda, MD 20817
301-530-4420 or 800-475-6473
www.sjogrens.org

Social Security Administration
800-772-1213
www.ssa.gov

United Network for Organ Sharing
700 North 4th St.
Richmond, VA 23219
888-894-6361
www.unos.org

Websites

There are so many websites that have information for people with lupus that to list them all would be longer than the rest of the book. So instead, in each category below you'll see some suggestions for websites that may be helpful. Remember, by the time you read this and try to reach the websites, some of them may no longer exist, and there may be many new ones. As always, use discretion in what you read, what you believe, and how you use the provided information.

LUPUS INFORMATION

Could I Have Lupus?
www.couldihavelupus.gov; 800-994-9662

Healing Well Community Support Resources
www.healingwell.com/lupus

Lupus Guide
www.informationonlupus.com

Lupus Guild: Improving Awareness About Lupus
www.lupusguild.org

The Lupus Network, Inc.
www.thelupusnetwork.org; 708-263-5720

ProHealth: Commerce with Compassion
www. prohealth.com/lupus; 800-366-6056

The US in Lupus
www.usinlupus.com; 855-874-6587

World Lupus Day
www.worldlupusday.org

GENERAL INFORMATION (ADULTS AND CHILDREN)

American Chronic Pain Association
www.theacpa.org

Americans with Disabilities Act
www.usdoj.gov/crt/ada; 800-514-0301

The Center for Children with Special Needs
http://www.cshcn.org/; 206-884-5735

Disaboom: Information and Resources for People with Disabilities
www.disaboom.com

Dry.Org—Internet Resources for Sjögren's Syndrome
www.dry.org

International Association for Medical Assistance to Travelers
www.iamat.org; 716-754-4883

Kids Health
www.kidshealth.org

National Institute of Allergy and Infectious Diseases (NIAID)
www.niaid.nih.gov

National Center for Medical Home Implementation
www.medicalhomeinfo.org/for_families/care_notebook

National Dissemination Center for Children with Disabilities
www.nichcy.org; 800-695-0285

National Women's Health Information Center
www.womenshealth.gov/faq/lupus.cfm; 800-994-9662

Nemours—A Children's Health System
www.nemours.org
10140 Centurion Parkway, Jacksonville, FL 32256
904-697-4100 (Corporate); Locations in: DE, FL, NJ, PA

Our Kids: Devoted to Raising Kids Special Kids with Special Needs
www.our-kids.org

Pacer Center: Champions for Children with Disabilities
www.pacer.org

Pain.com: Your Pain Management Resource
pain.com

Starbright World
www.starbrightworld.org

Stop Chronic Disease
stopchronicdisease.com

Teens Health
teenshealth.org/teen

University of Maryland Health System: Your Child: Development & Behavior Resources
www.med.umich.edu/yourchild

U.S. Pain Foundation
www.uspainfoundation.org

WebMD
www.webmd.com

SOCIAL NETWORKING

The most popular social networking services in the world are:

>   Facebook (www.facebook.com)
>   Twitter (www.twitter.com)

After these sites, the most popular in the United States are:

>   LinkedIn (www.linkedin.com)
>   MySpace (www.myspace.com)

According to Wikipedia, among the most popular social networking services in other parts of the world are:

>   Orkut and Hi5 in South America and Central America
>   Nexopia (mostly in Canada)
>   Friendster, Mixi, Multiply, Orkut, Wretch, renren and Cyworld (Asia and the Pacific Islands)
>   Twitter, Facebook, Orkut, and LinkedIn (India)
>   Decayenne, Tagged, XING, Badoo, and Skyrock (in parts of Europe)

StudiVZ (mostly in Germany)
iWiW (mostly in Hungary)
Bebo, VKontakte, Hi5, Hyves (mostly in the Netherlands)
Nasza-Klasa (mostly in Poland)
Tuenti (mostly in Spain)

HEALTH AND OTHER NETWORKING

Care Pages
www.carepages.com

Chronic Chick Talk, Life with Lupus & Fibromyalgia
www.chronicchicktalk.com

Daily Strength
www.dailystrength.org/c/Lupus/support-group

DxLupus
www.DxLupus.org

The Free Library
www.thefreelibrary.com

Healing Well, Community Support Resources
www.healingwell.com/lupus

The Health Care Blog
www.thehealthcareblog.com

Imedix: Health Information, Medical Questions & Patient Community
www.imedix.com

Inspire: Autoimmune Diseases Support Group
www.inspire.com/groups/autoimmune-diseases

Inspire: Lupus Support Group
www.inspire.com/groups/lupus

Kids Health
www.kidshealth.org

MD Junction: Online Support Groups
www.www.mdjunction.com/lupus

Starbright World: Share Connect Support
www.starbrightworld.org

Stop Chronic Disease
www.stopchronicdisease.com

Teens Health
www.teenshealth.org/teen

We Have Lupus
www.forum.wehavelupus.com/forum.php

SUN-PROTECTIVE CLOTHING
www.coolibar.com
www.exofficio.com
www.LLBean.com
www.SierraTradingPost.com
www.solareclipse.com
www.solartex.com
www.sungrubbies.com
www.sunprecautions.com
www.sunprotectiveclothing.com
www.sunveil.com

FINANCIAL AND PRESCRIPTION ASSISTANCE

Disability Lawyers.Com
www.disabilitylawyers.com

Disability Resources
www.disabilityresources.com

Medicare
www.medicare.gov; 800-633-4227

National League of Cities Prescription Discount Card Program
www.nlc.org/inside_nlc/MEMBERSHIP/prescription_discount_program.aspx
Provides discount savings to individuals in participating cities.

Partnership for Prescription Assistance
www.pparx.org; 888-477-2669

Patient Access Network
www.patientaccessnetwork.org; 866-316-7263

RxAssist
www.rxassist.org; 401-729-3284

RxHope
www.rxhope.com; 877-267-0517

Social Security Disability Help
www.socialsecurity-disability.org/disabling-conditions/
    lupus-and-social-security-disability

Social Security Disability Secrets
www.disabilitysecrets.com

PRESCRIPTION DISCOUNT PROGRAM INFORMATION

www.drugcardamerica.com; 888-299-5383
www.esunhealth.net; 866-662-1351
www.freedrugcard.us; 866-410-4225
www.pscard.com; 888-516-2535
www.rxfreecard.com; 800-886-8412
www.togetherrxaccess.com; 800-444-4106
www.yourrxcard.com; 866-561-1926

PROFESSIONAL MEDICAL ORGANIZATIONS

American Academy of Dermatology
www.aad.org

American Academy of Neurology
www.aan.com

American Academy of Ophthalmology
www.aao.org

American College of Cardiology
www.cardiosource.org

American College of Chest Physicians
www.chestnet.org/accp

American College of Gastroenterology
www.acg.gi.org

American College of Physicians
www.acponline.org

American College of Rheumatology
www.rheumatology.org

American Society of Hematology
www.hematology.org

CLINICAL TRIALS AND RESEARCH

Alliance for Lupus Research
www.lupusresearch.org; 800-867-1743

The Center for Information and Study on Clinical Research Participation (CISCRP)
www.ciscrp.org; 877-MED-HERO

Centerwatch
www.centerwatch.com/patient/trials.html

Clinical Connection
www.clinicalconnection.com; 800-887-0639

Clinical Trials
www.clinicaltrials.gov

CRISP Database
www.crisp.cit.nih.gov

Johns Hopkins Medicine, Division of Rheumatology
www.hopkinsmedicine.org/rheumatology/clinics/lupus_center.html; 410-955-9114

Lupus Clinical Trials Consortium
www.lupusclinicaltrials.org

Lupus Foundation of America, Inc.
www.lupus.org; 202-349-1155

Lupus Research Institute
www.lupustrials.org; 877-95-TRIAL

Mayo Clinic
www.mayoclinic.org; 507-284-2511 (MN) or 904-953-2000 (FL)

National Institutes of Health (NIH)
www.nih.gov; 301-495-4484
www.clinicaltrials.gov

Search Clinical Trials
www.searchclinicaltrials.org

UCLA Division of Rheumatology
www.rheumatology.ucla.edu; 310-825-9447

CAMPS FOR CHILDREN WITH CHRONIC ILLNESS

Association of Hole in the Wall Camps
www.holeinthewallcamps.org; 203-562-1203
228 Saugatuck Ave.
Westport, CT 06880
Lists national and international locations.

Camp Boggy Creek
www.boggycreek.org; 352-483-4200
30500 Brantley Branch Rd.
Eustis, FL 32736

Camp ChiMer (Kidney)
www.kidney.org; 800-489-9585
Lake Doniphan
Excelsior Springs, MO 64024

Camp Del-Ja-Ri at Camp Alexander Mack
www.campdeljari.org; 574-658-4831
1113 E. Camp Mack Rd.
Milford, IN 46542

Camp Korey at Carnation Farm
www.campkorey.org; 425-844-3100
28901 NE Carnation Farm Rd.
Carnation, WA 98014

Camp Sunshine
www.campsunshine.org; 207-655-3800
35 Acadia Rd.
Casco, ME 04015

MCGHealth
www.mcghealth.org; 706-721-0211
1120 15th St.
Augusta, GA 30912-5563

The Painted Turtle
www.thepaintedturtle.org; 310-451-1353
P.O. Box 455
Lake Hughes, CA 93532

Victory Junction
www.victoryjunction.org; 336-495-2076
4500 Adam's Way
Randleman, NC 27317

DIETARY SUPPLEMENTS AND COMPLEMENTARY OR ALTERNATIVE MEDICINE

Alternative Health News Online
www.altmedicine.com

Alternative Medicine Review
www.thorne.com/altmedrev/index.html

American Holistic Medical Association
www.holisticmedicine.org; 216-292-6644
23366 Commerce Park, Suite 101B
Beachwood, Ohio 44122

American Medical Student Association
www.amsa.org; 703-620-6600

Federal Trade Commission
www.ftc.gov/bcp/menus/consumer/health.shtm (Diet, Health & Fitness page)
877-FTC-HELP

Food and Drug Administration (FDA), Center for Food Safety & Applied Nutrition
www.cfsan.fda.gov
Provides "Tips for the Savvy Supplement User: Making Informed Decisions and Evaluating
    Information" and safety information on supplements.

Food and Drug Administration, Office of Dietary Supplements
www.fda.gov; 301-827-6242

MedlinePlus
www.nlm.nih.gov/medlineplus/complementaryandalternativemedicine.html

National Institutes of Health, National Center for Complementary and Alternative Medicine
    (NCCAM)
www.nccam.nih.gov; 888-644-6226

National Institutes of Health, National Library of Medicine
www.nlm.nih.gov/services/dietsup.html

National Institutes of Health, Office of Dietary Supplements
www.ods.od.nih.gov

Natural Standard
www.naturalstandard.com

WholeHealthMD.com
www.wholehealthmd.com

A CLOSING POEM:
HOPE IS A KITE

Hope is a kite
Flying high on the wind
Bringing smiles and cheer
To the faces of all.

Hope is a kite
Drifting lazily through the sky
Never being brought down
By the branches of a tree.

Hope is a kite
Traveling with the sun
And following the moon
Far beyond the sky's limits.

Hope is a kite
Gliding on the breeze
Giving people, young and old
The strength to go on.

BRIANNA S., AGE TWELVE

INDEX

MORE TITLES IN THE
"COPING WITH" SERIES

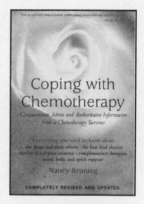

978-0-89529-791-4
U.S. $20.00 / $25.00 CAN

978-0-89529-856-0
U.S. $15.95 / $22.50 CAN

978-1-58333-131-6
U.S. $20.00 / $25.00 CAN

All available from Avery.

AVERY a member of Penguin Group (USA) | www.penguin.com